ILLUSTRATED ENCYCLOPAEDIA OF DERMATOLOGY

ILLUSTRATED ENCYCLOPAEDIA OF DERMATOLOGY

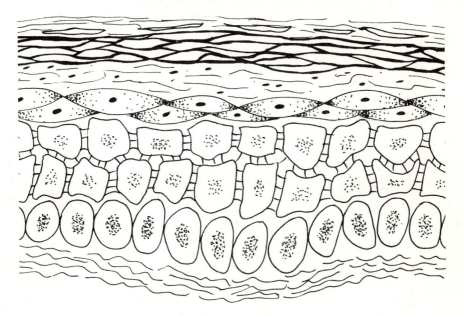

LIONEL FRY

Consultant Dermatologist, St Mary's Hospital, London W2

FENELLA T. WOJNAROWSKA

Dermatology Registrar, St Mary's Hospital, London W2; present address Senior Registrar, St John's Hospital for Diseases of the Skin, London WC2

PARVIN SHAHRAD

Associate Professor, Iran National University, Tehran, Iran; present address Luton and Dunstable Hospital, Bedfordshire, UK

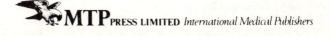 **MTP** PRESS LIMITED *International Medical Publishers*

Published by
MTP Press Limited
Falcon House
Lancaster, England

ISBN: 0-85200-309-9

Printed in Great Britain by
Butler & Tanner Ltd, Frome and London

CONTENTS

PREFACE

This book will, it is hoped, fill the gap between current, smaller texts on dermatology and the standard, large reference books. It should be helpful to those embarking on a career in dermatology and to general practitioners and primary physicians with a special interest in this field.

In this book the emphasis is on clinical aspects of skin diseases, and it is assumed that the reader has some knowledge of the anatomy and physiology of the skin. The differential diagnosis of each disorder is extensively discussed and sex predilection and age of onset are illustrated diagrammatically. As in other branches of medicine, treatments are now frequently changing and these are fully covered. Aetiological factors in skin disorders are now becoming clearer and separate sections on this subject are discussed for each disease. Prognosis and natural history are not always adequately covered in texts on dermatology, so these topics are set out under separate headings.

A small number of the illustrations have been loaned from colleagues and institutions, and we gratefully acknowledge this assistance from the following: The Wellcome Museum of Medical Science; Photographic Department, Institute of Dermatology, St John's Hospital; Dr Roger Clayton; Dr W. H. Jopling; and Dr P. Rodin.

We are also grateful to the staff of MTP for their assistance in preparing this book, and to Mrs Helen Martin for coping so admirably in transforming our handwriting into a typed manuscript.

1 ACANTHOSIS NIGRICANS

This curious condition exists in several forms, which differ in their causes.

Presentation The age at which acanthosis nigricans develops depends on the cause. Men and women are equally affected except in the inherited type.

The areas involved are the sides of the neck, the axillae, groins and palms of hands. The skin becomes thick, with pronounced ridging, and papillomatous, giving a velvety or in severe cases a warty appearance. The skin is dark brown or black (Figure 1.1).

Four types are distinguished:

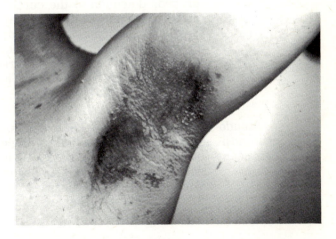

Figure 1.1 Acanthosis nigricans of the axilla, showing warty hyperpigmentation

1

True benign acanthosis nigricans

This may be present at birth or appear during childhood or at puberty. It often worsens at puberty and thereafter is static or may regress. It is inherited as a dominant, but is more common in female children. There are no other disorders associated with it.

Benign acanthosis nigricans

This type is associated with other diseases but not with malignant disease.

It may develop in childhood as part of certain genetically determined syndromes.

Benign acanthosis nigricans may develop in childhood, adolescence or adult life in association with a number of endocrine disorders.

These disorders include syndromes with hypo- and hypersecretion by the pituitary, polycystic ovaries and Cushing's syndrome. These cases are difficult to distinguish from pseudo-acanthosis nigricans occurring in dark-skinned, obese subjects. Many of the patients with endocrine disorders are obese.

The acanthosis nigricans is usually mild.

Malignant acanthosis nigricans

This develops in adult life usually in late middle age or old age. It is a manifestation of malignancy, usually carcinoma of the stomach, or sometimes of breast or lung. Other adenocarcinomas and lymphomas are more rarely the cause. Acanthosis nigricans may precede detection of the carcinoma by 5 years, or may appear only in the terminal stages.

Malignant acanthosis nigricans is much more severe and extensive than other forms. The intertriginous areas, mucous membranes and the palms and soles may be involved. The lesions are very warty and black.

Pseudo-acanthosis nigricans

This is a disease of obese adults. The obesity may be nutritional or hormonal in origin. The patients are usually brunette or dark. All intertriginous areas may be affected. The skin becomes thick and dark, and there may be numerous skin tags. Histologically it is indistinguishable from true acanthosis nigricans.

Differential diagnosis

The most important distinction to make is between true and pseudo-acanthosis nigricans in an adult. Post-inflammatory hyperpigmentation is distinguished by the normal texture of the skin.

Diagnosis and investigations In adults underlying carcinoma or endocrine disorder should be sought.

Aetiology It is believed that a humoral agent causes acanthosis nigricans.

Treatment Removal of the cause, i.e. carcinoma or endocrine disorder, will result in return to normal. Pseudo-acanthosis nigricans will improve with weight loss.

Natural history The childhood types may improve after puberty, the adult ones only with removal of the cause.

2 ACNE

Acne vulgaris is very common during the teenage years. Most adolescents (90%) have some manifestation of acne, and it is a problem in about 50% of these. The sex incidence is equal.

Acne presents between the ages of 10 and 30. The peak incidence is mid-teens in girls (14–17), and late teens in boys (16–19) (see Figure 2.1).

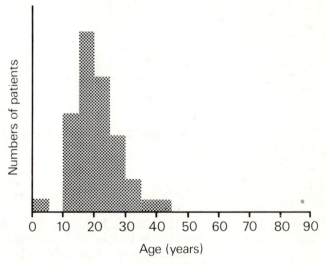

Figure 2.1   The age distribution of acne

Acne is localized to the face and upper trunk and shoulders (see Figures 2.2 and 2.3). The chin and forehead are often the first sites to be involved. The area around the eyes and eyelids is spared. In older women the beard area is predominantly affected. Premenstrual flares of acne are often confined to the chin. The upper trunk, chest, back and shoulders and upper arms are involved. Acne rarely extends below

5

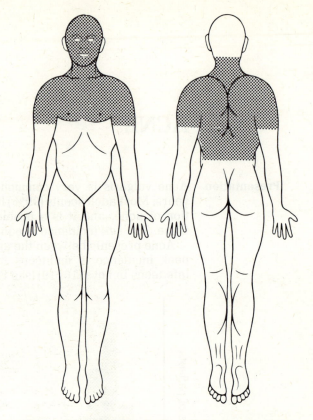

Figure 2.2   The distribution of acne on the body

the waist. The face and trunk may be affected independently.

The initial lesion is the comedone. When the orifice is visible and plugged with a horny plug it forms an open comedone – a blackhead. If the orifice is closed it forms a small white papule – the closed comedone. Inflammation around these causes erythematous papules (Figure 2.4), pustules, and in severe cases cysts (Figure 2.3) and nodules, which persist for many weeks. There may be associated seborrhoea manifest as greasy skin and hair. There may be post-inflammatory hyperpigmentation. Scarring often occurs with depressed, pitted scars (Figure 2.5) or keloids. Keloids occur particularly on the trunk (Figure 2.6).

Acne fulminans This is rare. Severe cystic acne in teenage boys
(acute febrile (Figure 2.3) may be accompanied by fever and joint
acne) pains. There is leukocytosis and a raised ESR.
Erythema nodosum may also occur.

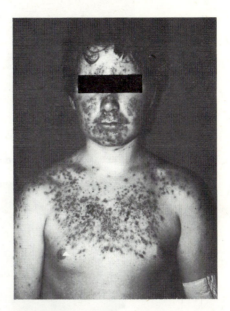

**Figure 2.3   Severe cystic acne in a
typical distribution. This patient had
acute febrile acne**

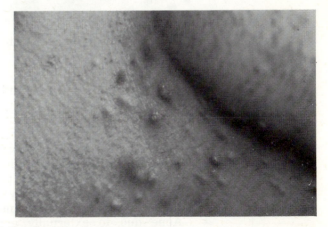

**Figure 2.4   Lesions of acne: open and closed come-
dones, pustules and papules**

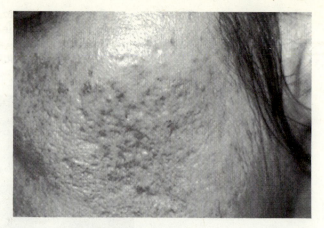

Figure 2.5   The comedones and pitted scars of acne

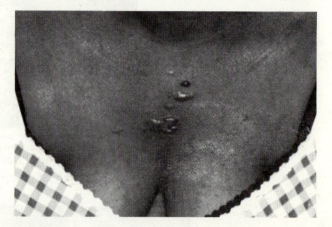

Figure 2.6   Keloids due to acne in the typical site on the chest

Differential diagnosis

Rosacea is often confused with acne, but the erythema and papules are confined to the face, and there are no comedones. Peri-oral dermatitis is confined to the peri-oral or peri-orbital areas; there are papules but no comedones. Negro males often suffer pseudofolliculitis barbae, a folliculitis due to growth of hairs back into the skin; the pustules are confined to the beard area. Occasionally the small pustules of follicular seborrhoeic eczema may cause confusion.

Acne due to externally applied chemicals is localized to the site of application and comedones predominate (see below).

Diagnosis and investigations   The typical appearance of acne rarely requires biopsy to identify it.

Endocrine investigation is indicated in women with severe acne (resistant to therapy), facial hirsutes and infrequent menses. They may have polycystic ovaries. The serum testosterone is at the upper end of the normal range, its urinary excretion (measured as 17-oxosteroids) is increased and the sex hormone binding globulin low. Amenorrhoea and virilization of the external genitalia suggest an androgen-secreting tumour.

Aetiology   Acne is a disease of the sebaceous gland and its duct. Only a few of the thousands of sebaceous glands present on the face need to be involved to produce severe acne. The primary event is disputed. It may be obstruction of the sebaceous duct due to alteration of the lining cells, abnormal sebum production with excess quantities or altered composition rendering it more inflammatory, or bacterial colonization with *Propionibacterium acnes* modifying the sebum or directly releasing mediators of inflammation. All three mechanisms may be involved.

Obstruction of the duct by a horny plug forms a comedone. A sebaceous gland that cannot discharge its sebum becomes distended and excites a foreign body reaction with much inflammation. Rupture of the gland into the dermis causes intense inflammation and cysts and nodules are formed.

Hormonal factors   The sex hormones, both naturally occurring and synthetic, have a profound effect on acne. Androgens induce and exacerbate acne. Many women experience a premenstrual flare of acne. Acne usually remits during pregnancy. The acne of certain women is due to excess testosterone production, high free plasma testosterone due to low sex hormone binding globulin, and increased peripheral uptake. The serum testosterone may be normal because increased urinary excretion compensates. The androgen may be ovarian, in association with polycystic ovaries, or adrenal in origin.

The oral contraceptive pill influences acne. There is often an improvement in acne when a high oestrogen pill is taken. The androgenic, anti-oestrogen activity of the newer synthetic progesterones, e.g. norgesterol, exacerbates acne.

Corticosteroids, endogenous or exogenous, whether given systemically or topically, can induce acne.

Drugs Phenobarbitone, isoniazid, bromides and iodides can all induce acne or worsen it.

Treatment

Topical therapy

Washing Washing makes very little difference.

Keratolytics Keratolytics are beneficial for the superficial pustules and comedones. Salicylic acid is effective, many of the newer commercial preparations contain benzoyl peroxide, which is an efficient keratolytic. The keratolytic should be applied each night after washing the face. Slight erythema and peeling is desirable, and the frequency or strength of the application should be increased until this results. The choice of cream, gel or lotion should be determined by the patient's preference, as his co-operation is essential.

Antibiotics Topical clindamycin is widely and successfully used in the USA. It is applied as a 1.5% solution each night. Systemic absorption is low.

Retinoic acid Topical retinoic acid is most successful for comedones. In addition to its irritant effect, it alters sebaceous duct keratinization. It is applied each night until mild erythema and peeling are produced, the frequency being adjusted to avoid too severe a reaction. It takes 6–8 weeks to produce an improvement. Severe irritant reactions and hyperpigmentation are the major side effects.

Ultraviolet light Natural sunlight, provided the heat and humidity are not too great, or artificial ultraviolet light are often beneficial to acne. This is partly due to the peeling effect. The tan renders the erythema much less obvious, so that the cosmetic appearance improves. The patient's morale benefits from the tan.

Intralesional steroids These, given by a syringe or dermojet into large cysts, reduce the inflammatory reaction and speed resolution. Scarring may be reduced.

Systemic therapy

Diet | There is no place for diet in the management of acne.

Antibiotics | Antibiotics have the major role in the treatment of acne. Each suitable antibiotic is successful in about 70% of patients; lack of success with one does not preclude success with another. Therapy must be prolonged. There is little response before one month, and improvement continues for three months. Thereafter the dose should be reduced every 2–3 months. Many patients require a maintenance dose every two to three days for many years in order to remain free of acne.

Antibiotics are more successful in treating pustules, nodules and cysts than comedones.

Tetracycline in a dose of 500 mg once daily on an empty stomach is the most widely used antibiotic. Side-effects are rare. It should not be given to pregnant women or those at risk of pregnancy, because of adverse effects on fetal teeth and bones, and possible teratogenic effects.

Erythromycin 500 mg b.d. or *Co-trimoxazole* one tablet b.d. are useful alternatives. Either may succeed when tetracycline has failed.

Clindamycin 150 mg daily is often successful in cases which are resistant to therapy with other antibiotics. Its use should be reserved for the most severe, because of the small risk of necrotizing enterocolitis.

Dapsone in high doses 100–300 mg daily is used for severe cases of acne, particularly cystic acne unresponsive to other forms of treatment.

Corticosteroids in moderate doses (prednisone 10–30 mg daily) will suppress acute febrile acne, and severe cystic acne. In low doses (prednisone 5 mg nocte) they suppress adrenal androgen production and improve androgen induced acne.

Anti-androgens | The anti-androgen cyproterone acetate is used in the treatment of women with excess androgen production. It is given clinically in doses of 100 mg daily combined with oestrogen 50 μg for the first ten days of the menstrual cycle, and the oestrogen is continued for the next 12 days. The cyproterone acetate opposes the peripheral effect of androgens. The oestrogen is essential to prevent conception and feminization of the male fetus. In addition it wipes out ovarian production of androgen and by raising the sex hormone binding globulin lowers the plasma free testosterone.

Oral contraceptives

Oral contraceptives containing high doses of oestrogens (50 μg) are beneficial to acne. The new low dose pills, with 30 μg of oestrogen in combination with an androgenic progesterone, often induce or exacerbate acne. Norgesterol (Eugynon 30, Microgynon 30) is particularly to be avoided in those women prone to acne.

Retinoids

Aromatic retinoids have shown good results in recent trials. Their use, however, in women will be limited by their teratogenic effects.

Natural history and prognosis

In the vast majority of people, acne is a mild and short-lived condition. Most of those with acne are free of disease by their early twenties. In a few it persists into the thirties and forties. Premenstrual flares of acne may persist until the menopause. The acne often subsides despite the persistence of seborrhoea.

ACNE CONGLOBATA

Presentation

This severe chronic disfiguring form of acne may arise in pre-existing acne, or in patients whose acne has remitted. It commences between the ages of 16 and 30. Males predominate. There is often a strong family history.

The trunk, including the buttocks, upper arms and thighs, is involved. There are many comedones, often multiple and grouped. There is an abnormal, severe inflammatory response to this, with abscess formation and discharging interconnecting sinuses. Cysts and inflammatory nodules are numerous, and these may ulcerate and become necrotic. There is severe scarring often with keloid formation.

There may be associated hidradenitis suppurativa of apocrine glands in axillae, groins and breast.

Acute febrile acne may occur with acne conglobata.

Differential diagnosis

The clinical picture is unique.

Diagnosis and investigations Leukocytosis and a raised ESR accompany acute febrile acne.

Aetiology It is not known why some individuals mount such a severe inflammatory response to acne. A defect in cell-mediated immunity has been reported.

Acute febrile acne is thought to be an immune complex hypersensitivity response.

Treatment Very longterm (years) antibiotic therapy with tetracycline 500 mg daily, co-trimoxazole 1 tablet b.d. or erythromycin 500 mg b.d. is indicated. Prednisone 10–30 mg daily is very helpful in the short term, and provides dramatic relief of symptoms in acute febrile acne. Dapsone 100–300 mg daily may be helpful.

Natural history and prognosis Acne conglobata may persist for decades, often into the 50s. Squamous cell carcinomas may arise in scarred lesions.

INFANTILE ACNE

Presentation Typical acne can occur in infancy and childhood.

It usually commences in the first two years of life. It is much more common in male children (m : f = 4 : 1). There are papules, pustules and comedones.

Differential diagnosis The chief sources of diagnostic confusion are comedone naevus, which is asymmetrical and lacks pustules, and exogenous acne due to acnegenic applications, e.g. topical steroids or oils. Micropapular eczema may occasionally cause confusion.

Diagnosis and investigations The morphology of the lesions usually makes the diagnosis obvious.

Occasionally it is the presenting symptom of virilizing syndromes (congenital adrenal hyperplasia, androgen secreting tumours), sexual precocity, or Cushing's syndrome, so a general physical examination is essential. Biochemical studies for urinary 17-oxo- and oxogenic steroids are indicated in such cases.

Aetiology It is thought that adrenal or testicular androgens are involved.

Treatment Topical applications are often helpful (see p. 9) as superficial lesions predominate.

Systemic erythromycin can be given in low doses. Tetracyclines must *not* be given because of the damage to teeth.

Natural history and prognosis Most children will be free of acne by 5 years; many earlier.

ACNE DUE TO EXOGENOUS FACTORS

Presentation Acne due to exogenous factors, climatic, mechanical or chemical, occurs most frequently in those with a past or present history of acne.

It can occur at any age and in both sexes. The age and sex distribution is determined by the method of exposure.

Tropical acne This occurs in hot humid conditions. It can occur at any time during adult life under suitable conditions. It is more common in those with a past history of acne. Men predominate. It is chiefly seen in men working in hot, humid conditions, and in soldiers in the tropics. It is presumed that hydration of the skin obstructs the sebaceous duct. The only treatment is removal from tropical conditions.

Mechanical acne This occurs under headbands, bra straps and any situation in which there is occlusion and friction.

Chloracne The chlorinated aromatic hydrocarbons cause acne in those exposed to them. They are present in fungicides, herbicides, insecticides and wood preservers, and are used during the manufacture of electrical cables. People exposed to them either topically, or by ingestion or inhalation, develop chloracne. This occurs in men in occupations manufacturing these compounds or those people accidentally exposed. The lesions are found chiefly on the face and neck, but the trunk and limbs can be affected. There are many comedones, and papules and pustules also develop.

The acne may persist for years after exposure.

Oil acne   Cutting oils, mineral oils and vegetable oils induce acne, primarily comedones (Figure 2.7), at the site of contact with the skin. Exposure is usually occupational.

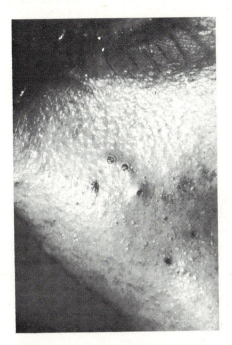

Figure 2.7   Comedones of exogenous acne

Acne cosmetica   Greasy hair pomades, brilliantines, vegetable cosmetic oils and greasy creams can all produce acne at the site of application (Figure 2.7).

Acne medicamentosa   Strong topical steroids can often induce comedones and pustular acne when applied to the face or trunk.

Differential diagnosis   All these types of acne must be differentiated from acne vulgaris. Comedones predominate. Confusion may arise with senile comedones occurring in sun-damaged skin.

Aetiology   Oils may cause obstruction of the sebaceous duct, as does hydration. The mechanism by which chloracne occurs is not known.

Natural history and prognosis   Slow resolution occurs after removal of the offending substance. Topical keratolytics or retinoic acid may speed resolution of comedones.

All these agents exacerbate existing acne, and may make treatment of acne vulgaris difficult.

3 AMYLOIDOSIS

Amyloid is a protein with some mucopolysaccharide. There are a number of causes for deposition of amyloid in the skin. However, it is convenient to consider amyloidosis under the clinical presentations rather than the biochemical. Amyloid may be formed only in the skin and this gives rise to a condition termed lichen amyloidosis. Amyloid may also be deposited in the skin in systemic amyloidosis. Systemic amyloidosis may be primary or secondary to underlying disease. Deposition of amyloid in the skin does not usually occur in secondary amyloidosis.

CUTANEOUS AMYLOIDOSIS (LICHEN AMYLOIDOSIS)

Presentation The disorder commonly affects middle-aged (Figure 3.1) persons of either sex. The lesions are firm

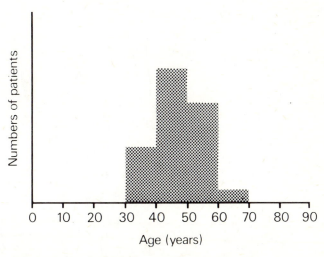

Figure 3.1　Age of onset of lichen amyloidosis

17

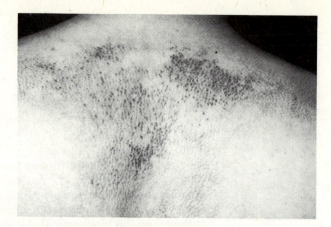

Figure 3.2   Brown papules of lichen amyloidosis

yellowish-brown papules 1–3 mm. They usually have a shiny surface and are discrete (Figure 3.2). The common sites of involvement are the fronts of the legs, the extensor surfaces of the arms and the lower back (Figure 3.3). Occasionally the lesions are larger and present as nodules or plaques.

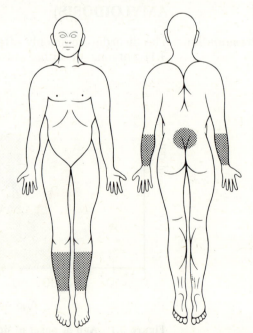

Figure 3.3   Common sites of cutaneous amyloidosis

Differential diagnosis Lichenified eczema may be papular and is common on the lower legs. The yellow colour of the lesions may be suggestive of xanthomata. Hypertrophic lichen planus on the front of the legs may also have similar appearances to the nodular variety. Granulomatous disorders have also to be considered.

Investigations A biopsy will be necessary to establish the diagnosis and special stains for amyloid should be requested.

Aetiology Unknown.

Treatment There is some benefit from the use of potent topical steroids or injecting the lesions with steroids.

Natural history and prognosis The lesions persist indefinitely. There are no systemic complications.

SYSTEMIC AMYLOIDOSIS

Presentation About a quarter of patients with systemic amyloidosis develop skin lesions. The sexes are equally affected and the commonest age of onset is middle age. The lesions are small papules which have a yellowish colour. Occasionally nodules and plaques will develop. Purpura may be associated with the skin lesions. The commonest sites of involvement are the eyelids, central area of the face, lips and tongue. Occasionally the tongue enlarges due to a diffuse infiltration with amyloid. If the larynx is involved hoarseness may develop.

Differential diagnosis The yellow papules and plaques have to be distinguished from xanthomata. The purpuric element is absent in xanthomata. Benign tumours of the sweat glands and hair follicles occur on the face, but they are not usually the yellow colour of amyloid deposits. Usually when the skin lesions are present other organs such as the liver and spleen will also be involved and palpable.

Investigations A biopsy with special stains for amyloid will give the diagnosis. The bone marrow usually shows plasma cell hyperplasia.

Aetiology   The cause is unknown. The abnormality appears to be in the bone marrow where the hyperplasia of the plasma cells is associated with production of an abnormal protein.

Treatment   None is available which alters the course of the disease.

Natural history and prognosis   Death usually occurs within 2 years of onset of the disease. The cause of death is often heart failure from involvement of the cardiac muscle. Myelomatosis often develops and may itself be responsible for death.

4 BEHCET'S DISEASE

Presentation Behcet's disease characteristically presents with the triad of oral and genital ulceration and a uveitis. The disorder usually first presents in young adults, but may begin in childhood, or middle age (Figure 4.1). It is approximately five times as common in males as females (Figure 4.2).

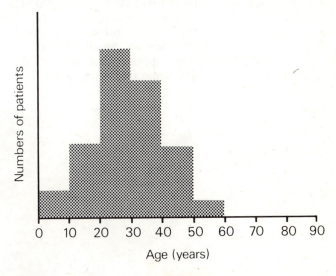

Figure 4.1   Age of onset of Behcet's disease

The lesions usually appear in the mouth and genitalia simultaneously although occasionally involvement at one site may precede the other. The mouth ulcers are round or oval with a yellow base surrounded by an erythematous edge. The ulcers are painful and may extend to the oesophagus. In the male the genital lesions usually affect the scrotum

21

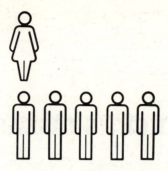

Figure 4.2 Behcet's disease is more common in males (5 : 1)

(Figure 4.3) and in the female the labia majora. Characteristically the ulcers are shallow and vary from a few mm to a few cm. Other skin lesions are present in nearly two-thirds of patients, and vary in their morphology. Small papules and pustules occur (which are sterile) and characteristically this type of lesion occurs at sites of trauma such as venepuncture. These lesions may affect any part of the skin. In addition, small, deeper, erythematous nodules may appear and are similar in appearance to erythema nodosum.

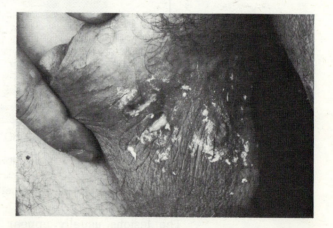

Figure 4.3 Ulcers on the scrotum in Behcet's disease

The eye lesions present as irritation, photophobia or impaired vision. Conjunctivitis may occur, but more commonly there is a uveitis, vitreous opacities and an anterior hypopyon may be present.

Other organs that may be involved are the central nervous system, joints, and veins. The central nervous system involvement is variable and may simulate multiple sclerosis. Arthritis and venous thrombosis may also occur.

Differential diagnosis

The oral lesions have to be distinguised from pemphigus, severe aphthosis, recurrent herpes simplex and erythema multiforme. In Behcet's disease the associated genital lesions and eye involvement should distinguish the disease from the other causes, but erythema multiforme may also affect the eyes and genitalia; however the latter disease is more acute and self limiting.

Investigations

Skin and mucosal biopsies

These usually show non-specific inflammatory changes, but occasionally there is thrombosis of the small vessels.

Haematology

Occasionally there is a leukocytosis and eosinophilia.

Intradermal injection of normal saline

This often produces a small papule at the site of injection and is a useful test in confirming the diagnosis.

Aetiology

The cause of Behcet's disease is unknown. A virus aetiology has been postulated in the past but there has been no satisfactory confirmatory evidence.

Treatment

There is no specific treatment for Behcet's disease. Systemic corticosteroids offer the best hope of controlling the disease process, but unfortunately they are not always effective.

Prognosis

The prognosis is variable. Patients with central nervous system involvement tend to have a poor prognosis and the disease may well kill the patient in a matter of months or a few years. If the disease is limited to the mouth, skin and eyes, the disorder may last for many years and even burn itself out eventually.

5 DEFICIENCY STATES

PELLAGRA

Presentation Pellagra may occur at any stage and in either sex if the diet is deficient in nicotinic acid. Pellagra consists of the triad, dermatitis, diarrhoea, and dementia. The rash occurs in the exposed areas (Figure 5.1).

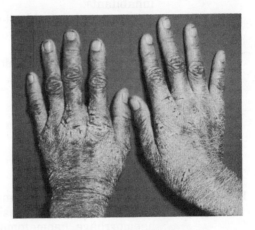

Figure 5.1 Pellagra occurs in exposed areas

It commences as a red scaly rash and as it subsides after a few days, it leaves hyperpigmented skin. In chronic cases the skin becomes thickened, scaly and a dark red colour.

In pellagra the skin lesions appear before the diarrhoea and mental symptoms.

Differential diagnosis Other photosensitive eruptions have to be considered. These include photosensitive eczema, porphyria, drug induced photosensitive rashes, and systemic lupus erythematosus. Hartnup disease occurs in

25

children and is due to malabsorption of amino acids, particularly tryptophan. The rash is the same as that in pellagra.

Investigations None are usually necessary to establish the diagnosis. In Hartnup disease the urinary and faecal amino acids should be measured.

Aetiology Pellagra is due to a deficiency of nicotinic acid and/or tryptophan in the diet. Nicotinic acid can be synthesized from tryptophan in the presence of B vitamins. In Hartnup disease tryptophan transport in the jejunum and kidney tubules is impaired and this leads to a deficiency of tryptophan.

Deficiency of nicotinic acid is seen in persons who do not drink milk or eat meat and eggs. This occurs most commonly in the underdeveloped countries where these foods are too expensive for many inhabitants.

The drug isoniazid interferes with nicotinic acid metabolism and may give rise to pellagra.

Treatment Oral nicotinamide or nicotinic acid will result in clearance of the lesions.

Progress The skin lesions are reversible with specific therapy.

SCURVY

Presentation Scurvy may present at any age if vitamin C intake is inadequate. The skin lesions include perifollicular haemorrhage, haematomas and subsequently brown pigmentation, particularly on the legs, due to haemosiderin. Follicular hyperkeratosis and broken hairs are seen on the limbs. Bleeding gums are seen in patients with teeth and who have poor oral hygiene. Other symptoms include depression, lethargy, anorexia and pain in the joints due to haemarthrosis.

Differential diagnosis The perifollicular haemorrhage must be distinguished from other causes of purpura. Follicular hyperkeratosis on the upper and outer arms and fronts of the thighs is very common in young adults and does not signify any pathological state.

Investigations   The vitamin C saturation test may be carried out to establish the diagnosis.

Aetiology   In Western Europe and the USA, scurvy is usually seen in food faddists and old people who do not eat fruit, salads and uncooked vegetables. It may be seen in the underdeveloped countries due to poverty and poor diet.

Treatment   Oral vitamin C.

Prognosis   The skin changes are reversible with adequate vitamin C intake. In chronic cases so-called woody oedema of the legs with discolouration, may occur.

KWASHIORKOR

Presentation   Kwashiorkor appears between the ages of 6 months and 5 years. The skin lesions present as reddish-brown scaly patches anywhere on the body. They may show either post-inflammatory hyper- or hypopigmentation. The hair may become a reddish-brown colour. Inflammatory changes of the mucous membranes are common, particularly around the mouth and eyes.

The non-dermatological features include muscle wasting, pot-belly and oedema. There is failure to thrive.

Differential diagnosis   The skin lesions are only part of a generalized disorder, and the non-dermatological features usually suggest the diagnosis.

Aetiology   Kwashiorkor is due to protein malnutrition.

Treatment   Correction of dietary deficiencies.

IRON DEFICIENCY

The dermatological disorders attributed to iron deficiency include hair loss, pruritus, koilonychia and changes in the oral mucosa.

The hair loss which is reported due to iron deficiency is a diffuse loss and is said to occur predominantly in young women. The haemoglobin concentration may be normal but the serum iron and tissue stores are low. The hair loss is reversible with treatment.

Iron deficiency is a rare cause of generalized pruritus. No rash is present and the pruritus subsides when the iron deficiency is corrected.

The typical change of iron deficiency affecting the oral mucosa is that of atrophic changes of the epithelium of the tongue. The tongue has a smooth appearance with loss of the filiform papillae.

6 DERMATITIS HERPETIFORMIS

Presentation Dermatitis herpetiformis is essentially a disease of adults; it is extremely rare in childhood. It may occur in the late teens, but it most commonly begins in the third and fourth decades (Figure 6.1). However, it may appear for the first time later in adult life. Males and females seem to be equally affected.

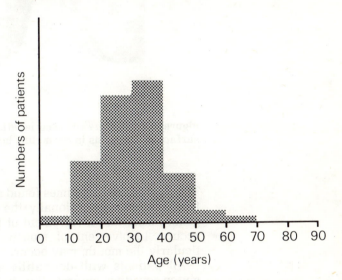

Figure 6.1   Age of onset of dermatitis herpetiformis

The characteristic lesion is a small blister on an urticarial base. The lesions are often grouped, hence 'herpetiform'. The lesions are intensely irritating and thus are scratched by the patient. Thus, it is common not to find blisters when the patient is examined, but ony excoriations, the blisters having been destroyed by scratching. The commonest site of

29

involvement is the elbows and extensor surface of the forearms (Figure 6.2). Other common sites are the knees, buttocks, and scapular regions of the back (Figure 6.3).

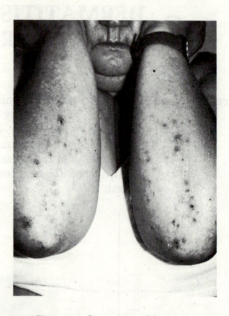

Figure 6.2   Blisters and excoriated lesions on the extensor surface of forearms in dermatitis herpetiformis

The lesions are sometimes found at sites of pressure from clothing. Occasionally the disorder becomes generalized, and involvement of the scalp and face occurs. Involvement of mucous membranes, particularly the mouth, may occur.

All patients with dermatitis herpetiformis have gluten-sensitive enteropathy, but there is clinical evidence of this in only 10–20% of patients.

Differential diagnosis   Other diseases which may present with blisters have to be distinguished from dermatitis herpetiformis. Pemphigus occurs usually in middle aged and elderly patients. The blisters tend to be larger than those found in dermatitis herpetiformis, and are flaccid. There is usually no irritation in pemphigus. Pemphigoid is a disease of elderly patients. As in der-

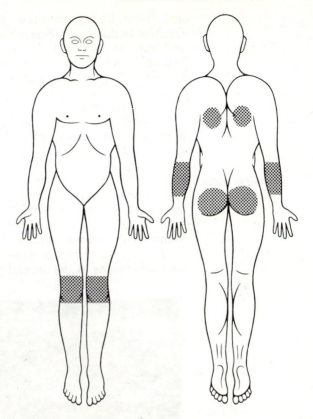

Figure 6.3   Common sites of onset of dermatitis herpeti-formis

matitis herpetiformis, the blisters are often situated on an urticarial base, and may be very irritating. The blisters in pemphigoid tend to be larger than in dermatitis herpetiformis, and do not affect any particular area as in dermatitis herpetiformis. Erythema multiforme characteristically affects the hands, and 'target' lesions may be present to help in the diagnosis. Erythema multiforme is not usually an irritating disorder, and is self limiting.

Papular urticaria (insect bites) is intensely irritating and may be very persistent, particularly if the source of insects is not removed. Papular urticaria is most often found on exposed areas, e.g. lower legs in women, but is sometimes difficult to distinguish from dermatitis herpetiformis.

Non-blistering diseases such as scabies, eczema

and 'neurotic excoriations' may all present difficulties in diagnosis. Eczema is often very irritating and may be localized to the elbows and forearms. Scabies is a very irritating condition like dermatitis herpetiformis, and commonly affects the buttocks. Neurotic excoriations are lesions induced by patients, but they complain of intense irritation. The sites are usually different from dermatitis herpetiformis, namely upper back, upper arms and thighs.

Investigations
Skin biopsies

It is more important to take a biopsy from the *uninvolved* skin than from a lesion. A biopsy should be taken from the *uninvolved* skin for immunofluorescent studies. Characteristically IgA deposits are found in the dermal papillae (Figure 6.4). A biopsy from a lesion shows a sub-epidermal blister and microabscesses in the dermal papillae.

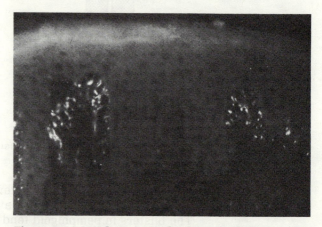

Figure 6.4   IgA deposits in the dermal papillae

Haematology

Because patients with dermatitis herpetiformis have a gluten-sensitive enteropathy, they may be iron and/or folate deficient. Thus, a full blood count, serum iron, serum folate and red cell folate studies are necessary.

Gastro-intestinal biopsy

As the enteropathy is mild, tests of function of the small intestine are frequently normal. An intestinal biopsy is necessary, however, to determine the degree of involvement of the intestine, and is necessary before treatment with a gluten-free diet.

Aetiology   Until ten years ago nothing was known about the cause of dermatitis herpetiformis. However, in the late 1960s it was shown that patients with dermatitis herpetiformis had a small intestinal enteropathy which was identical to that found in coeliac disease, and it has now been shown that the skin eruption is also gluten dependent. If patients are treated with a gluten-free diet their dapsone requirements gradually fall, and a large proportion will eventually no longer require dapsone. However, as with the intestine, if gluten is re-introduced into the diet the rash returns within a few days. At present it is not known how gluten causes damage to the small intestine, or how it produces the skin lesions. It is probable that there is some underlying immunological abnormality in patients with dermatitis herpetiformis, as the anti-reticulin antibody and anti-nuclear antibodies are found in a significant proportion of patients. The histocompatible antigen HLA-B8 is found in over 80% of patients with dermatitis herpetiformis, which is the same incidence as that in coeliac disease.

Treatment   The rash of dermatitis herpetiformis can be controlled by dapsone. The dose required varies from one patient to another. It may be as high as 300 mg per day, or as little as 50 mg twice a week. Dapsone is certainly not a cure, and the rash returns when the drug is stopped. Unfortunately, dapsone is not without side effects, the most serious of which is haemolytic anaemia. If this is severe the drug must be stopped. Dapsone also causes methaemoglobinaemia. This is important in elderly patients as, if severe, it may precipitate angina pectoris. Occasionally patients cannot take dapsone because of headaches. Other drugs which may control the eruption are sulphapyridine and sulphamethoxypyridazine.

Possibly the treatment of choice is a gluten-free diet. However, for this to be effective the diet has to be strict, and if patients cannot adhere to a strict diet, the treatment will be ineffective. A gluten-free diet does impose a number of social restrictions on the patient's life. It must be emphasized that the benefit of a gluten-free diet on the rash will not be apparent for many months. The average duration for a patient to be able to stop taking dapsone after commencing a gluten-free diet is two years. However, the dose of dapsone required for control of the rash will begin to fall after approximately six months.

At present, treatment of dermatitis herpetiformis, whether by drugs or diet, must be considered to be lifelong.

Prognosis   Dermatitis herpetiformis is a chronic disorder and less than 10% of patients have a spontaneous remission. Even in those patients with a remission the disease may appear again. If patients are able to adhere to a strict gluten-free diet they are able to enjoy good health, and are symptom free. Reintroduction of gluten to the diet will cause a relapse of the disease.

7 DERMATOMYOSITIS

Dermatomyositis is a clinical syndrome of a characteristic rash coupled with myositis. The cutaneous or muscular signs may dominate the clinical picture, although in some patients the cutaneous involvement may be minimal. There are no cutaneous signs in the majority of cases of polymyositis.

There are differences between the disease in children and adults; the disease in children has a more pronounced vasculitis and is not related to malignancy.

Presentation Childhood cases usually present before the age of 10; adult cases are more common much later in life. Women present chiefly between 40 and 50, men a

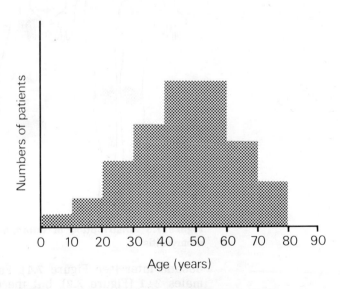

Figure 7.1 The age of onset of dermatomyositis

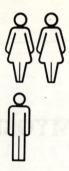

Figure 7.2   Sex ratio in dermatomyositis

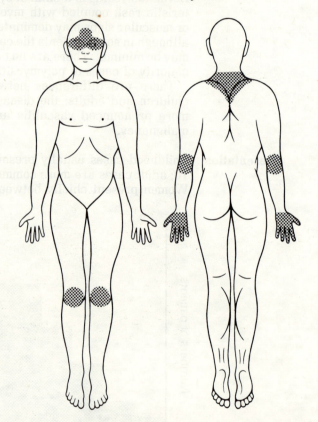

Figure 7.3   Distribution of cutaneous lesions of derm-atomyositis

decade later (see Figure 7.1). Females outnumber males 2 : 1 (Figure 7.2), but the disease in men is more commonly associated with a neoplasm. The disease occurs in all races, but is most common in Negroes.

There have been many reports of an increased incidence of carcinoma in patients with dermatomyositis. The incidence depends on the age of the patients. There is no association between carcinoma and dermatomyositis in childhood or in young adults. In older patients there is an association, and among old men as many as 50% may have carcinoma. The commonest organs implicated are lung, ovary, uterus, breast and stomach. Removal of the tumour may result in remission of the dermatomyositis.

Cutaneous lesions The most typical distribution is the face, especially the upper eyelids; knuckles and finger joints; elbows and knees (see Figure 7.3).

The face There is a violet colouration of the eyelids, forehead and cheeks (Figure 7.4). There may be associated

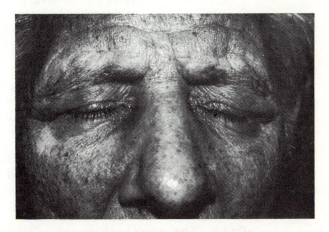

Figure 7.4 Erythema and oedema of eyelids in dermatomyositis

oedema. Erythema, telangiectasia and scaling may be present on the forehead and cheeks.

Sometimes there is erythema of the scalp and diffuse hair loss.

The hands Characteristically the knuckles, dorsum of the interphalangeal joints and nail fold are involved, with

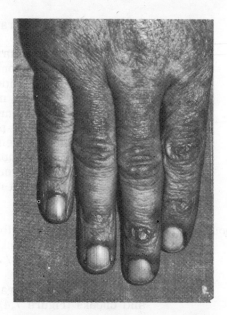

Figure 7.5   Hands of patient with dermatomyositis showing erythema of the knuckles and nail folds, and nail fold infarcts. Perifollicular papules are also present

violaceous or red plaques (Figure 7.5), these may be smooth and shiny or scaly. The whole back of the hand may be involved. There may be red perifollicular papules. Oedema of the hands is common.

The nail folds in addition to the above mentioned plaques may be ragged and show thrombosed telangiectasia (Figure 7.5). Splinter haemorrhages occur.

Trunk   The upper back may show telangiectasia, red scaly plaques or perifollicular papules.

Vasculitic ulcers occur on the trunk.

Arms and legs   The knees and elbows often are involved with violet or red scaly plaques. The limbs may have extensive involvement, with scaly plaques or with perifollicular papules. Oedema of the limbs may be very striking. Vasculitic ulcers occur.

As the rash resolves there may be atrophy and hypo- or hyperpigmentation.

Occasionally there is a diffuse scleroderma-like change.

Calcification of the soft tissues may occur and is a good prognostic sign. Calcinosis cutis of the elbow, hand and knee joints occurs more rarely (Figure 7.6).

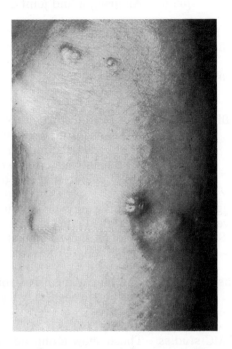

Figure 7.6   Subcutaneous deposits of calcium

Muscles   All muscle groups may be involved. The proximal muscle groups are usually the first involved. Truncal muscles and muscles of speech, swallowing and respiration may all be affected. Weakness of the respiratory muscles may be fatal. The oesophagus may be involved.

There may be pain and tenderness of the affected muscles. The weakness may be mild or so profound that the tendon reflexes are lost. Wasting is often severe.

Oedema often overlies affected muscles.

Calcification of the muscles can occur.

Heart   Cardiac muscle can be affected, manifest as cardiac failure or dysrhythmias.

Lungs	The lungs may be involved by failure of the respiratory muscles, aspiration pneumonia or fibrosing alveolitis. The latter has a very poor prognosis.
Joints	Arthralgia and joint effusions are common.
Raynaud's phenomenon	This occurs in a third of patients.
Constitutional symptoms	Fever and weight loss may be marked.
Differential diagnosis	The full blown picture is unmistakable. Mild cutaneous cases may suggest a contact eczema because of the distribution on the eyelids. Systemic lupus erythematosus can be difficult to differentiate. The violet colour suggests dermatomyositis.
Diagnosis and investigations *Skin biopsy*	Results may be confusing, giving an appearance similar to lupus erythematosus. Direct immunofluorescence shows deposits in blood vessels of IgG and/ or IgM and C_3 in some cases.
Muscle biopsy	The biopsy must be from clinically involved muscle as the disease is very patchy. It is diagnostic if positive.
EMG studies	These show a characteristic pattern.
Blood tests	The ESR may be elevated. There may be hypergammaglobulinaemia and positive rheumatoid factor, ANF and false positive WR. The muscle enzymes creatinine phosphokinase (CPK), aspartate transaminase (AST, SGOT) and aldolase may be raised, but can be normal.
Urine tests	Urinary creatine excretion is always raised. Myoglobinuria may be present.
Respiratory function tests	These tests should be done, particularly if there is weakness of the respiratory muscles.
Chest X-ray	These should be done to detect any lung involvement or an occult neoplasm.
Search for carcinoma	This should be undertaken in all patients past middle age.

Aetiology   Dermatomyositis is thought to be an auto-immune disease, probably cell mediated. It seems to be triggered by carcinomas, viral infections and immunization in some patients.

Treatment
General measures   Bed rest is necessary in the acute stage. Physiotherapy is essential to minimize wasting and prevent contractures.

Systemic therapy   Moderate to high dose steroids (prednisone 50–100 mg daily) are given initially and then reduced to a maintenance dose and eventually tailed off. If there is no response to steroids, cytotoxics such as azathioprine, cyclophosphamide or methotrexate are required.

   If a carcinoma is present, and is resectable, it should be removed, and in about two-thirds of patients this will result in remission of the dermatomyositis.

Natural history and prognosis   Treatment has reduced the mortality of childhood dermatomyositis from 30 to 10%, although many have gross residual damage. The mortality for adults has fallen from 50 to 25%. Those that die do so within the first two years from lung problems. Some eventually achieve complete remission.

8 DERMATOSES DUE TO INSECTS

SCABIES

Presentation   A common skin disease resulting from infestation of the skin by the organism *Sarcoptes scabiei* var. *hominis*. It has a worldwide distribution, affects both sexes and is most commonly seen in infants, children and young adults (Figure 8.1).

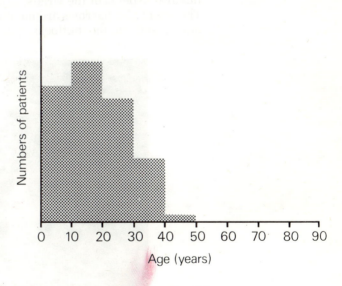

Figure 8.1   Age incidence of scabies

The first symptoms appear more than two weeks after infestation, the main complaint being generalized irritation which is more severe at night. The pathognomonic lesion is a burrow. The typical burrow is a greyish coloured, scaly, tortuous and linear lesion up to 1 cm in length (Figure 8.2). There

43

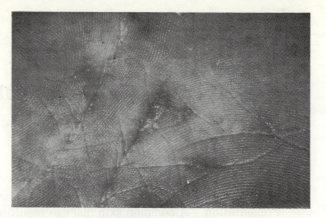

Figure 8.2   Burrows on hands in scabies

may be a small vesicle at one end and where the
mite is present. The burrow occurs on the palms,
flexural aspects of the wrists, and interdigital folds.
The insect also burrows around the axillary folds and
navel, and on the buttocks, perianal area, penis,

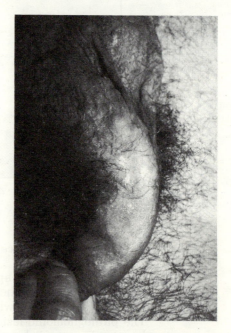

**Figure 8.3   Nodular lesions on the
penis and scrotum in scabies**

scrotum, and around the nipples, but here they present as reddish-brown scaly nodules (Figure 8.3). In infants and young children, burrows may be found on the soles, neck and face.

The generalized eruption which occurs on the trunk and limbs consists of small red papules, and is thought to be due to sensitization from the contents of the burrows. Secondary infection of the burrows may occur and clinically this presents as pustules.

Differential diagnosis

Scabies must be differentiated from generalized pruritus in which there is no visible skin cause, but there may be secondary changes due to scratching. The absence of burrows confirms the diagnosis.

Secondary eczematous changes, which may be seen in scabies, can be distinguished from primary eczema by the presence of burrows and a history of possible contact and the demonstration of the acarus.

Dermatitis herpetiformis may present as numerous small excoriated papules and if the buttocks are one of the main sites of involvement, the eruption is similar to that of scabies. The presence of burrows on the hands and genital area may be the only distinguishing feature.

Pediculosis corporis and pubis may also present with widespread irritation. In pediculosis pubis, nits are present on the pubic hairs.

Investigations

The most satisfactory way to confirm scabies is by finding the acarus or an egg on microscopy. To demonstrate this, a burrow is gently scraped with a blunt blade, and the contents examined by the low power of a microscope. Demonstration of the acarus is not necessary to establish the diagnosis if the clinical features are suggestive of the diagnosis.

Aetiology

The infection is caused by *S. scabei* var. *hominis* mites. The gravid female burrows in the keratin where she lays the eggs. When these are hatched the mites migrate from the burrow to the surface of the skin.

The generalized eruption is thought to be an immune response to the contents of the burrow, but which particular object is not known. The mite cannot survive away from the skin for more than a few hours and hence the transmission is by close bodily contact.

Treatment It is important that the topical application used in treatment is applied to the whole of the body surface below the head. All the members of the household and intimate friends should be treated simultaneously. The commonest preparations are γ-benzene hexachloride lotion 1% and benzyl benzoate BP.

The method of treatment is as follows: after bathing, the lotion is applied to the whole body except the head and neck, and this is repeated after 24 hours without a previous bath, and on the 3rd day the patient takes a bath. Patients should be warned that it may take several days for the irritation to subside, and the papular lesions especially on the genitalia may persist for months, although the patients are no longer infectious.

Course and prognosis The disease is persistent in the majority of patients until treated. It may lessen in severity or be mild in those with immunity to the infection.

NORWEGIAN SCABIES

A rare clinical pattern of scabies which causes epidemics in hospitals for the mentally retarded and in immune deficient patients. A large number of mites are present in the skin. Clinically there is generalized scaling and erythema of the skin with gross hyperkeratosis of the palms, soles and elbows. Irritation may be minimal or absent.

PEDICULOSIS (LICE)

Sucking lice are wingless insects, which can infest humans and cause pediculosis. There are three clinical forms depending on the species.

Pediculosis capitis

This is found worldwide with a higher incidence in pre-school children. Poor hygiene is a predisposing factor.

Presentation The characteristic feature is severe irritation of the scalp due to the parasite biting the skin. It is more severe on the back of the scalp and nape of the neck. Severe excoriation of the scalp causes secondary infection which presents as crusted and scabbed lesions. Secondary infection may be so severe as to cause constitutional upset. Exudation of the lesions in the scalp causes matting of the hair. Lice may be seen on the hair, but the nits (oval eggs) are more easily found. They are seen as small whitish-yellow objects 0.5 mm long, firmly cemented to the hair shaft, looking like scales, but they cannot be removed from the hair, other than by sliding them along the hair shaft to the end of the hair.

Differential diagnosis Pediculosis capitis must be differentiated from scalp infections, impetigo, seborrhoeic eczema and psoriasis of the scalp. The diagnosis is established by finding the mite or nits. Microscopic examination of the nit shows an encapsulated organism.

Aetiology This disease is caused by infestation with *Pediculis humanus capitis*, the head louse. The egg or nit hatches in 8 days. Infestation is usually transmitted indirectly by using an infested comb, hat or brush.

Treatment When secondary infection is severe, systemic antibiotics are required. Treatment of the infestation is either with topical γ-benzene hexachloride solution which is applied to the hair and scalp after washing and left for 24 hours, or with 0.5% malathion solution, which is similarly used but left for 12 hours.

The hair must then be shampooed and combed thoroughly to remove the nits. Treatment should be repeated after a week.

Pediculosis corporis

Presentation Pediculosis is rare in the western world and is usually only seen in vagabonds. It may, however, still be seen in some poor communities in other parts of the world. The lesions which may be present are pinpoint redness due to bites, small papules, weals and excoriations. Patients with long standing infestation may present with hyperpigmentation, secondary infection and eczematous changes. Lice and eggs are not usually seen on the skin, but are found in the seams of clothing. The diagnosis is established by finding the lice in the clothing.

Aetiology This disease is due to *Pediculus humanus corporis* infestation. Usually 10–15 organisms are found on an individual. The eggs which are cemented to the hair or clothing hatch in 8 days. Transmission is by close contact with infested clothing or bedding.

Treatment Treatment is with 1% γ-benzene hexachloride cream. Clothing and bedding should be thoroughly disinfected with γ-benzene hexachloride lotion or powder before laundering.

Pediculosis pubis

Presentation An infection found throughout the world affecting both sexes, mostly adults, but it can occur in children on the eyelashes and eyebrows.

   The presenting feature is severe irritation in the pubic area. However if the hair elsewhere on the body is also affected then the irritation may be felt on the trunk and thighs in males and axillae in both sexes. Excoriation and secondary infections may be found on examination. The diagnosis is established by finding the lice or more commonly the nits. The latter can be seen adhering to the hairs.

Aetiology Pediculosis pubis is usually transmitted by sexual contact and rarely from clothing or bedding. Infants are affected on the eyebrows and lashes from contact with an infected parent.

Treatment 1% γ-benzene hexachloride cream or lotion should be applied to the affected areas, and left for 24 hours, or a 0.5% malathion solution left for 12 hours. It is important to treat the sexual partners.

   If there is involvement of eyelashes or eyebrows this should be treated by an ophthalmologist.

PAPULAR URTICARIA

Presentation The skin lesions are caused by hypersensitivity to insect bites. It is most common in young children, especially those from poorer families, and occurs mainly during the summer season. It affects both males and females. The onset of the disease is usually between the ages of 2 and 6 years.

The most common presentation is urticarial papules. They usually occur on the exposed areas, such as the legs and arms, but rarely on the face. They may also be found on non-exposed areas. The lesions are a few mm in diameter and are discrete, but occur in groups. The lesions often take several days to resolve and are intensely irritating. Occasionally the lesions may persist for months. In severe reactions to the bites the urticarial lesions may progress to blister formation (Figure 8.4) and may be as large as a few cm. The diagnosis is based on seasonal attacks, the clinical appearances and the distribution of the eruption. A change in the environment results in recovery.

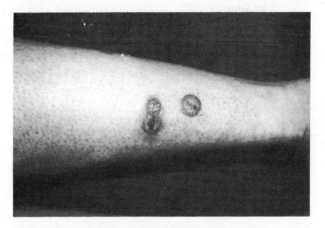

Figure 8.4   Bullous lesions due to insect bites

Differential diagnosis   Papular urticaria must be differentiated from scabies; in the latter, burrows may be found on the hands and wrists and the common sites for the papules are the genital area and buttocks. A history of infection in a close friend or family is common in scabies, but rare in papular urticaria. Atopic eczema, particularly if lichenified and papular, may resemble papular urticaria. In eczema there is often a past of family history of atopy, and the rash may also be found in the flexures. Prurigo nodularis, which is an excoriated papular eruption, occurs in older patients.

Aetiology The lesions are caused by hypersensitivity response to insect bites. There may be family history of similar problems in the parents or siblings.

Treatment Treatment during the attacks is symptomatic with systemic antihistamines and topical steroids. If secondary infection occurs antibiotics are necessary. A short course of systemic corticosteroids may be considered if the lesions are very widespread. Ideally the source of the insects should be identified and domestic animals which are a common source should be treated by a vet. Insecticide powders containing pyrethrum are effective in treating furniture and bedding. Insect repellants may be of some help.

Prognosis There may be repeated attacks over a few years, but the child eventually grows out of the problem. Each attack usually clears spontaneously in a few days or weeks, but occasionally will last for months.

9 DRUG ERUPTIONS

Presentation
It would be justifiable to say that all drugs are capable of causing skin lesions, and that any drug may cause any type of rash. However, certain drugs are more likely to cause certain types of skin eruptions often imitating disease entities. No history of skin disease today is complete without asking the patients whether they take any drugs, self-prescribed ones included. Many drugs bought without prescriptions are capable of causing rashes. Apart from the history of recent drug intake there are other clues that the eruption may be drug induced. The rash is usually of sudden onset and symmetrical. The extent of the eruption varies, it may be localized to the limbs or trunk, or it may be generalized. Occasionally there is constitutional upset at the same time as the rash appears. Depending on the drug involved and the mechanism of production of the skin lesions the time taken from drug intake to development of the rash will vary from a few hours to a few weeks.

Urticaria and angioneurotic oedema
The commonest drugs to cause urticarial reactions are the penicillins and salicylates. The rash may commence within hours or as long as six weeks after drug intake. Occasionally there is associated swelling of the tongue and laryngeal tissues and in these instances the disorder may prove fatal unless treatment is readily available.

Purpura
This is usually produced as a result of damage to the capillaries by the drug, and like purpura from other causes, it is commonest on the lower limbs due to increased venous pressure (Figure 9.1). The drugs most likely to cause purpura are the barbiturates, thiazide diuretics, phenothiazines, isoniazid and para-aminosalicylic acid. Carbromal (a hypnotic).

51

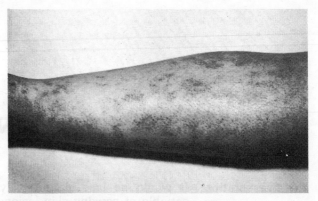

Figure 9.1   Purpura due to a phenothiazine

produces a distinctive pattern of purpura; the purpuric lesions are small and there is often surrounding erythema and pigmentation.

Maculopapular erythemas

These eruptions tend to be extensive (Figure 9.2) and eventually become scaly. The eruption may begin either on the limbs or trunk, and is one of the commoner types of rash due to drugs. Occasionally this

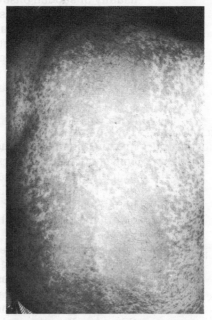

Figure 9.2   Extensive maculopapular eruption due to ampicillin

type of rash may become confluent and resemble an exfoliative dermatitis. Antibiotics, most commonly ampicillin and co-trimoxazole, cause this type of eruption. Other drugs which are frequently associated with this rash are barbiturates and phenothiazines.

Bullous eruptions   Non-specific bullous eruptions occur most commonly with barbiturates, sulphonamides, iodides and bromides. The blisters tend to be large and tense and may involve any part of the body, although the limbs seem commoner than elsewhere.

Pigmentation   Brown macular pigmentation on the upper cheeks, forehead, nose and upper lip, sometimes referred to as chloasma or melasma, is characteristically seen in pregnancy. It also occurs with the contraceptive pill and hydantoin. The pigment is melanin.

A diffuse yellow colour is produced by the antimalarial drug meparine. It can be distinguished from jaundice as the sclerae are not usually affected.

Exfoliative dermatitis   This is a generalized redness and scaling of the skin. It classically is a complication of gold therapy in the treatment of arthritis. It is also produced by sulphonamides, sulphonylureas, and phenylbutazone. It may occur with heavy metals, but these are rarely used today.

Lupus erythematosus   The typical cutaneous lesions of lupus erythematosus of the butterfly rash on the face and other exposed areas is produced by a number of drugs. These include hydrallazine, procainamide, griseofulvin, penicillin, reserpine, phenylbutazone and some oral contraceptives. The serological tests for lupus erythematosus are usually positive, but the disease is not so severe as in the idiopathic variety and there is usually no renal disease.

Acneiform eruptions   This is a papular and pustular eruption usually affecting the face and upper trunk, but comedones are not always present. The drugs most likely to cause this type of rash are systemic steroids, androgens, oral contraceptives (which have a relatively low oestrogen but high progesterone content), iodides, bromides and isoniazid.

Lichenoid eruption   This rash is very similar to lichen planus. The lesions are violaceous and tend to leave residual pigmentation. However, on occasions the rash occurs in confluent rather than discrete papules and is sometimes referred to as lichenoid eczema. The trunk is commonly involved in lichenoid rashes due to drugs. The antimalarial drugs, meparine, chloroquine and quinine, cause this type of eruption. In addition, thiazide diuretics, heavy metals, phenothiazines and methyldopa may precipitate this rash.

Erythema multiforme

Classical erythema multiforme even progressing to the Stevens–Johnson syndrome may be caused by barbiturates, gold, phenylbutazone, sulphonamides, sulphonylureas, and phenytoin.

Erythema nodosum

Typical erythema nodosum may be drug induced and the usual drugs to be implicated are the sulphonamides and sulphonylureas.

Psoriasiform eruptions

Although true psoriasis may be induced by withdrawal of corticosteroids or by giving chloroquine in susceptible individuals, a psoriasiform eruption has been described due to β-adrenergic blocking drugs (Figure 9.3). The drug which frequently caused this eruption was practolol and this has been withdrawn.

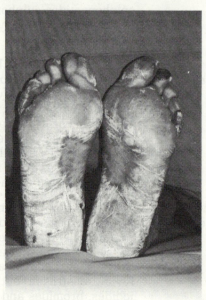

Figure 9.3 Hyperkeratotic scaly eruption due to a β-blocker

However, there are now reports of other 'β-blocker' drugs causing similar eruptions. The hands, feet and extensor surfaces of the limbs are mainly affected, although in severe forms the disorder could become generalized.

Photosensitivity A number of drugs which normally cause no skin reactions may do so if the patients are exposed to sunlight. The eruption, confined to exposed areas, is usually that of an acute eczema, with erythema, scaling (Figure 9.4) and in some cases crusting and

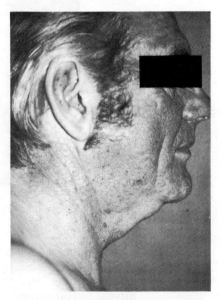

Figure 9.4   Photosensitive eruption due to tetracycline

exudation. The drugs most likely to cause photosensitivity are the tetracyclines, particularly demethylchlortetracycline, sulphonamides and the phenothiazines, particularly chlorpromazine. The latter produces a slate grey scaly eruption on the exposed areas.

Oral contraceptives *per se* do not cause photosensitive eruptions, but in susceptible individuals they may precipitate certain types of porphyria which results in a bullous eruption in the exposed areas.

Fixed drug This is a curious phenomenon in which the eruption
eruptions occurs at the same site or sites each time the drug is

taken. The lesion may be solitary, and is well demarcated. It usually commences as a red patch and then
becomes urticarial and on occasions, even bullous.
The lesion heals by crusting and scaling and characteristically leaves an area of pigmentation which
may be persistent (Figure 9.5). The diagnosis usually
comes to mind if the drugs are taken intermittently

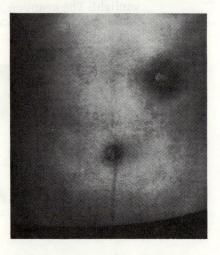

Figure 9.5   Fixed drug eruption

and on each occasion the lesion occurs at the same
site. The drugs which are most likely to cause a fixed
drug eruption are phenolphthalein (found in lax-
atives) barbiturates, sulphonamides, quinine, tetracyclines and phenylbutazone.

Infectious   If patients with infectious mononucleosis are given
mononucleosis   ampicillin they all develop a rash. The eruption is a
and ampicillin   generalized erythematous eruption with some punctate purpura.

Differential   The differential diagnosis of a drug rash is often
diagnosis   from the disease it is mimicking. The erythematous
maculopapular eruption has to be distinguished
from pityriasis rosea if only the trunk is involved,
and from some forms of secondary syphilis. The
bullous eruptions may be similar to pemphigoid, particularly in the elderly. Exfoliative dermatitis often
appears the same as erythroderma due to psoriasis

or endogenous eczema. In the latter two diseases there is usually a preceding history of the disorder. The diagnosis of a drug eruption is usually made from a history of recent or current medication.

Investigations   At present there are no worthwhile tests that will prove that a rash is due to a particular drug. If there is any doubt about the diagnosis then investigations into the alternative diagnosis should be carried out.

Aetiology   The mechanism by which drugs cause skin lesions is not fully understood in the majority of instances. It is probable that the pathogenesis is either allergic or a direct toxic effect. In the allergic situation the drug acts as an antigen and the body produces antibodies to this, and an antigen–antibody reaction then occurs in the skin with complement activation and subsequent tissue damage. The second mechanism is a direct toxic effect of the drug on the tissues with resultant damage and inflammation. Obviously the host is the important factor in the production of drug eruptions, because the incidence is relatively low compared to the numbers taking the drug. It would appear that the production of the rash is an idiosyncratic response by the host, whether it be allergic or toxic.

Treatment   The most important part of the treatment is to stop the offending drug. If patients are taking several drugs then ideally all drugs should be stopped. If this is not practical because some of the drugs are life saving, then those not absolutely necessary should be stopped. It should also be remembered that some drugs or groups of drugs are more likely to cause skin eruptions than others, and obviously these are the ones to be discontinued. Those most likely to produce rashes are antibiotics, salicylates, other anti-inflammatory agents, particularly those related to phenylbutazone, thiazide diuretics, and heavy metals. If the patient has been taking several drugs and they are stopped, then the drugs should be reintroduced one at a time, once the rash has cleared. It should be remembered that as the mechanism of production of the rash is unknown, it may take days or weeks before the rash reappears following the administration of the drug.

If it is known that a particular drug is responsible

for the rash then this drug should be avoided in the future. There have been reports where a drug would seem to have been responsible for a rash and then when given again no eruption developed. This may have been due to tolerance developing, or that there were particular circumstances (possibly due to the disease) in the host at a given time which were such that a rash is produced, but that this set of circumstances is not present again the next time the drug is given.

Cross-sensitization does occur between drugs of similar chemical formulae. Thus, if one form of penicillin causes a rash then all penicillins should be avoided. It is advisable that patients wear a disc around their neck or wrist listing the drugs to which they are known to be sensitive.

Actual positive treatment is rarely required in drug eruptions, the rash fading within days once the drug is discontinued. However, there are instances when the rash is persistent or severe when therapy is required. As the eruption is essentially an inflammatory response in the skin, steroids are the most effective drugs, whether the eruption is bullous, lichenoid, or an exfoliative dermatitis. If the disease is widespread, systemic steroids will be required. Prednisone 20–30 mg daily is usually sufficient, but if the disease is severe, such as the Stevens–Johnson syndrome or an exfoliative dermatitis, higher doses will be required. If the eruption is urticarial, systemic antihistamines are indicated.

Natural history and prognosis   The majority of drug eruptions clear within a few days of discontinuing the drug. Exceptions do occur such as persistent urticaria following penicillin, and exfoliative dermatitis following gold. As a general rule morbidity and mortality are low, but death may occur in angioneurotic oedema, or associated with the Stevens–Johnson syndrome, and exfoliative dermatitis. Providing the offending drug is avoided in the future, the patient should have no further trouble as regards the skin.

10 DYSKERATOTIC DISORDERS

Disorders associated with abnormal keratinization include very common lesions such as callosities and corns and rare genetic syndromes. The abnormalities may be generalized or limited to specific parts of the body. The classification is usually based on clinical features and depends on the type of lesion produced and the site.

KERATOSIS PILARIS

Presentation This is a very common condition, so common in fact that it is sometimes considered physiological rather than pathological. It is more common in females than

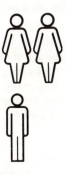

Figure 10.1   Keratosis pilaris is more common in females

males (Figure 10.1). It usually commences in childhood or adolescence. The lesion is excess formation of keratin at the site of the follicular orifice. Clinically

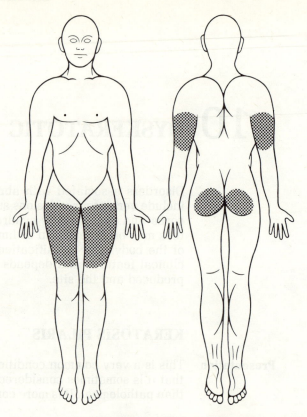

Figure 10.2   Common sites of keratosis pilaris

this presents as small rough papules. The commonest sites are the backs of the upper arms, front of the thighs and buttocks (Figure 10.2). Less commonly is it seen on the lower legs and face. Occasionally the lesions have an erythematous background, particularly when the condition is extensive on the back.

Differential diagnosis   The distribution of the eruption and age of the patient suggests the diagnosis. Sometimes keratosis pilaris is part of a more generalized disorder of keratinization such as ichthyosis.

Investigations   None.

Aetiology   The aetiology is unknown but genetic factors have been implicated.

Treatment Keratolytic agents are helpful. The commonest used is salicylic acid in a cream base. The concentration required to improve the condition varies from 2 to 10%. Other substances which may be used are 10% urea cream, or 10% sodium chloride in a cream or ointment base.

Natural history and prognosis Keratosis pilaris tends to clear in the majority of patients in adult life, although the age at which this occurs varies. It often persists in the third decade, but its incidence declines slowly after this age.

CALLOSITIES

Presentation Callosities are localized areas of hyperkeratosis usually in response to trauma. They may occur as plaques, or as papules which are often pressed into skin from pressure, particularly on the soles where these may be called corns. The lesions are hard and often have a yellow colour. The size varies from a few millimetres to a few centimetres. The commonest site is the soles of the feet. However, callosities may occur anywhere due to mechanical trauma, as seen on the hands due to various sports or occupations.

Differential diagnosis The commonest disorder which has to be distinguished from callosities is viral warts, particularly on the soles of the feet. Not infrequently the pressure from the wart causes hyperkeratosis and callosity formation, and the wart may be virtually buried in this excess keratin. The true callosity and wart can be distinguished by paring of the lesion with a scalpel. The wart will show a well demarcated area and cleft surface and possibly capillary bleeding points. The callosity may show a central area of shiny, compact keratin, but it does not have the clefted appearance that the wart exhibits. Punctate keratoses occur on the palms and soles, but are not confined to areas of trauma. The lesions are usually smaller and on the palms do not show surrounding hyperkeratosis.

Aetiology Apart from the obvious response of the skin to repeated mechanical trauma, it seems that some persons have an inherent tendency to callosities particularly on the soles of the feet.

Treatment   Obviously if possible the source of the problem should be removed. However, once they develop callosities are often self perpetuating as they increase the pressure on the surrounding skin with a production of more keratin. The lesions should be pared regularly, if necessary by a chiropodist. This lessens the pressure on the surrounding skin. Keratolytic ointments may be helpful, usually 10% salicylic acid ointment is used.

Natural history and prognosis   If the callosities are associated with a particular occupation or sport, then the lesions will persist until the sport or occupation is stopped. On the soles of the feet, once formed they may be self perpetuating.

PUNCTATE KERATOSIS

Presentation   Punctate keratoses may occur in adolescence or adult life and will depend on the cause of the problem. The sexes are equally affected. They commence as small circumscribed areas of hyperkeratosis (Figure 10.3).

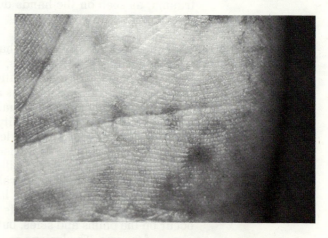

Figure 10.3   Punctate keratoses on the palm

They are raised but often have a concave smooth surface. The size varies from 2 to 5 mm. The lesions occur classically on the palms and soles.

Differential diagnosis Punctate keratoses have to be distinguished from callosities and viral warts. Callosities are usually localized to pressure areas, and viral warts have a clefted surface and capillary bleeding points, which may be seen when the lesion is pared.

Investigations There have been reports that there is an increased incidence of internal malignancies in association with punctate keratoses. This may be due to the fact that arsenic may cause cancer as well as the punctate keratoses. Simple screening tests such as a chest X-ray, stools for occult blood, and ESR may be justified.

Aetiology Punctate keratoses may be due to arsenic, usually given as medication 20–30 years prior to the lesions appearing. Punctate keratoses may also occur as part of an inherited disorder. In the latter cases, the lesions are often larger than those due to arsenic.

Treatment Topical keratolytic agents such as 10% salicylic acid ointment may soften and flatten the lesions, but the treatment is purely symptomatic.

Natural history and prognosis The lesions whatever the aetiology tend to be persistent. If the keratoses are due to arsenic then skin malignancies can be expected to occur. Arsenical punctate keratoses are considered to be premalignant themselves, but the skin malignancies may occur elsewhere on the body.

KERATODERMA

Keratoderma is thickening of the skin with the predominant feature being excess keratin formation. The keratodermas may be subdivided into the erythrodermas, in which the palms and sole are spared, and the palmoplantar keratodermas.

There are two recognized syndromes of erythrokeratoderma, both of which are rare.

Erythrokeratoderma variablis

Presentation This disorder usually presents in the first two years of life. The lesions are red and hyperkeratotic plaques of varying shapes. They usually begin on the limbs or buttocks but the face may also be involved.

Differential diagnosis   Psoriasis usually does not occur in this age group and in psoriasis the lesions are not so persistent and respond to treatment. Ichthyosiform erythroderma is usually more widespread and shows an increased severity of the condition in the flexures of the limbs.

Investigations   Biopsy.

Aetiology   The disorder is considered to have a genetic basis, and the gene is thought to be an autosomal dominant one.

Treatment   Topical steroids may be helpful in suppressing the erythematous part of the disorder, and keratolytics, such as salicylic acid ointment, will remove some of the excess keratin.

Symmetrical progressive erythrokeratoderma

Presentation   The disorder may commence at any time during infancy or childhood. The lesions are sharply demarcated, symmetrical hyperkeratotic plaques. They may begin on the backs of the hands and fingers, dorsa of the feet, fronts of the legs. Small patches may appear elsewhere on the body.

Differential diagnosis   The disorder has to be distinguished from psoriasis which usually begins at an older age. Ichthyotic conditions tend to be generalized rather than localized.

Investigations   Biopsy.

Aetiology   Thought to be genetic, autosomal dominant.

Treatment   Keratolytic agents such as 5–10% salicylic acid ointment, or 10% urea cream.

Natural history and prognosis   The disorder tends to be persistent, but does not become extensive.

KERATODERMA OF THE PALMS AND SOLES

Presentation Increased keratin on the palms and soles is not in itself a diagnosis, it is in fact a manifestation of several different skin disorders and the appearances will to a certain extent depend on the cause. The skin may be rough (Figure 10.4), or relatively smooth. The age of onset will also depend on the cause. Some of the inherited conditions will present in infancy, whilst acquired forms will develop later in life.

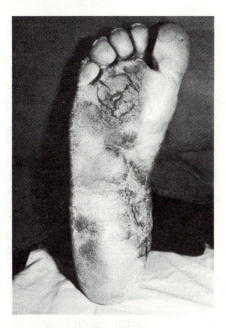

Figure 10.4 Keratoderma of the sole. Thick keratin and fissures

Differential diagnosis Many of the infantile forms of keratoderma on the palms and soles have skin lesions elsewhere and a family history of the disorder may be present. Occasionally the keratoderma is not uniform but of a particular pattern, such as punctate or linear (Figure 10.5). The diagnosis will depend on these features. Secondary or acquired keratoderma may be a manifestation of psoriasis, eczema, Reiter's disease, lichen planus, syphilis or yaws. The

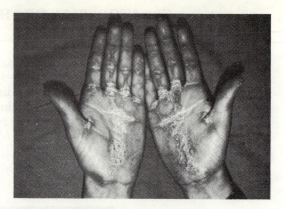

Figure 10.5   Inherited linear keratoderma

diagnosis is usually suggested by the history and lesions at other sites.

Investigations   A biopsy is not usually very helpful.

Aetiology   The syndromes which appear in infancy are of a hereditary nature.

Treatment   Keratolytics are the only treatment. On the palms and soles, the concentrations have to be greater than elsewhere as there is usually more keratin. Salicylic acid up to 15% may be necessary, or urea up to 20%. Sodium chloride 10–15% is sometimes effective when salicylic acid and urea are not.

Natural history and prognosis   The hereditary conditions tend to be persistent although some may improve in adult life. One type of keratoderma of the palms and soles is associated with carcinoma of the oesophagus. In this type of keratoderma the skin lesions usually appear between the ages of 5 and 15, and the carcinoma appears in the fourth or fifth decades. The prognosis of the secondary keratodermas is that of the primary disease.

KNUCKLE PADS

Presentation   The age of onset is usually between 15 and 30 and there is no sex predilection. The lesions begin as flat scaly plaques over the dorsa of the interphalangeal

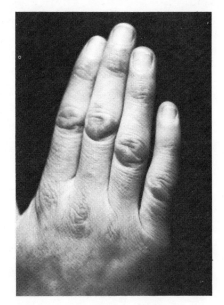

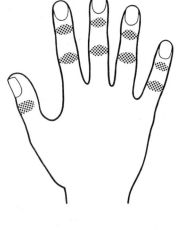

Figure 10.6 Knuckle pads

Figure 10.7 Distribution of knuckle pads

joints (Figure 10.6). The usual distribution of knuckle pads is shown in Figure 10.7.

Differential diagnosis
Viral warts have a clefted surface and thrombosed capillaries presenting as black dots may be seen in viral warts. Capillary bleeding points may be visible when the warts are pared. Granuloma annulare in the papular stage may have a similar appearance and occur at the same sites.

Investigations
If the diagnosis is in doubt, a biopsy will be helpful.

Aetiology
In some patients there is a family history of the condition suggesting that genetic factors are an important cause of the lesions. The lesions are due to thickening of the connective tissue to form fibromatous swellings. The overlying skin is hyperkeratotic, but the primary defect appears to be in the dermis.

Treatment
Surgery is the only possible treatment.

Natural history and prognosis
The lesions are persistent, and apart from the cosmetic appearance are not important.

11 ECZEMA

Eczema and dermatitis are used synonymously to describe a particular pattern of skin reaction to various different stimuli.

There are two major groups of eczema, exogenous and endogenous or constitutional. The differentiation is important to the patient, as exogenous eczema can be prevented by removing the cause. The presence of one type of constitutional eczema is associated with an increased incidence of other types of endogenous eczema and with exogenous eczema.

The appearance of an eczema is not specific to any one type of eczema. The appearance depends on severity, chronicity and site.

The major symptom of eczema is pruritus.

EXOGENOUS ECZEMA

There are three types of exogenous eczema: irritant, allergic contact eczema and photosensitive eczema. Photosensitive eczema is discussed separately (Chapter 33).

Irritant eczema

All people are susceptible to irritant eczemas. Many irritant eczemas are occupational.

There are two classes of irritants:

Strong irritants. Strong acids, alkalis, caustics and detergents cause an acute toxic contact eczema. This may be so severe that necrosis or even corrosion is produced. All people exposed will react with only a short exposure.

Weak irritants. Many substances encountered at work and in the home are weak irritants (see Table 11.1). Their irritant effects are enhanced by prolonged contact, i.e. failure to wash them off; occlusion by rings, protective gloves, or napkins; washing with harsh cleansers; inadequate drying of the hands, and cold winds.

Table 11.1   Weak irritants

Bleaches
Cleansers
Cutting oils
Detergents
Enzymes (e.g. biological washing powders and body secretions)
Plants (e.g. orange peel)
Soaps
Solvents
Weak acids
Weak alkalis

Patients with atopic eczema are very vulnerable to irritant eczema. A pre-existing eczema is often worsened by irritants.

Presentation   Irritant eczema occurs at all ages and in both sexes. In infancy and incontinent old age, urine and faeces, occluded by napkins and rubber pants, can induce or exacerbate napkin eczema. Saliva from drooling or lip biting and licking does the same. Housewives, particularly the mothers of young children, encounter numerous irritants, and suffer from chronic hand eczema. This may be superimposed on an endogenous eczema. Occupational exposure to irritants is frequent; the harsh solvents used to clean the skin often compound the damage.

Most irritant eczemas occur on the hands, as they are exposed to the irritants (Figure 11.1). Both the palms and backs of the hands are affected. Volatile irritants, e.g. ammonia, will affect the face. The perineum and buttocks are affected in napkin eczema.

Strong irritants cause erythema, oedema, papules, vesicles and bullae. There may be necrosis and ulceration.

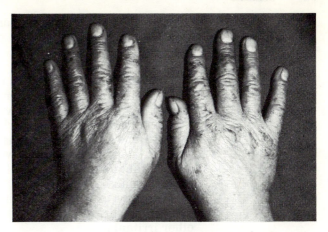

Figure 11.1   Occupational irritant eczema

Weak irritants initially cause drying and cracking of the skin. Continued use causes eczema, there is erythema, oedema scaling and fissuring. Papules and vesicles are rare.

Differential diagnosis   Irritant eczemas can be difficult to distinguish from endogenous hand eczema and acute allergic contact eczema. Atopic eczema affects the palms and backs of the hands, and its presence elsewhere particularly in flexures is the main distinguishing feature. However, people whose atopic eczema is inactive as well as those with active eczema are more susceptible to irritant eczema. Discoid eczema is distinguished by the localized plaques with surrounding normal skin, pompholyx by its intermittency, localization to sides of fingers and palms, and the presence of blisters. Allergic contact eczema almost never affects the palms.

Aetiology   Irritants cause damage by degreasing the skin; they gain access to epidermal cells causing separation of the cells and damage to the membranes and cytoplasm which may lead to cell death. The influx of inflammatory cells releases mediators, and oedema and inflammation result.

Diagnosis and investigations   The history, particularly occupational exposure to irritants, is important. Sometimes visits to the place of work are necessary, particularly if occupational compensation is involved.

Patch testing to potential contact allergens (see below) may be necessary to exclude an allergic eczema.

Treatment   The most important part of the treatment is removal of the irritant, or if this is impossible to minimize contact by protective gloves, washing off after contact, and the use of mild skin cleansers, e.g. emulsifying ointment. The hands must be protected with emollients and gloves in cold weather.

Moderate strength topical steroid ointments speed healing.

It is many months before the skin is completely healed and during this period it is very vulnerable to other irritants.

Natural history and prognosis   Removal of the irritant results in permanent healing. Sometimes this is impossible. Housewives cannot give up housework, and it may be impossible to change a job. A compromise may be necessary and reduced exposure to irritants and the use of mild steroids may improve the eczema to a level acceptable to the patient.

Major improvement is rapid, but complete healing takes months.

Allergic contact eczema

Certain elements and compounds have the ability to act as contact allergens and to evoke an allergic contact eczema (also known as contact hypersensitivity).

The development of contact allergy requires the sensitizer to be present on the skin and to be absorbed into the dermis.

Strong sensitizers need few applications to induce hypersensitivity. A single application is usually sufficient, and there is a reaction one week later. All immunologically competent persons exposed to these allergens will react. DNCB (dinitrochlorbenzene) is such a compound and is used as a test of cell mediated immunity.

Weak sensitizers are much more commonly encountered. Only a small number of those exposed become sensitized. It is not known why some indi-

Table 11.2 Common contact allergens

Substance	Source
Antibiotics (bacitracin, neomycin, soframycin, etc.)	Antibiotic creams, powders and dressing
Antihistamines (Antihisan, Caladryl)	Proprietary anti-itch creams
Antiseptics	Dettol, Germolene
Balsams	Perfumes in cosmetics and polishes, etc.
Chromate	Cement
	Leather
	Matches
Cobalt	Cement
Colophony	Soaps
	Sticking plaster
Dyes (paraphenylene, diamine etc.)	Hair dye
	Clothing
Lanolin	Cosmetics, ointments
Local anaesthetics	Pain and itch-relieving creams, sprays, suppositories, etc.
Nickel	Jeans' studs, jewellery, underwear fastenings, zips
Plants	Chrysanthemums, poison ivy, poison oak, primula
Preservatives (Parabens, etc.)	Creams, ointments, etc.
Rubber – domestic	Elastic, gloves, shoes
– commercial	Tyres (unusual because palms affected)

viduals are susceptible. Prolonged exposure, even decades, may be necessary to induce hypersensitivity.

Absorption of the allergen and hence sensitization is promoted by moisture, e.g. sweating, a humid environment, occlusion under protective gloves, dressings, etc. Areas with thin skin, the eyelids, flexures and backs of hands are most often affected. Degreased and chapped skin which has lost its protective layer of sebum, or broken skin, from eczema or varicose ulceration, is more liable to sensitization.

The common sensitizers are shown in Table 11.2. Many of these are iatrogenic exposures. When combined with topical steroids the allergy is partially suppressed but the continuance of the eczema points to the cause. Contrary to the belief of many patients and doctors, washing powders almost never cause contact allergies.

Presentation

Contact allergy is very rare below the age of 15 and in extreme old age. This is presumed to be due to diminished cell mediated immunity in the young and very old. Contact allergy is common between those two extremes of age. Population testing showed an incidence with a peak of 10% in middle aged women.

The sex incidence depends on the allergen. Nickel sensitivity is most common in women, rubber allergy is prevalent in both sexes, chromate and cobalt sensitivity is common in men because of their exposure during cement mixing and laying.

The distribution of the eczema corresponds to the sites of exposure to the allergen. Areas of thin skin are affected initially. The eyelids are the first region of the face to be affected. Sensitizers in contact with the hands affect the skin between the fingers and the backs of the hands. The palms are not affected as their thick horny layer prevents absorption. There is spread to adjacent sites, e.g. from backs of hands to wrists. Distant sites may be involved particularly the eyes and antecubital fossae. A severe contact eczema may become generalized.

Certain patterns of eczema suggest particular allergens. Eczema of the ear lobes, neck, wrists and umbilicus (Figure 11.2) often with secondary spread to the eyelids suggests nickel allergy. Rubber glove dermatitis presents with eczema of the backs of the hands and wrists with a clear upper limit. Allergy to

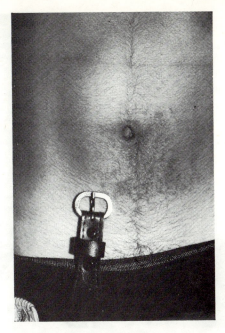

Figure 11.2   Contact allergic eczema due to nickel buckle

rubber tyres causes allergic eczema of the palms, at the place where they are gripped; this site is very rare with other allergens.

Cosmetics contain many potential allergens, perfumes, dyes, preservatives and lanolin. When sensitization occurs the eyelids are involved first, the rest of the face later. Nail varnish allergy does not affect the nails but areas touched by the fingers, e.g. eyelids (Figure 11.3) and neck. Hair dyes may sensitize after one or two applications or after years of use. A mild reaction affects the eyelids, neck and ears, severe reactions the face (Figure 11.4), neck and shoulders. The scalp is less affected. Clothing eczemas due to dyes or special finishes commence in moist occluded areas, popliteal and antecubital fossae and axillae, the vault being spared.

Occupational allergic hand eczemas affect the backs of the hands and lower arms.

Airborne allergens, from plants, powders, matches and volatile materials affect the face and neck.

The first sign of a contact allergic eczema is erythema and oedema. Facial oedema may be so

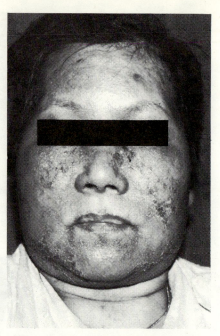

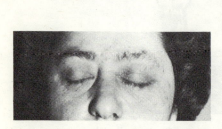

Figure 11.3   Contact allergic eczema of eyelids due to nail varnish

Figure 11.4   Acute contact allergic eczema due to hair dye

severe that the eyes are closed. There may be marked weeping of the serum and crusting. Papules and vesicles appear a little later. Bullae may be present in acute cases. Chronic contact eczema causes erythema and scaling.

Differential diagnosis

Irritant and endogenous eczemas may be confused. Eczema of the eyelids may be due to atopic eczema or seborrhoeic eczema, but the past history and involvement of other sites e.g. scalp and flexures or intertriginous area enable the distinction to be made in many cases.

Diagnosis and investigations

The diagnosis should be confirmed by patch testing. The patient is tested to a standard battery of common sensitizers, and any of the substances in the patient's environment that are under suspicion. The patches are applied to the back and outer arms under occlusion for 48 hours (Figure 11.5). The patches are removed at 48 hours and read at 2−3 and 5−7 days. A negative response is no reaction.

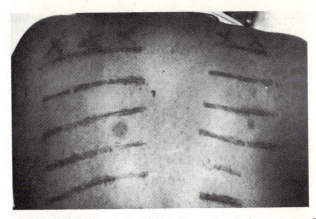

Figure 11.5 Sites of application of patch tests and positive patch test

Erythema is a weak positive, vesicles or bullae a strong positive. A response first appearing at one week may be primary sensitization.

Patch testing should never be done in a severe acute eczema as it will cause an exacerbation. High dose systemic steroids or application of topical steroids to the back in the previous month may give false negatives.

Aetiology Allergic contact eczema is a Type IV hypersensitivity reaction. The allergen penetrates the epidermis and is processed by the Langerhans cell (the epidermal equivalent of a macrophage), and presented to T lymphocytes in an antigenic form. Production of T lymphocytes directed against the antigen occurs in draining lymph nodes, the T cells then migrate back to the epidermis and react with antigen bound to Langerhans cells. Lymphokines and other mediators of inflammation are released, and a severe inflammatory response occurs.

Treatment Very severe contact eczema requires systemic steroids in moderate dosage prednisone 30 mg) as a short course. Potassium permanganate soaks are useful for acute weeping or bullous eruptions. Weak topical steroids should be applied twice daily to the face and diluted potent steroids to the body. Creams should be used for weeping eczema; ointments if it is dry.

The cause must be identified and avoided.

Natural history and prognosis

There is a very rapid response to therapy; most patients are much better within a few days. However, it may take months for the eczema to completely resolve.

Occasionally, occupational exposure is unavoidable and protective clothes and face masks have to be used in conjunction with a weak topical steroid.

ENDOGENOUS ECZEMA

The endogenous eczemas occur in constitutionally predisposed individuals. They may be exacerbated by external factors but are *not* due to them.

There are many kinds of endogenous eczema (see Table 11.3). They differ in their pattern of distribution and the ages susceptible.

Table 11.3   Endogenous eczemas

Type	Ages susceptible
Atopic eczema	Infancy, childhood
Seborrhoeic eczema	Infancy, adults
Discoid eczema	Adults
Pompholyx eczema	Adults
Lichen simplex	Adults
Asteatotic eczema	Old age
Varicose eczema	Middle–old age

Atopic eczema

Twenty to thirty per cent of the population are potentially atopic. They have a genetically determined predisposition to atopic eczema, extrinsic asthma, rhinitis and conjunctivitis. In only a small number (5%) of these individuals will atopic eczema develop.

Atopic eczema is also known as infantile eczema because of its onset in infancy, or flexural eczema because of its distribution, with a predilection for the flexures.

Presentation

Atopic eczema presents early in life (Figure 11.6). It is rare before one month of age. Most infants (60%)

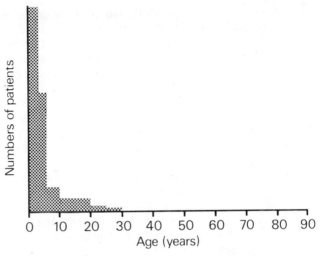

Figure 11.6   Age of presentation of atopic eczema

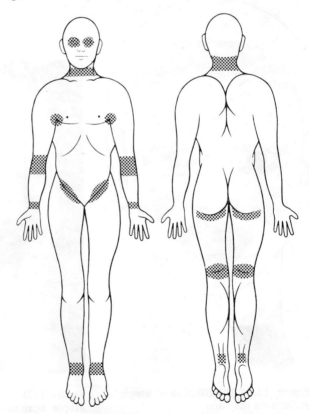

Figure 11.7   Distribution of atopic eczema

present between two months and one year. In 90%
the eczema is manifest by 5 years. The remaining
10% present later, even as young adults; however it
is very rare for atopic eczema to commence after 30.
In about 10% of patients it remits and then recurs
much later.

Both sexes are affected.

Atopic eczema occurs in all races. It is more common in urban environments. The highest incidence is
in recently urbanized groups, e.g. West Indians
emigrating to London.

The distribution of the eczema changes with age.
The eruption is symmetrical. In babies the face and
trunk are chiefly affected. In early childhood it
assumes the characteristic flexural distribution
(Figure 11.7). The face is involved particularly around

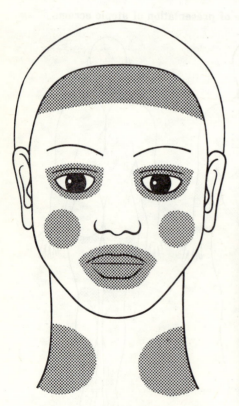

**Figure 11.8   Distribution of atopic
eczema on the face**

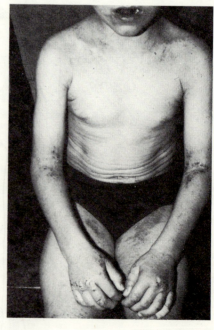

**Figure 11.9   Flexural distribution of
atopic eczema. The eczema is red,
scaly and crusted**

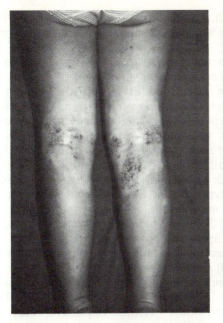 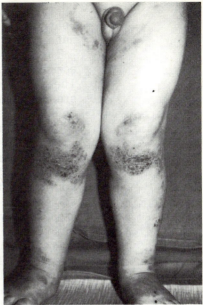

Figure 11.10 Flexural atopic eczema. There is erythema, excoriations and post-inflammatory hypopigmentation

Figure 11.11 Atopic eczema with 'reverse pattern' on the knees

the eyes and mouth, the cheeks and forehead (Figure 11.8). The scalp may be affected. The flexures are involved, the neck, antecubital fossae, popliteal fossae, gluteal folds, ankles and wrists (Figures 11.9 and 11.10). There may be eczema of the trunk. Anogenital involvement can cause pruritus vulvae and ani. The hands, both the backs (Figure 11.9) and palms, are often involved. Involvement of the nail fold causes ridging of the nails.

In Negro children it is common to see 'the reverse pattern' with the extensor surfaces of the knees (Figure 11.11) and elbows involved.

Any area of the body can be affected. In a few the eczema becomes generalized and erythroderma results. This is more likely to occur in adults than infants.

The lymph nodes draining any eczematized area can become enlarged, this can be very marked and cause great parental alarm. Resolution occurs with clearing of the eczema.

The most distressing symptom of eczema is the intolerable itch. Intense pruritus precedes the appearance of any skin lesion. Excoriations are a prominent sign.

The lesions are diverse in morphology. Typically eczematous areas are red and scaly (Figure 11.9). These may be excoriated (Figure 11.10), weeping or crusted (Figure 11.11). It is very rare to see vesicles. Small red papules are common. In Negro children micropapules and papules may predominate. The scalp may be scaly. The repeated scratching gives rise to lichenification. These are plaques of thickened skin with exaggerated skin ridges. Lichenification occurs typically on the neck and flexures. In adolescents and adults repeated scratching is associated with excoriated papules and nodules giving a pebbly appearance to the skin.

Postinflammatory hypo- and hyperpigmentation (Figure 11.10) are common.

Facial pallor and an extra crease under the lower eyelid are said to be stigmata of atopic eczema. The skin is often dry. White dermographism is characteristic of atopic eczema: firm stroking of an erythematous area produces a white line, probably due to vasoconstriction.

Atopic eczema is often improved by a change of environment: holidays with sunlight and sea bathing, or hospital admission. However, a few patients are made worse by sunlight. Most atopic eczema patients worsen during the winter probably because of the 'chapping' effect of the cold. Infections and emotional stress cause deterioration of the eczema.

Complications
Bacterial infection

Staphylococcal infection of atopic eczema is common, and causes discomfort, pain, weeping and crusting of the eczema. Streptococcal infections are also common, and cause pustules and erythema accompanied by pain, tender lymphadenopathy, and systemic symptoms of constitutional upset, and pyrexia.

Viral infections

These occur more frequently in children with atopic eczema than in normal children. They have a high incidence of viral warts and molluscum contagiosum.

Kaposi's varicelliform eruption is a serious consequence of infection with vaccinia virus or herpes simplex. Infection with vaccinia is acquired either by smallpox vaccination or contact with a recently vaccinated person. The virus becomes disseminated, and umbilicated vesicles appear and there is lymphadenopathy, fever and systemic upset. This can be fatal. Children with atopic eczema and household contacts should *not* be vaccinated against smallpox.

Ocular manifestations Patients with atopic eczema are prone to develop cataracts and keratoconus.

Atopic manifestations There may be other manifestations of the atopic state, viz. extrinsic asthma, urticaria and drug allergy, seasonal hay fever and conjunctivitis.

Differential diagnosis In infancy the distinction between seborrhoeic eczema of infancy and atopic eczema can be difficult, the earlier age of onset and localization to the scalp and intertriginous areas point to the former. Atopic eczema is suggested by a positive family history of atopy.

An acute contact eczema with secondary spread to eyelids and antecubital fossae can closely resemble atopic eczema in adults. The family history and distribution give the clues.

Diagnosis and investigations
Intradermal tests Immediate skin tests (Type I) to intradermal allergens may be positive. This reflects the atopic state. The allergens giving positive tests have no relevance to the eczema.

Blood tests These reflect the atopic state and are not specific to the eczema.

Eosinophilia, raised serum IgE and positive RAST (radio-allergen absorption tests) may all be found.

Aetiology It is thought that the tendency to atopy may be inherited separately from the factors governing which organs are affected.

There are two main theories concerning the aetiology of the atopic state:

Mucosal IgA deficiency This theory proposes that there is a transient deficiency of mucosal IgA during the first few months of life. The absence of IgA in the intestinal mucosa and lumen allows allergens present in food to enter the blood stream. These then stimulate IgE antibodies and possibly other immune mechanisms. In normal infants intestinal IgA neutralizes these antigens.

The mechanism by which the eczema is produced is unknown. It is postulated that prolonged and exclusive breast feeding by eliminating potential allergens at this crucial time may reduce the incidence of atopy. Its occurrence in a few cases despite breast feeding has been attributed to allergens in the maternal milk (from the mother's food) or inhaled allergens.

T-lymphocyte deficiency   Atopics have diminished cell mediated immunity as shown by increased susceptibility to virus infections, diminished susceptibility to allergic contact eczema, and diminished responses to tests for delayed hypersensitivity.

Atopic children have reduced absolute and relative numbers of T lymphocytes. This deficiency can be shown in potential atopics before one month of age, when there are no manifestations of atopy. It is postulated that the deficient T cells are regulator lymphocytes (possibly T-suppressor cells), and over-production of IgE in response to allergens occurs.

The mechanism causing the eczema is not understood.

Treatment
Environmental manipulation
Climate   Exposure to cold winds and low temperatures should be avoided because of the drying and cracking effects that these have on the skin.

Holidays with warmth, sun and sea bathing are often very beneficial. About six weeks are needed for the full response to be obtained.

Ultraviolet light   Many patients benefit from sunlight or from artificial ultraviolet light. PUVA therapy (psoralens and long range ultraviolet light) has been used with benefit in a few cases.

The patients that are exacerbated by sunlight should avoid it.

Clothing   Wool and man-made fibres cause pruritus and should be avoided. Cotton or silk should be worn next to the skin.

Psychological stress   This should be minimized, but it is usually impossible to do so. Often clearing of the eczema improves the psychological state.

Diet   Exclusive breast feeding in infancy reduces the incidence of atopy during the first year of life; it does not completely abolish it, and it is not known whether it will have a long term effect. It is thought that allergens in cows' milk, eggs and other foods may have a deleterious effect on atopic eczema. Exclusion diets with total exclusion of milk, all milk products, beef, eggs and chicken with substitution of soya bean based milk has been reported to improve the eczema in some atopic children. However, this diet requires obsessional parents and a very docile cooperative child. Many patients cannot manage the diet.

Topical therapy
Topical steroids

These have greatly changed the treatment of atopic eczema. They should be used intensively when the eczema is present and discontinued when the skin is clear. Hydrocortisone should be used on the face; more potent steroids cause thinning and erythema. It is also useful for the body in infants. It is applied two to three times daily. The ointment greases the skin and has a longer duration of action than the cream. Diluted potent steroid ointments should be used on the body in severe childhood eczema and adult eczema. The weakest dilution that is effective should be used. Full strength potent steroids may be needed for lichenified patches.

Urea

Urea 10% in a cream or ointment hydrates the skin, reduces cracking and has an antipruritic effect. It can be combined with hydrocortisone. It is most helpful for the diffuse dry skin or ichthyosis. It is applied after bathing.

Crude coal tar

This is effective in eczema. It can be used as a topical application or mixed with emulsifying ointment (20% liquor Picis Carb. in emulsifying ointment) as a soap substitute. The emulsifying ointment helps to grease the skin and is helpful on its own as a soap substitute. Coal tar impregnated bandages are useful for the legs.

Bath preparations

There are many soap substitutes and greasing agents for the bath. Twenty per cent liquor Picis Carb. in emulsifying ointment is one of the most effective, but is not always acceptable to patients and parents because of the smell and the difficulty in cleaning the bath. Plain emulsifying ointment can be used as a soap substitute. Various oils or oatmeal preparations can be added to the bath to soothe and grease the skin.

Topical antibiotics	These may be required for superficial skin infections. Sensitization may occur so use should not be prolonged.
	Terra-Cortril is helpful for painful cracks and fissures.
Systemic therapy Steroids	Systemic steroids in high doses will suppress atopic eczema. However, as the disease is very chronic, long-term steroid therapy is required; this is undesirable in children and young adults and they are very rarely used. Growth stunting is an unacceptable side-effect in young children.
Antihistamines	Antihistamines at night are helpful in reducing the pruritus and by inducing drowsiness enable the child to sleep through the night.
Antibiotics	As skin infections in eczema are often widespread and extend below the epidermis, systemic antibiotics are required. Erythromycin is the antibiotic of choice.
Natural history	Remissions of atopic eczema occur at any age. Ninety per cent are clear by 10–12 years, but 10% recur often during the teenage years. Most patients are clear by 30 years.
	Late onset, reverse pattern, associated asthma, family and social problems all make the prognosis worse.

Seborrhoeic eczema

This is a very common eczema; many people have minor degrees of seborrhoeic eczema. There are two clinical types: seborrhoeic eczema of infancy and the adult form. Areas rich in sebaceous glands or intertriginous areas are most often affected.

Seborrhoeic eczema of infancy

This has other names according to the site chiefly affected. Cradle cap is the name given when the scalp is the area affected. Involvement of the napkin area is termed 'nappy rash', 'napkin eczema' or 'diaper dermatitis'.

Presentation   It begins very early in life (Figure 11.12), before atopic eczema. Many cases begin in the first month of life and most within the first three months. The areas affected are the scalp (cradle cap), the

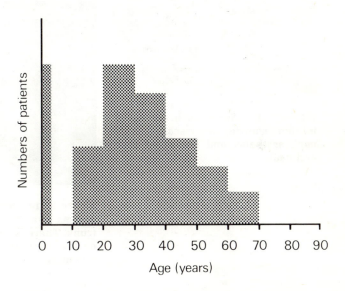

Figure 11.12   Age of onset of seborrhoeic eczema

cheeks, the folds of the neck (Figure 11.13), the axillae, and the folds of the elbows and knees. The napkin area is often the first and most severely involved area. This is thought to result from the combination of constitutional predisposition to seborrhoeic eczema combined with the irritant effect of urine and faeces on the skin. There is often spread from the napkin area to the trunk (Figure 11.14). The seborrhoeic eczema may become generalized.

The scalp is often red and covered in scales; these may be fine and white, or thick and greasy. The face and trunk show erythema and scaling (Figures 11.13 and 11.14). Under the napkin and in folds the skin is red, moist and macerated (Figure 11.14). Occasionally there may be very pronounced scaling in the

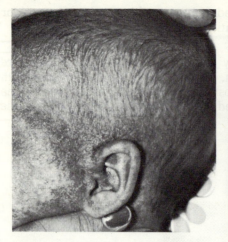

Figure 11.13 Seborrhoeic eczema of infancy, showing scaly scalp (cradle cap), erythema and scaling of face and neck

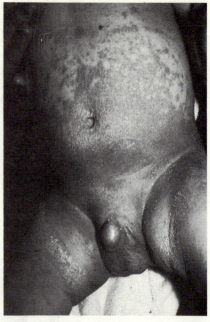

Figure 11.14 Spread of seborrhoeic eczema from the napkin area to the trunk. There is erythema and scaling on the trunk, the napkin area is red and moist

napkin area and the rash is then termed psoriasiform. Pruritus does not seem to be a significant feature. Secondary infection of the napkin area with candida is very common; this gives rise to 'satellite lesions', small pustules extending beyond the rash.

Differential diagnosis   Atopic eczema may be difficult to distinguish; the family history, later onset, different distribution and pruritus distinguish it.

Diagnosis and investigations   Swabs confirm the presence of candida.

Aetiology   Seborrhoeic eczema is of unknown cause. The irritant effect of wet napkins is able to evoke it in those constitutionally predisposed.

There is no predisposition to seborrhoeic eczema in later life.

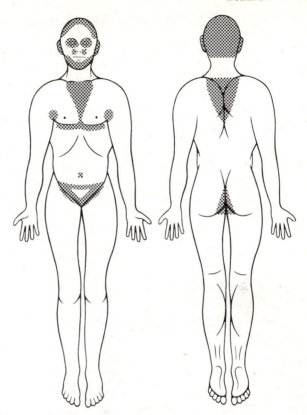

Figure 11.15   Distribution of seborrhoeic eczema

Treatment   This eczema is very rewarding to treat. Cradle cap is best treated by applying a mild keratolytic (1% sulphur and 1% salicylic acid in aqueous cream) overnight to the scalp and shampooing it off the next day. Applications 2–3 times per week are usually sufficient to keep the scalp clear. The face and body should be treated with a weak topical steroid (1% hydrocortisone). This is best applied in combination with nystatin in the napkin area, because candida is such a frequent secondary invader. Emulsifying ointment should be used as a soap substitute. The napkins should be changed frequently and left off for several hours each day. Treatment should be reapplied each time the napkin is changed.

Natural history and prognosis   The prognosis is very good. Most children are clear by 18 months. It does not predispose to adult seborrhoeic eczema.

Adult seborrhoeic eczema

Mild forms of this endogenous eczema are very common. Dandruff and intertrigo are often manifestations of seborrhoeic eczema.

Presentation   Seborrhoeic eczema commences at any age from teenage onwards. Young adults are often affected (Figure 11.12).

Both men and women are affected.

The distribution of seborrhoeic eczema is shown in Figures 11.15 and 11.16. Any or all of these sites may be affected. The scalp and ears are common sites, both behind the pinna and in the external auditory meatus. The face is often affected (Figure 11.16); the eyebrows, around the eyes, and nasolabial folds are typical sites. The areas around the lips, forehead

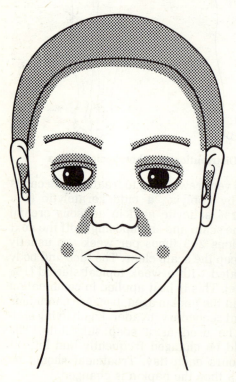

Figure 11.16 Distribution of seborrhoeic eczema on the face

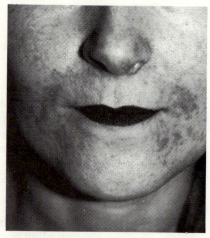

Figure 11.17 Seborrhoeic eczema of the nasolabial and circumoral areas. There is erythema and scaling

and cheeks may also be involved (Figure 11.17). The centre of the chest, the centre of the back, over the scapulae and between the shoulder blades are involved. All the intertriginous areas: axillae, under the breasts, umbilicus, abdominal fold, groins, perineum, vulva, glans penis and foreskin (Figure 11.18) and the perianal area, can be affected.

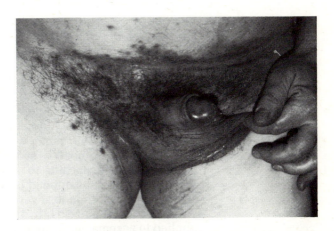

Figure 11.18   Seborrheoic eczema of the abdominal fold, groins and glans penis. These areas are moist and red

Severe cases can become generalized.

Seborrhoeic eczema is red and scaly (Figure 11.17). The scalp may show fine white scaling, or there may be greasy yellow scales on a background of erythema. Severe cases may have thick crusted scales and weeping. The eczema on the face and trunk is red and scaly, often in well circumscribed patches (Figure 11.17). Involved intertriginous areas are red and moist, often with maceration (Figure 11.18). The edge is ill-defined. There is a rare follicular form, with tiny perifollicular pustules.

Seborrhoeic eczema is often very itchy.

Stress and fatigue make seborrhoeic eczema worse. Sunlight is often beneficial.

Differential diagnosis   Severe seborrhoeic eczema of the scalp or intertriginous areas may be difficult to distinguish from psoriasis. Fungal infection of the groins can give rise to a red scaly rash.

When the eyelids alone are involved an allergic contact eczema should be excluded.

Diagnosis and investigations

Secondary infection of intertriginous areas should be excluded by taking swabs for bacteria and candida.

Scrapings should be examined for fungus.

Patch testing should be carried out if an allergic contact eczema is considered.

Treatment

The scalp is best treated by the application of keratolytics to the scalp overnight, and shampooing them off the next day. Two per cent salicylic acid and 2% sulphur in aqueous cream is effective; the strength can be increased to 5%. Resistant cases may require Ung. Cocois Co. (coal tar solution 10%. sulphur 5%, salicylic acid 5%, camphorated oil 10%, coconut oil 30%, and emulsifying ointment to 100%), used in the same way. Applications 2–3 times a week are usually sufficient, the frequency being adjusted according to severity. Lotions of potent steroids may be applied between hair washes if scaling and irritation is severe.

Weak topical steroids (hydrocortisone) should be applied to eczema on the face, twice daily, until healing occurs.

Intertriginous areas should be treated with a moderate strength steroid cream. Antiseptic paints, e.g. 1% aqueous gentian violet, magenta paint, are useful in intertriginous areas, as they are drying and prevent secondary infection. They should be applied morning and evening, the topical steroid can be applied after drying of the paint. Moderate strength steroid ointments should be used on the trunk.

Natural history and prognosis

This eczema runs a very chronic course, often persisting indefinitely. There are periods of relapse and remission. Different areas may be affected at different times.

Discoid eczema

This endogenous eczema is common. It may be associated with pompholyx eczema (see below).

It is also known as nummular eczema.

Presentation   It affects young adults. Although it does occur in children it is rare before 20. It most commonly presents between 20 and 40 years, but may commence in old age. Both sexes are affected.

The extensor surfaces of the limbs (Figure 11.19), the hands and feet, particularly the dorsal surfaces, are involved. Involvement of the nail folds causes nail ridging. The face is rarely affected.

The lesions are symmetrical, well defined and coin-like in both size and shape (Figure 11.19). Sometimes they are many centimetres in diameter. There may be few or many lesions.

The lesions are well defined scaly plaques. The acute lesions may have papules and exude serum (Figure 11.19). This eczema is often very itchy.

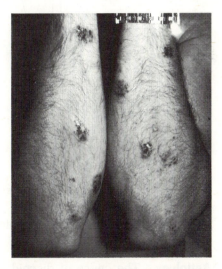

Figure 11.19   Discoid eczema: coin-like lesions on the extensor aspect of the arm. The eczema is red and crusted

Differential   Lichen simplex is solitary and lichenified.
diagnosis   A few lesions may resemble ring worm, but the lack of central clearing distinguishes it.

Plaques of mycosis fungoides can resemble discoid eczema, but are persistent.

Diagnosis and   A biopsy shows eczema and will exclude mycosis
investigation   fungoides.
Skin biopsy

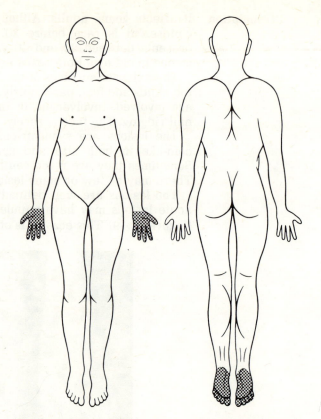

Figure 11.20   The distribution of pompholyx eczema

Scrapings   Scrapings for mycological examination exclude fungus.

Aetiology   The cause of discoid eczema is unknown, as is its relationship to pompholyx eczema.

Treatment   Topical steroids are very efficacious. The lesions usually respond to a short course of moderate strength steroids. Sometimes very potent steroids are necessary.

Antihistamines are sedative and helpful at night.

Natural history and prognosis   The severity of the disease is variable. Many young women have a few dry scaly, pruritic patches on their upper arms, which cause little discomfort or cosmetic disability. Some patients have severe, numerous and extensive lesions. The response to treatment is good, but recurrence occurs. Often there may be months or years of activity and then remission.

Pompholyx eczema

This is one of the most incapacitating of the endogenous eczemas. This is because of its localization to the palms and soles so that both work and walking are difficult.

Pompholyx eczema is also known as dyshidrotic eczema because it is often associated with excess sweating. It may be subdivided on the basis of its site into cheiropompholyx on the hands and podopompholyx on the feet.

Presentation   Adults are most commonly affected. It usually presents in young adults, but may commence at any age. It is rare in childhood.

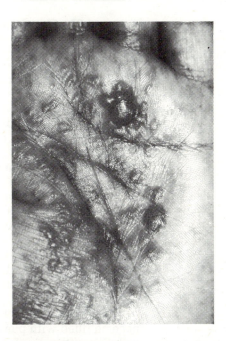

Figure 11.21 Acute pompholyx eczema of the palm, showing vesicles and bullae.

Both men and women are affected.

The eruption is usually, but not invariably, symmetrical. Either the hands or feet, or both, may be affected (see Figure 11.20). The sides of the fingers, palms (Figures 11.21 and 11.22), and occasionally the dorsum of the fingers are affected. Similarly the

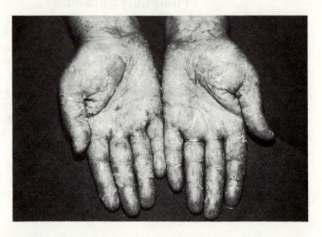

Figure 11.22 Chronic pompholyx eczema of the palms and fingers. The skin is red and scaly. A fissure is present on the palm

toes, tips, sides and dorsum, and the soles are affected on the feet. Often the eruption may be confined to one small area. In severe cases the eczema may spread to the backs of the hands or dorsum of the feet, and up the arms or legs. Rarely it may become generalized.

The initial lesions are small vesicles. These may expand and coalesce to form large bullae (Figure 11.21), resolve, or gradually dry up. These usually persist for 1–2 weeks. The next stage is prolonged and may last for many weeks. The chronic stage is not always preceded by the blisters, or they may not always be noticed. In this stage the palms and soles are dry and scaly and painful fissures form (Figure 11.22). The nails become ridged if the nail fold is involved.

Secondary infection is common. The blisters become filled with pus and there may be associated cellulitis with pain, fever and lymphadenopathy.

Attacks are often precipitated by heat or emotion, probably by induced sweating.

The chief symptoms are intense pruritus. When the vesicles are erupting, puncture of them may give relief. Pruritus persists in the chronic stage and the fissures are painful.

Discoid eczema may be present on the limbs and trunk.

Differential diagnosis The vesicles may be confused with an acute fungal infection or with the pustules of pustular psoriasis.

The chronic dry scaly stage resembles irritant and atopic eczema, psoriasis or fungal infections. The other eczemas are differentiated by the involvement of the backs of the hands. There may be nail involvement with characteristic pitting or onycholysis in psoriasis, or psoriasis elsewhere. Fungus and psoriasis are much less itchy.

Diagnosis and investigations Fungal infection should be excluded by taking scrapings for mycological examination.

Swabs for bacterial culture may be necessary if secondary infection is suspected.

Aetiology The cause of this endogenous eczema is unknown. A relatively high proportion of women with pompholyx have positive patch tests to nickel, and in some of these patients exacerbations can be related to a recent high nickel intake, often caused by boiling acidic fruits in stainless steel saucepans. A low nickel diet has been advocated as a therapy.

It has been suggested that pompholyx of the hands can be a reaction to a fungal infection of the feet. These cases are exceptionally rare.

Treatment The acute blistering stage is best treated with potassium permanganate soaks (1 : 8000) for 15 minutes three times a day. This dries up the eczema and prevents infection. After the soaks, the eczema should be allowed to dry and then a weak steroid applied. The dry, cracking phase requires moderate to very potent steroid ointments, greasing agents, e.g. emulsifying ointment or 20% liquor picis carb. in emulsifying ointment as a soap substitute, the proprietary preparation Terra-Cortril or Tinct Benz. Co. are helpful for the fissures.

Systemic antihistamines allay the pruritus and are sedative. Systemic steroids may be required in severe attacks, moderate doses (prednisone 30 mg daily) are usually sufficient. some patients have such severe and persistent pompholyx that maintenance low dose systemic steroids (prednisone 10 mg daily) are necessary to enable them to live a normal life.

Systemic antibiotics are necessary for secondary infection.

Natural history and prognosis

Pompholyx is a very variable condition. Its severity ranges from an isolated attack every few years, to months of recurrent attacks, or a severe persistent incapacitating condition. In some patients it is lifelong.

Lichen simplex

This can be regarded as a localized form of atopic eczema.

Presentation

Lichen simplex occurs mainly in adults. Women are affected more often than men. There is often a personal or family history of atopy.

The lesions are usually single. Common sites are the nape of the neck (Figures 11.23 and 11.24), less commonly the forearms, wrists, shins and ankles. The plaques vary in size from a few to many centimetres. They are well defined and lichenified with thickened epidermis and exaggerated skin ridges (Figure 11.24). They are often reddish purple and may be hyperpigmented. Papules may be present giving a pebbly appearance.

The plaques are intensely itchy and a cycle of itch, scratch and inflammation leading to more itch is set up. Stress has an adverse effect.

Differential diagnosis

Discoid eczema (see above) causes pruritic eczematous plaques and if a single lesion is present may cause confusion, but lichenification is absent. Hypertrophic lichen planus on the legs is distinguished by the purple colour and Wickham's striae.

Lichen amyloid on the lower limbs may be very itchy; its symmetrical distribution and rippled appearance differentiate it from lichen simplex.

Diagnosis and investigations

Skin biopsy is occasionally necessary to confirm the diagnosis.

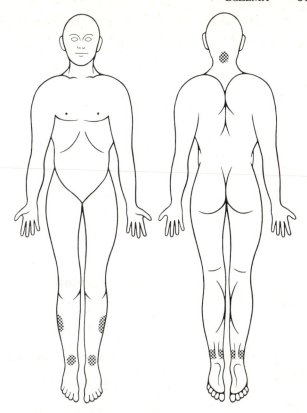

Figure 11.23   Lichen simplex: common sites

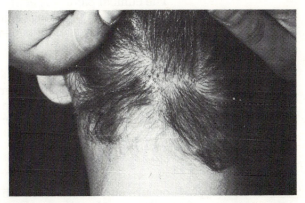

Figure 11.24   Lichen simplex on the occipital region, a typical site

Aetiology   Atopics have a low threshold for pruritus, but the cause of the local pruritus is unknown. Constant scratching in response to the itch causes lichenification of the atopic skin.

Treatment   It is difficult to interrupt the cycle of itch and scratch. The very potent topical steroids are usually the most successful. Intralesional steroids will speed resolution. Occlusion with coal tar bandages is often successful, but it is unpopular with patients.
Systemic antihistamines are useless.

Natural history and prognosis   Lichen simplex may resolve with treatment, but recurrence at the same or a different site is common. Permanent resolution usually occurs in old age.

Asteatotic eczema

Asteatotic eczema is also known as eczema craquelé, xerosis or winter itch.

Presentation   This is a disease of the elderly. Both sexes are affected.
It occurs chiefly in winter, and is very common in old people brought into hospital and subjected to much scrubbing and bathing.
The legs, particularly the shins, are chiefly affected, it can extend to the thighs (Figure 11.25) and arms and trunk.
The clinical picture is characteristic. There is fine dry scaling and cracking (Figure 11.25), the cracks are red. This gives an appearance like crazy paving or crazed china.
It is itchy.

Differential diagnosis   The appearance is characteristic. However, as it often occurs after hospital admission it is falsely attributed to drugs administered.

Diagnosis and investigations   None are relevant.

Aetiology   It occurs only in the constitutionally predisposed. It may be considered as a very excessive chapping effect. Cold temperatures chap the skin, harsh soaps,

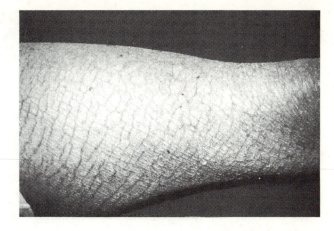

Figure 11.25   Asteatotic eczema on the thigh showing scaling and 'crazy paving' appearance.

and frequent washing degreases it, central heating dries it out. The combination of all these irritants and the constitutional predisposition produces asteatotic eczema.

Treatment   Topical steroids diluted in white soft paraffin reduce the itching and heal the skin. Greasing agents, e.g. emulsifying ointment, should be used as soap substitutes.

Natural history and prognosis   Healing of the skin is rapidly achieved and continued use of greasing agents usually prevents recurrence.

Varicose eczema

Varicose eczema is also known as hypostatic eczema.

Presentation   The middle aged and elderly are affected.

Men and women are both affected, although women predominate.

The eczema commences on the inner aspect of the shin, just above the medial malleolus (Figure 11.26). It often spreads to involve the whole of the shin, and when severe the other leg, arms and trunk will be involved.

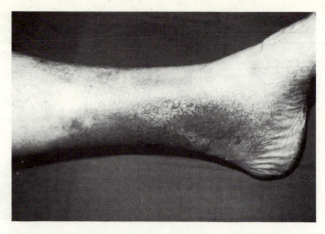

Figure 11.26   Varicose eczema at the typical site. There is erythema, scaling and pigmentation

There is initially itching. The rash commences as dry scaly skin, it may become erythematous (Figure 11.26) and purpuric. Thick greasy scales may accumulate. The skin heals but becomes thin, shiny and hyperpigmented.

Slight trauma results in breaking of the skin and an ulcer ensues.

There is often associated oedema of the leg.

Complications
Ulceration   The thin skin, with poor blood flow due to high back pressure and poor 'run off', is easily damaged and heals slowly, so that ulceration results. Bacterial infection often further delays healing.

Allergic contact eczema   The thin broken skin of varicose eczema or ulceration, combined with occlusive dressings provides optimum conditions for allergic contact sensitization. The chronic use of topical antibiotics as creams, dressing or powders, or of topical local anaesthetics or antihistamines is common, and often results in acute disseminated contact eczemas.

Irritant eczema   A similar disseminated eczema may result from the use of irritants, e.g. keratolytics or proprietary antiseptics. Patients use very harsh and inappropriate remedies. These exacerbate the eczema.

Autosensitization   Prolonged severe varicose eczema may become generalized.

Differential diagnosis	Localized varicose eczema is typical.
Diagnosis and investigations	The cause of the hypostasis must be sought. Venography may be necessary to determine if a surgical cure of the hypostasis is possible. Ulcers should be swabbed for secondary bacterial infection.
Aetiology	Hypostasis may result from varicose veins or the post-phlebitic leg. It is not clear why poor tissue perfusion and high venous pressure cause eczema.
Treatment *General*	Hypostasis should be minimized by elevation of the leg and support stockings or bandages. Raising the foot of the bed by 9 inches is easily done. Surgical intervention to obliterate the varicose veins should be undertaken when possible.
Topical treatment	Weak topical steroids (hydrocortisone or 10 times dilutions of potent steroids) should be applied twice daily. Any potential sensitizers should be avoided. Coal tar bandages are very effective in healing the eczema and providing support, but are poorly tolerated by many patients.
Natural history and prognosis	The prognosis is poor unless the cause of the hypostasis is eliminated. Varicose ulcers require a cooperative and motivated patient if permanent healing is to be achieved.

AUTOSENSITIZATION

This can occur with any eczema whether endogenous or exogenous.

Presentation	A severe local eczema becomes disseminated. There is symmetrical spread to distant sites. It may become generalized. There are characteristic patterns; e.g. varicose eczema often spreads to the arms, nickel sensitivity to the eyes.
Differential diagnosis	It may be difficult to differentiate between endogenous eczema with autosensitization or with superimposed allergic contact eczema.

Aetiology   In a few patients a delayed type response to their own epidermal antigens has been demonstrated.

Treatment   Systemic and/or topical steroids will be required to control the eczema.

Natural history and prognosis   This is determined by the prognosis of the triggering eczema.

12 ENDOCRINE DISORDERS AND THE SKIN

Endocrine disorders have diverse effects on the skin, and occasionally patients with endocrine disorders present to the dermatologist.

There are certain cutaneous markers of endocrine disease that are not organ specific:

Acanthosis nigricans Acanthosis nigricans developing in a young person, particularly if obese, suggests an underlying endocrine abnormality; often the pituitary is at fault (see page 1).

Vitiligo Vitiligo is an auto-immune disease and may be occasionally associated with other more serious auto-immune diseases (see page 299). When present it suggests that the disease of an endocrine gland is auto-immune.

The other changes seen in endocrine disease are specific for certain hormones.

Thyroid disease
Pretibial myxoedema Pretibial myxoedema is usually located on the front of the shins, but can arise elsewhere. There is localized thickening of the skin, which is often purplish in colour (Figure 12.1).

It is sometimes associated with thyroid acropachy (Figure 12.2) and exophthalmos.

It is caused by the action of long acting thyroid stimulator (LATS) and is found in hypothyroidism, hyperthyroidism and euthyroid patients.

Hypothyroidism Hypothyroid patients have dry, cold, puffy skin. There is often a yellow tinge to the skin due to carotinaemia. They sweat little. The hair is coarse, and hair loss from the vertex and eyebrows is common. Xanthelasma are occasionally present.

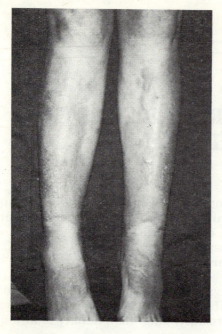 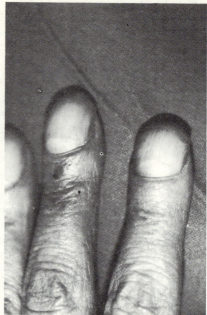

Figure 12.1 Pretibial myxoedema: red plaques of thick skin on the shins and feet

Figure 12.2 Thyroid finger clubbing associated with thyroid disease

Thyrotoxicosis

Thyrotoxic patients have a warm moist skin. They sweat excessively. Onycholysis, i.e. separation of the distal part of the nail from the nail bed, may occur (Figure 12.3). The hair is fine and often thinned, particularly anteriorly.

The adrenal cortex
Addison's disease

There is marked pigmentation in Addison's disease. The skin becomes darker, particularly on light exposed areas, and there is dark brown pigmentation of the buccal mucosa, lips (Figure 12.4), nipples, genitalia, sites of friction, e.g. knees, elbows, palms and soles, scars and darkening of pigmented naevi.

These changes result from the hypersecretion of ACTH by the pituitary.

Cushing's syndrome

Excess glucocorticoids, whether endogenous or iatrogenic, produce a very characteristic picture. The skin is atrophic, and the blood vessels are easily visible through the epidermis giving the skin a red colour. The skin is fragile, and heals poorly. The

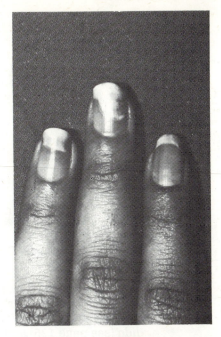

Figure 12.3   Onycholysis in association with thyroid disease

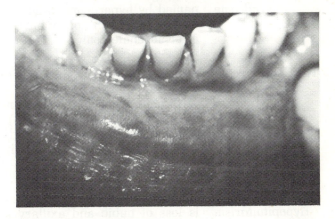

Figure 12.4   Pigmentation of the lips in Addison's disease

blood vessels rupture easily and purpura and bruises are common. Striae which retain their red colour are common and widespread (Figure 12.5). These changes are all due to loss of collagen fibres.

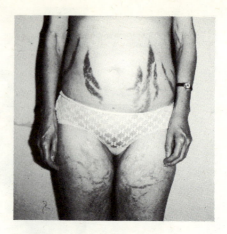

Figure 12.5   Striae in Cushing's syndrome

Acne is common among those who are acne prone. Hirsutism is often marked.

The skin is unusually susceptible to infection by *Candida* (see page 125) and fungus (see page 149).

Nelson's syndrome Cushing's syndrome of pituitary origin may be accompanied by hyperpigmentation as seen in Addison's disease. Pigmentation often becomes very marked after adrenalectomy.

The parathyroids Hypoparathyroidism gives rise to dry scaly skin and
Hypopara- dry brittle hair.
thyroidism Chronic mucocutaneous candidiasis of mouth, fingers and nails (Figure 12.6), and intertriginous areas is sometimes associated with hypoparathyroidism, and more rarely with other endocrine disorders.

The pituitary When the pituitary gland become underactive there
Hypopituitarism is loss of pubic and axillary hair, the scalp hair becomes thin. The skin is dry and wrinkled and pale.

Acromegaly Acromegaly causes the skin to become thick and greasy, the features become coarse. Sweating is increased.

Acne does not result from the seborrhoea of acromegaly.

The ovaries

*Polycystic ovary
syndrome
(Stein–Leventhal
syndrome)*

This may present with greasy skin, severe acne and hirsutes. These are the result of overproduction of androgens.

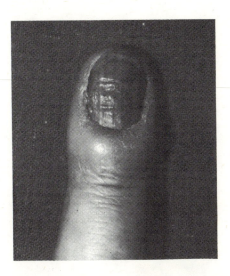

Figure 12.6 Hypoparathyroidism: chronic candidiasis of nail fold and nail plate

The pancreas
Diabetes

See page 233.

Glucagonoma

Necrolytic migratory erythema is a recently described, very distinctive marker for the rare glucagon secreting alpha cell tumours.

The patients are usually postmenopausal women, between 50 and 60. The rash involves the trunk, particularly intertriginous areas, and the perineum, and limbs. Trauma and friction may initiate lesions. There may be a severe stomatitis. The rash is annular, showing an advancing red edge with bullae, erosions and crusts and central healing.

There is associated weight loss, diabetes and a normochromic anaemia. Glucagon levels are very high.

Removal of the tumour cures the rash.

13 EPIDERMOLYSIS BULLOSA

Epidermolysis bullosa is a term used to include a number of hereditary disorders which present with blisters early in life. The term literally means separation of the epidermis from the underlying skin with blister formation. There are a number of classifications of epidermolysis bullosa based either on clinical or genetic grounds. Clinically there are two main types, one of which only has blisters on the skin and does not lead to scarring (the so-called simple type), and the other, sometimes referred to as the dystrophic type, is associated with scarring and involvement of the mucous membranes. Both types are rare.

Presentation
Simple type

The blisters are not usually present at birth but appear when the child starts to crawl. The blisters appear at sites of trauma, i.e. the hands, feet and knees (Figure 13.1). The blisters are tense and last a few

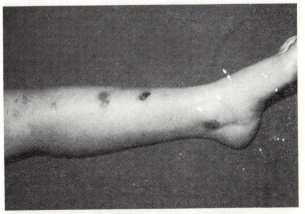

Figure 13.1 Erosion, blister and healing lesions in epidermolysis bullosa

111

days and heal without scarring. The tendency to form blisters appears to lessen in adult life.

Dystrophic type This may be further subdivided into those infants in which blisters are present at birth and those in whom the blisters develop later. When blisters are present at birth the disease is more severe, and in this type there is involvement of the mucous membranes. The blisters heal to leave thin scars. In the severe form the digits may be bound together by the scar tissue. Blisters and erosions develop in the mouth and these lead to scarring. The larynx and oesophagus are also affected, the latter involvement often gives rise to an oesophageal stricture, one of the most severe complications of the disease. Later in life malignant change may occur in the mucous membranes severely affected.

In the severe form there is deformity of the teeth and nails. The latter are dystrophic and ultimately the nail bed may be destroyed leading to absence of the nails.

Differential diagnosis Other diseases which may present with blisters in young children include severe reactions to insect bites; however, these are not necessarily at sites of trauma. In very young infants impetigo, which may present as large blisters and eroded areas, has to be considered. A rare disorder known as toxic epidermal necrolysis which also affects very young infants and which presents with large eroded areas has to be considered in the differential diagnosis of the dystrophic type of epidermolysis bullosa.

Investigations A skin biopsy will show a blister in the region of the basement membrane. In the so-called 'simple type' the primary site of pathology is above the basement membrane in the basal cells of the epidermis. In the dystrophic varieties the blisters are subepidermal and involve the basement membrane and upper dermis. This is best shown by electron microscopy.

Swabs for bacteriology should be taken to exclude infective conditions which have to be considered in the differential diagnosis.

Aetiology The various forms of epidermolysis bullosa are all considered to be genetically determined. The blisters occur due to defects at the region of the dermo–epidermal junction, which results in minor trauma giving rise to blister formation. In the dystrophic variety the pathology involves the upper dermis and therefore scarring results.

Treatment   In the simple non-scarring form of the disease there is no effective treatment and none is usually required. Topical or systemic antibiotics are sometimes necessary to control secondary infection.

In the dystrophic forms of the disease, systemic corticosteroids can be helpful in controlling the severity of the disorder and are indicated when there is severe involvement of the oral cavity and oesophagus.

Natural history and prognosis   The simple non-dystrophic forms are persistent in childhood and adolescence, but there is a tendency for the condition to improve in adult life.

In the dystrophic form, if severe, the child may die in infancy because of severe involvement of the mouth, larynx and oesophagus. In less severe forms patients may reach adult life, but there is a risk of leukoplakic carcinomata.

Genetic counselling is important and fetal skin biopsy for electron microscopy will show the abnormality, and permit termination of affected pregnancies.

14 ERYTHEMA MULTIFORME

Erythema multiforme is a polymorphic but characteristic eruption that occurs in response to many different stimuli.

Presentation Any age may be affected. The most serious form known as Stevens–Johnson syndrome occurs most frequently in children and young adults. Three times more males than females are affected by the Stevens–Johnson syndrome (Figure 14.1).

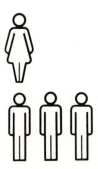

Figure 14.1   Sex ratio of Stevens–Johnson syndrome

The eruption is very symmetrical and usually peripheral. The hands, both dorsum and palms (Figure 14.2), are a characteristic site; sometimes the rash is confined to the hands. The dorsa and soles of the feet, knees, forearms and elbows are affected, more rarely the trunk and face.

The mucous membranes, the conjunctiva, mouth and genitalia are involved in severe cases. In very severe cases the gastro-intestinal, respiratory and urinary tracts are involved.

The rash is polymorphic (Figure 14.3). The initial lesions are red macules; these may become papular. They spread outwards and the centre may become purple or purpuric, forming the diagnositic target or iris lesion (Figures 14.2 and 14.3).

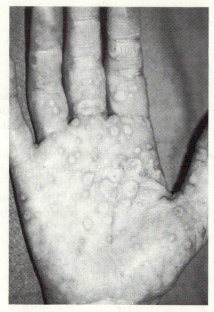

Figure 14.2 Erythema multiforme on the palm: target lesions are present

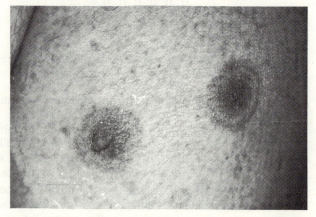

Figure 14.3 Polymorphism of erythema multiforme: target and bullous lesion

Vesicles and bullae may develop (Figure 14.3). These can occur in target lesions, which then have a central bulla, encircled by a ring of vesicles.

The mucous membranes develop bullae which soon rupture to form erosions and crusts (Figure 14.4).

The cutaneous lesions may itch.

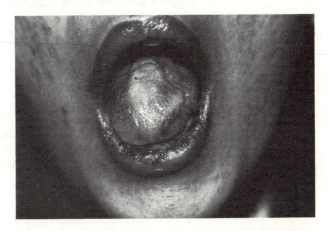

Figure 14.4   Erosions and crusts on the lips and tongue

Stevens—Johnson syndrome This is a very severe form of erythema multiforme. The onset is sudden with fever and constitutional symptoms, and the patient is very ill. The mucous membranes are affected with bullae and erosions. They become oedematous and crusted (Figure 14.4). There may be panophthalmitis. Respiratory tract involvement causes cough and dyspnoea, urinary tract involvement retention or frequency. Arthritis may occur.

Cutaneous lesions may be present, but are not invariably so.

Differential diagnosis Toxic erythema is not raised and bullous, and urticaria is monomorphic, but both can resemble early mild erythema multiforme. Bullous erythema multiforme may so closely resemble pemphigoid that only immunofluorescence will distinguish them. However, erythema multiforme affects a much younger age group.

Stevens—Johnson syndrome is differentiated from oral pemphigus and Behcet's syndrome by the sudden severe onset.

Diagnosis and investigations
Skin biopsy

Biopsy may be necessary to confirm the diagnosis. The bullae are sub-epidermal. Immunofluorescence is negative.

Blood tests

Viral titres or bacterial titres may be helpful in establishing the cause. Opsonization defects are found in some patients with recurrent herpes simplex and erythema multiforme.

Other tests

Throat swabs and swabs from herpes simplex-like lesions may confirm the cause.

Aetiology

Erythema multiforme is a vasculitis confined to the skin and mucous membranes.

The cause is unknown in about half of the cases. Viral infections, particularly herpes simplex, are most commonly implicated. The other causes are shown in Table 14.1. Erythema multiforme commences one to three weeks after exposure to the precipitating cause.

Table 14.1   Causes of erythema multiforme

Carcinoma

Drugs, particularly:
    Barbiturates
    Penicillin
    Phenylbutazone
    Sulphonamides

Infections
    Bacteria
    Fungi
    Mycoplasma
    Viruses – Herpes simplex

Pregnancy

Radiotherapy

Unknown (50%)

Treatment

Attacks are self limiting and in mild cases no treatment, or merely antihistamines to allay pruritis, is indicated.

High dose systemic steroids are helpful in reducing the severity of the attack. They are most frequently used for Stevens–Johnson syndrome.

The cause should be removed; however in cases of recurrent herpes simplex this may be impossible.

Natural history and prognosis   Erythema multiforme usually lasts a fortnight. The attacks are recurrent. There is a high (10%) mortality from Stevens–Johnson syndrome, and morbidity with damage to eyesight is also high.

15 ERYTHRASMA

Presentation   Erythrasma is a common and widespread chronic superficial infection of the skin. It is more prevalent in humid and warm climates. It may occur at any age although the peak of incidence is in early adult life. Males are more commonly affected than females (Figure 15.1).

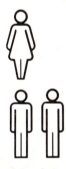

Figure 15.1   Sex ratio of erythrasma

The clinical lesions are characterized by well defined, superficial reddish-brown scaly patches (Figure 15.2). The lesion enlarges peripherally and becomes more brownish with wrinkling on the surface. The common sites are the groins, axillae, submammary area, anogenital skin and toe webs (Figure 15.3). In severe cases it may be generalized. The lesions may be asymptomatic or mildly itchy.

Differential diagnosis   Tinea cruris is a more inflammatory condition and advances down the thigh with a raised scaly edge. Tinea vesicolor tends to occur on the upper trunk but not the intertriginous areas. Intertrigo due to eczema or psoriasis tends to be a brighter red colour

121

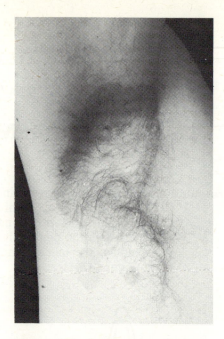

Figure 15.2   Lesions in erythrasma

and is more inflamed, and may give rise to fissuring of the skin.

Investigations   Wood's light (specific range of ultraviolet light) examination shows a pink colour. Bacteriological tests will confirm the diagnosis.

Aetiology   The causative agent is a diphtheroid gram-positive bacillus, *Corynebacterium minutissimum.*

Treatment   Systemic erythromycin and tetracycline will clear the lesions after a week. Fusidic acid ointment is also effective. Topical antifungal preparations have been used although they are not as successful as the above antibiotics.

Prognosis   Untreated erythrasma tends to be chronic. It may spread and become extensive but very rarely gives rise to symptoms apart from mild irritation.

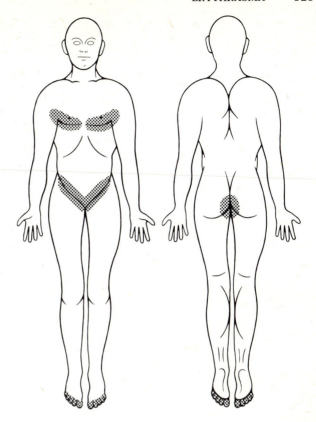

Figure 15.3   Common sites of erythrasma

16 FUNGAL INFECTIONS

Pathogenic fungi inhabit and eventually destroy keratin. The skin, hair or nails may be affected. The ability of the fungi to destroy keratin is thought to depend on enzymes produced by fungi. Different species of fungi affect different parts of the body. Some have the ability to live in hair or nails, and others have not. Most fungal infections are referred to as ringworm or tinea. The latter is a Latin word for a gnawing worm. The terms have been used because fungal infections tend to start as a small lesion and spread in an annular pattern. The centre of the lesion often clears giving rise to the classical red, scaly, annular lesion. In practice, however, many fungal infections do not present with annular lesions, and the clinical appearances of the disease will depend on the site of involvement and the species of fungus.

There are three main genera of fungi which produce the so-called ringworm disorders. These are *Trichophyton, Microsporum and Epidermophyton.*

Investigations The investigations for fungal infections are similar, irrespective of the site involved, and whether it is skin, hair or nails. In infections of the skin, the skin should be scraped with a blunt scalpel and it should be remembered that it is only the keratin which is required for examination. It is always best to collect specimens from the edge of a lesion as there is likely to be more fungus at this site. If blisters are present the roof of the blister should be taken for examination. In fungal infections of the scalp, hair as well as skin should be taken. Hair and skin should be collected by scraping the affected area with a scalpel. In nail infections the specimens should be taken from the edge or lower surface of the nail, by scraping the affected area with a relatively blunt metal instrument. A full thickness specimen of nail should also be taken. Scraping the top of the nail is not satisfactory as the fungus may be restricted to the lower surface of the nail. The specimens can be satisfactorily transported to the laboratory in a folded piece of paper, and stored like this for many weeks. The specimens of skin, hair and nail should be examined by direct microscopy and cultured.

Direct microscopy   The pieces of skin should be placed on a glass slide and one or two drops of 10% potassium hydroxide added. After 30 minutes most of the keratin will have dissolved and the hyphae are then visible.

Hair specimens should be left for one or two hours before being examined.

Full thickness specimens of nails should be left in potassium hydroxide for 12–24 hours to dissolve the keratin and allow the hyphae to be seen. If soft debris is obtained from the side of or under the nail, the specimen need only be kept in potassium hydroxide for 1–2 hours.

Culture   As direct microscopic studies may sometimes not show fungal hyphae (because of only a few hyphae being present or inexperience of the investigator), it is advisable to culture the specimens. Culture also allows identification of the species concerned. The culture medium usually employed is Sabouraud's medium. It takes up to two weeks to grow most fungi, and some take up to three weeks.

Wood's light   This is ultraviolet light filtered by a Wood's glass which allows transmission of ultraviolet light above 365 nm. Wood's light is of use in the diagnosis of fungal infections of the scalp. The hairs infected with certain species of fungus fluoresce a bright green. The two species which most commonly cause fluorescence in this country are *Microsporum audouinii* and *Microsporum canis*. However, the species *Trichophyton schoenleinii* which causes favus, produces fluorescence of hair, but the colour is a lighter green.

TINEA PEDIS
(FOOT RINGWORM: ATHLETE'S FOOT)

Presentation   Tinea pedis is uncommon in children. The disorder is most commonly seen in young and middle aged adults (Figure 16.1). It has a higher incidence in males than females (Figure 16.2). The fungi which most commonly cause infections of the feet are *T. rubrum, T inter-*

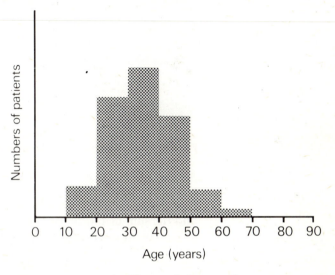

Figure 16.1   **Age incidence of tinea pedis**

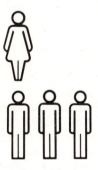

Figure 16.2   **Tinea pedis is more common in males (3 : 1)**

digitale and *E. floccosum.* The commonest presentation is scaling, maceration and fissuring of the skin in the clefts between the fourth and fifth toes. The infection usually spreads to involve the plantar surface of the toes (Figure 16.3).

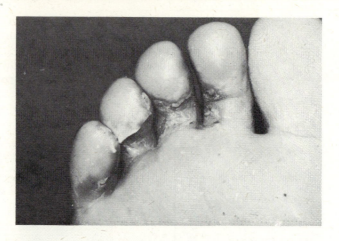

Figure 16.3   Fungal infection of the toes

All the toe clefts may be involved, but it is rare between the first and second toes. Occasionally the infection spreads on to the dorsal surface of the toes and dorsum of the foot proximal to the toes (Figure 16.4). The appearance in this situation is of redness and scaling, and occasionally there is a discernible, raised edge to the lesion with some clearing behind the edge. The infection may also spread to the sole of the foot. In this situation there is erythema and hyperkeratotic scaling. When the disorder affects the sole or dorsum, the involvement is invariably unilateral. Another clinical presentation is of an acute blistering eruption of the toes or soles of the feet, and commonly only a part of the sole is involved. This presentation of a fungal infection is more common in warm weather and is usually unilateral.

It is not possible to identify which organism is the cause of the skin lesions from the clinical appearance, and with regard to treatment it is of no importance. However, vesicular eruptions are more likely to be caused by *T. interdigitale* and *E. floccosum*.

Differential diagnosis   The commonest form of tinea pedis, i.e. the redness and scaling between the toes, has to be distinguished from simple maceration (intertrigo) and inter-

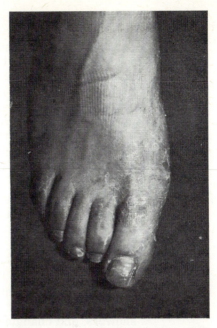

**Figure 16.4   Fungal infection. Red-
ness and scaling spreading from the
toes**

triginous psoriasis. Intertrigo and psoriasis tend to
be confined to the skin between the toes and do not
extend to the plantar surface of the toes. Lesions of
psoriasis are frequently present at other sites if
psoriasis is the cause of the lesions between the
toes. Mycological tests will be necessary to confirm
the diagnosis of a fungal infection if there is any
doubt. Erythrasma also presents with erythema and
scaling between the toes. It can be distinguished
from fungal infections by Wood's light examination,
which shows a pink fluorescence in erythrasma, and
by microscopy and culture of the affected skin.

   If the sole is involved with erythema and scaling,
the condition has to be distinguished from eczema
and psoriasis. In the latter two conditions the rash is
usually symmetrical, but in fungal infections it is invariably unilateral. Psoriasis tends to produce lesions with a sharply demarcated edge. If blisters are
present the fungal infection has to be distinguished
from acute pompholyx eczema. The latter is usually
symmetrical whereas fungal infections usually involve one foot. If the fungal infection becomes secon-

darily infected, pustules are present and the condition will then have to be distinguished from secondarily infected eczema or pustular psoriasis. In pustular psoriasis the area involved is usually discrete; it may be unilateral or bilateral, and the pustules are sterile. If there is involvement of the sole with a fungal infection there is invariably involvement between the toes, but this is less likely to occur in psoriasis and eczema, which should distinguish between the conditions on clinical grounds.

Investigations   Direct microscopy and culture of skin specimens.

Wood's light examination should be carried out if erythrasma is suspected. Erythrasma fluoresces coral pink.

Aetiology   Fungal infections of the feet are contracted from infected skin fragments. The infection is most likely to be caught from communal swimming pools, showers, and changing rooms. It would appear that some persons may have resistance to the infection as not all persons frequently using communal showers in a closed community, e.g. boarding school, will contract the infection. However, the factors which may protect some individuals are not fully understood.

Treatment   If the fungal infection is confined to the skin between the toes, only topical measures should be prescribed. Topical antifungal preparations such as Whitfield's ointment (benzoic acid 6% and salicylic acid 3%), clotrimazole 1% and miconazole nitrate 2% should be used after bathing for at least a month. If there is severe maceration a lotion such as magenta paint may prove more effective in clearing the rash and bring symptomatic relief.

In acute fungal infections, with blisters and exudation involving the toes and soles, potassium permanganate soaks 1 : 8000 for 15 minutes four times a day, should be prescribed. Weak topical steroid creams such as 1% hydrocortisone should also be used in the acute stage. If the infection involves the foot, apart from the skin between the toes, then a month's course of griseofulvin 500 mg daily is the most effective treatment.

Natural history and prognosis Fungal infections between the toes tend to be a persistent problem; although it is possible to clear the problem symptomatically, it tends to recur. This may in part be due to reinfection and partly due to failure to eradicate the fungus from the skin completely. Reinfection probably plays an important part because even after courses of griseofulvin which should clear the fungus, the relapse rate is high. The persistence of the infection between toes is probably due to the ideal conditions, warmth and moisture, that exist at this site. Because of the high relapse rate of the infection between the toes it is probably not justified to treat the infection with griseofulvin.

Fungal infections elsewhere on the feet have a better prognosis and although recurrences may occur, particularly in hot weather, the relapse rate is considerably less than that between the toes. It seems that certain individuals are more prone to infections spreading from between the toes to skin elsewhere on the feet, but what factors control the spread of infection are unknown.

TINEA CRURIS
(RINGWORM INFECTION OF THE GROINS)

Presentation Fungal infections of the groins are most commonly seen in young and middle aged adults (Figure 16.5).

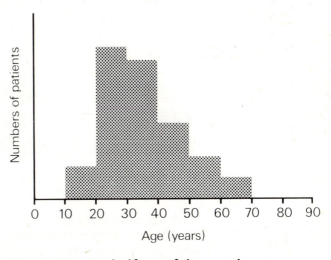

Figure 16.5   Age incidence of tinea cruris

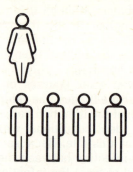

Figure 16.6 Tinea cruris is more common in males

It is predominantly a disorder of males; male to female 4 : 1 (Figure 16.6). The infection begins in the groins and spreads down the thigh or posteriorly to involve the buttocks. The patient becomes aware of the infection due to irritation. In the early stages there is erythema and scaling in the groin, but the infection quickly spreads (Figure 16.7). Thus by the time the patient seeks advice the lesion has extended

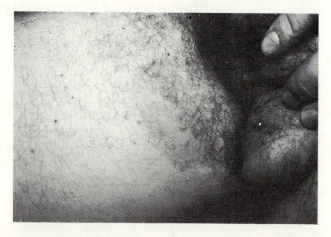

Figure 16.7 Tinea cruris. Reddish brown scaly rash spreading down the thigh

to the thigh or buttocks. There is usually a red, confluent scaly area with a raised edge. Occasionally there is clearing as the edge of the lesion advances, giving the typical ringworm appearance. The infection may be unilateral or bilateral. However, even in the latter the involvement is asymmetrical.

Differential diagnosis

The most common condition that has to be differentiated from fungal infections of the groins is seborrhoeic eczema (intertrigo) at this site. Seborrhoeic eczema is confined to where two skin surfaces are in contact and does not extend down the thigh. In seborrhoeic eczema the condition is invariably bilateral and symmetrical, and there is frequently involvement of the perianal skin. In infections with *Candida albicans* the eruption is usually confined to the groins, but small satellite pustules are present. Erythrasma usually presents as a reddish, confluent plaque extending from the groin to the thigh and perianal skin. Wood's light will show pink fluorescence in erythrasma. Psoriasis of the groins is invariably bilateral and symmetrical, and does not extend very far from the groins. There are usually lesions of psoriasis elsewhere.

Investigations

Specimens of skin should be taken for direct microscopy and culture. Wood's light examination should be carried out if erythrasma is suspected.

Aetiology

The warmth and moisture of intertriginous skin are predisposing factors which are ideal for the growth and survival of fungus. After the feet, tinea cruris is the second most common fungal infection. Patients with groin infection usually have tinea pedis, and the infection is probably transmitted by a towel. The condition is more common in tropical and semitropical climates, and this enhances the factors which predispose to the infection. The same species of fungus which cause tinea pedis cause infection in the groins, i.e. *T. rubrum, T. interdigitale* and *E. floccosum.*

Treatment

The most effective treatment for tinea cruris is a month's course of griseofulvin. The dose is 500 mg daily. Topical antifungal preparations such as Whitfield's ointment, clotrimazole and miconazole have a cure rate of approximately 80%. In the early stages and if maceration is present, magenta paint is helpful in alleviating irritation and even in clearing the eruption.

Natural history and prognosis   Tinea cruris responds well to both systemic and topical antifungal preparations and will clear completely. The problem tends to recur in certain individuals, particularly athletes, as they are more likely to be exposed to the fungus.

TINEA MANUUM
(RINGWORM INFECTIONS OF THE HAND)

Presentation   Ringworm infection of the hands is a disease of adults and there is no sex predilection. The commonest presentation is scaling of the palms and plantar aspects of the fingers. The scaling is usually very fine and there is accentuation of the skin creases. If the back of the hand is involved, there is often a papular, follicular eruption and there may be a red, scaly edge to a discoid lesion as in tinea coporis. The disorder is invariably unilateral.

Differential diagnosis   The scaling of the palm has to be distinguished from chronic eczema and psoriasis. In both the latter conditions the disorder is usually bilateral, whilst fungal infections tend to be unilateral. Psoriasis tends to be more erythematous and often presents as well demarcated patches rather than a confluent eruption. Taking scrapings of skin for mycological examination will give the correct diagnosis.

Investigations   Scrapings of skin for microscopy and culture.

Aetiology   T. rubrum is usually the species which infects the hand. Infection of the hands is relatively uncommon compared to foot infection. The source of infection would appear to be from the feet, as it is very rare to find infection of the hand without infection of the feet.

Treatment   Griseofulvin 500 mg daily for a month is the treatment of choice.

Natural history and prognosis   The disorder is effectively cleared by griseofulvin and recurrence is extremely rare.

TINEA CORPORIS
(RINGWORM INFECTION OF THE BODY)

Presentation Tinea corporis is relatively uncommon. It occurs both in children and adults and affects both sexes equally.

The typical lesion is a red, discoid or annular, scaly lesion (Figure 16.8). The edge of the lesion is raised and may be vesicular. Severe inflammatory changes

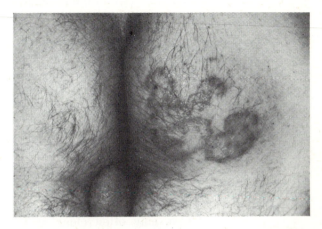

Figure 16.8 Typical annular lesion of a ringworm fungal infection

may occur and this depends on the host's response, and the species of fungus. Red scaly lesions occur with *T. rubrum* and *M. canis*, and acute inflammatory reactions are seen with *T. mentagrophytes* and *T. verrucosum*. In the latter infections there is no central clearing of the lesions and a severe pustular reaction may be present. If the affected area is hairy there is often a more severe inflammatory reaction, particularly around the hair follicles. Long standing infections may become very extensive and present as large confluent, red scaly areas, or a follicular, pustular reaction on a hairy limb.

Differential diagnosis The discoid scaly lesions have to be distinguished from discoid eczema. The eczematous eruption is usually symmetrical, whereas fungal infections are asymmetrical. The annular lesions have to be distinguished from a condition known as annular erythema. The only way a definite diagnosis may be made is by mycological tests. Resolving psoriasis often clears from the centre, giving rise to annular scaly lesions. There may well be other lesions of psoriasis elsewhere to help in establishing the diagnosis. Seborrhoeic eczema characteristically affects the centre of the chest and back between the shoulder blades and presents as red, scaly patches. However, there is no distinct raised edge to the lesions as may be seen in fungal infections. If there is any doubt as to the diagnosis, specimens should be taken for mycological examination.

Aetiology   All known pathogenic ringworm fungi may produce lesions on the trunk and limbs. The fungus may be contracted from another human or animals, usually cats, dogs or cattle. There may or may not be lesions elsewhere, i.e. between the toes or groins.

Treatment   Griseofulvin 500 mg daily for four weeks will clear the lesions. Topical antifungal preparations are not as effective.

Prognosis   Untreated, the lesions may persist indefinitely. Lesions associated with an acute inflammatory process may often clear spontaneously after a few weeks. The recurrence rate is very low. Reinfection appears to be low even if there is a fungal infection between the toes or in the groins.

TINEA CAPITIS (RINGWORM INFECTION OF THE SCALP)

Presentation   Tinea capitis is a disease of children and is very rare after puberty (Figure 16.9). Males are affected more commonly than females (Figure 16.10) 3 : 2.

The most common clinical appearance is of bald patches (Figure 16.11). Closer examination shows numerous short hairs of varying lengths, but usually less than 0.5 cm. The scalp is slightly scaly. The short hairs are due to the fact that the hair invaded by fungus breaks close to the surface of the scalp. The affected patches are of varying sizes, as the duration of infection is usually different between the various sites involved. Occasionally there are more severe inflammatory changes in the scalp and these

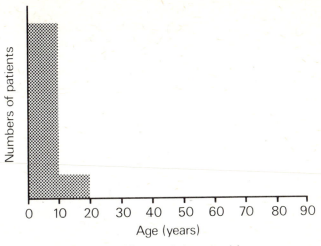

Figure 16.9   Age incidence of tinea capitis

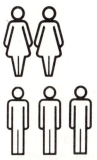

Figure 16.10   Tinea capitis is slightly more common in males (3 : 2)

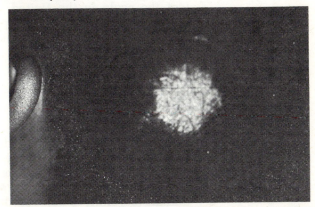

Figure 16.11   Bald patch in ringworm infection of the scalp

present as small pustules in the affected area. A very severe inflammatory response termed a 'kerion' sometimes occurs. The area affected is raised, has an irregular surface and pustules may be present. The hairs tend to fall easily in a kerion. If the inflammation is severe, scarring may follow.

Differential diagnosis

The most common disease that has to be distinguished from tinea capitis is alopecia areata. In the latter condition the scalp is normal and there is no scaling. The area may be completely bald and characteristically exclamation mark hairs (see page 178) may be seen at the edge of the bald area. Trichotillomania also presents as patchy hair loss. The hairs are broken close to the surface but there is no scaling of the scalp. Psoriasis and seborrhoiec eczema present as scaly patches in the scalp, but hair loss is rare.

Investigations

Wood's light examination will show green fluorescence of the affected hairs if the infection is due to *M. audouinii* or *M. canis*.

Specimens of skin and hair should be taken for microscopy and culture.

Aetiology

The hairs are invaded by the fungus which alters the structure of the hair, and as a result the hairs break. The scalp skin (keratin) is also invariably affected and hence the scaling. The commonest fungi to affect the scalp in the United Kingdom are *M. audouinii* and *M. canis*. Many species of fungi cause tinea capitis, and certain species predominate in different parts of the world.

Treatment

Griseofulvin is the only treatment that should be considered. The drug should be taken for six weeks.

Prognosis

Untreated the natural history depends on the degree of inflammation. The more severe the inflammation the more likely a spontaneous cure will occur. Griseofulvin has altered the prognosis considerably, and the morbidity is now very low. Scarring may occur after a kerion, and this may result in permanent hair loss, otherwise the hair will always regrow.

TINEA UNGUIUM
(RINGWORM INFECTION OF THE NAILS)

Presentation   Ringworm infection of the nails is a disease of adults and is very rare in children (Figure 16.12). Toe nails are more commonly affected than finger nails, and the problem is more common in males (Figure 16.13).

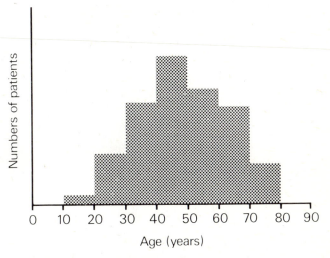

Figure 16.12   Age incidence of tinea unguium

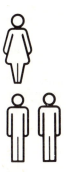

Figure 16.13   Tinea unguium is more common in males (2 : 1)

Fungal infections of the nails usually begin at the side of the nail plate. The involvement appears as a white or yellow discolouration (Figure 16.14). The infection then spreads towards the base of the nail.

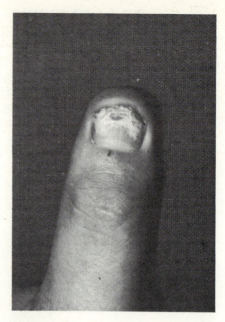

Figure 16.14 Fungal infection of the nail

The nail plate becomes thickened, and may crack and lift due to subungual hyperkeratosis. Alternatively the nail plate may become dystrophic and break with actual loss of the terminal part. Occasionally white opaque areas appear in the nail and this may be the only feature which the patient notices.

Fungal infections of the nails on both limbs are usually asymmetrical and usually only a few nails are involved. In fungal infections of the toe nails there is usually involvement of the skin between the toes. In ringworm fungal infections of the nail, the nail folds are normal.

Differential diagnosis Psoriasis is the commonest disorder that has to be distinguished from fungal infections of the nails. Both disorders cause dystrophy of the nail plate and subungual hyperkeratosis. Since both disorders are common the finding of lesions of psoriasis elsewhere does not necessarily establish that the nail abnormality is due to psoriasis. If pitting of the nails is present this is in favour of psoriasis, as pitting does not occur in fungal infections. Psoriasis of the nails is more likely to be bilateral and symmetrical, whereas fungal infections are usually asymmetrical.

Infection of the nail plate with *Candida albicans* is associated with inflammatory changes of the posterior nail fold, i.e. swelling and redness.

Severe alopecia areata is associated with nail dystrophy which in the late stages may be indistinguishable from a fungal infection. Eczema and lichen planus may produce abnormalities of the nails.

Investigations The hyperkeratotic tissue from under the nail plate and a full thickness clipping of nail should be taken for examination by microscopy and culture. It is more difficult to find the fungus in nail than in skin, and if the mycological tests are negative but the clinical suspicion of a fungal infection is high, then the tests should be repeated on new specimens.

Aetiology Ringworm fungus has the ability to grow in keratin, and nails are a form of keratin. In infections of the toe nails the source of the fungus is usually from involvement of the skin between the toes. Infection of the finger nails may or may not be associated with an infection of the toe spaces. The commonest species to infect the nails in the United Kingdom is *T. rubrum*, which is the commonest cause of tinea pedis. However, in other countries where *T. violaceum* and *T. tonsurans* are common causes of tinea capitis, these species most often cause nail involvement.

The reasons why only some patients with tinea pedis develop infections of the toe nails are not known. It would seem that some patients may have a resistance to the fungus. Likewise there is no satisfactory explanation as yet, as to why only some nails are affected and not all.

Treatment Griseofulvin is the only effective treatment. Finger nail infections usually respond well, and clear within six months. Toe nail infections do not respond so well, and the drug may have to be continued for up to two years. Different toe nails may respond in a dissimilar way; some clear whilst others do not. It was thought that this might be due to different rates of growth of the nails, but this has been shown not to

be the case. One of the reasons for failure of treatment may be non-compliance.

Prognosis Ringworm fungal infections of nails tend to be persistent. The problem is not always progressive and
the infection may remain limited to one nail or one
part of a nail for many years. It is rare however for
the infection to clear by itself. With treatment the
prognosis for finger nails is good, but variable for
toe nails. The incidence of reinfection of toe nails is
also relatively high compared to finger nails.

RINGWORM GRANULOMA
(MAJOCCHI'S GRANULOMA)

Presentation Majocchi's granuloma is a disease of adults and
more common in women.

The granuloma occurs on the limbs and is essentially a folliculitis. The disease presents as a plaque of
erythema and scaling on a limb with small nodules
or pustules around the hair follicles (Figure 16.15).
The lesion is invariably unilateral. The area involved may become extensive involving the whole of the
forearm or leg.

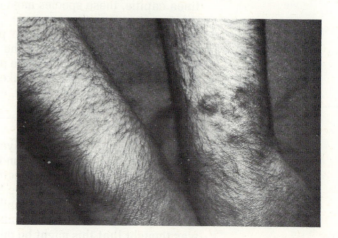

Figure 16.15   Fungal granuloma. Red infiltrated plaque

Differential diagnosis The disorder has to be distinguished from a bacterial folliculitis, and culture for bacteria from a pustule should be carried out. If no pustules are present other forms of granuloma may have to be considered. Infected eczema may present on the limbs, but eczema is usually bilateral and symmetrical.

Investigations Scrapings of skin for microscopy and culture. If negative a biopsy will reveal a granuloma and stains for fungal hyphae should be requested.

Aetiology The infection is caused by *T. rubrum* and the patient usually has an infection between the toes. The organism causes a folliculitis, and fragments of the infected hair are displaced into the dermis where they cause a foreign body granulomatous reaction.

Treatment Griseofulvin for six weeks cures the infection.

Prognosis Untreated the condition persists indefinitely. If there is severe dermal involvement there may be scarring and permanent hair loss.

FAVUS

Presentation Favus may be seen at any age but it is thought infections usually begin in childhood. The sexes are affected equally. The disorder is now rare in the United Kingdom, but it is common in the Middle East and is still present in parts of the USA and Canada. It is also common amongst the Bantu in South Africa where the disorder is known as 'Witkop' (Whitehead).

The commonest site to be involved is the scalp, but the lesions produced are different from those produced by other ringworm fungi (page 136). In the initial stages there is erythema of the scalp with matting of the hair, but no definite hair loss. In a more severe infection there is hair loss and scutula formation. A scutulum is a yellow cupshaped crust consisting of a dense mass of mycelia and epithelial debris. The cup faces upwards and is pierced by a hair. The scutula will eventually join up and form a massive yellow crust. In the most severe infections there is hair loss and atrophy of the skin. Once atrophy occurs the hair loss is permanent.

Occasionally there is involvement of the glabrous skin and nails. The nail infection is indistinguishable from that caused by other ringworm fungi. In infections of the skin, yellow scutula are formed as in infections of the scalp.

Differential diagnosis   Seborrhoeic eczema and psoriasis have to be distinguished from the early and mild infections which have erythema of the scalp. Mycology will be necessary to establish the diagnosis. Once hair loss and scarring of the scalp occurs, other causes of cicatricial alopecia have to be considered, e.g. discoid lupus erythematosus and lichen planus.

Investigations   Wood's light examination shows a pale green fluorescence of the hairs. Microscopy of the hair and skin will reveal hyphae, but culture of the organism is particularly slow.

Aetiology   Favus is caused by the fungus *T. schoenleinii*. It is contracted from an infected person. This species of fungus is the commonest cause of tinea capitis in some Eastern countries.

Treatment   Griseofulvin for 6–8 weeks will clear the infection.

Prognosis   If treatment is initiated at an early stage, before there is scarring, then the prognosis is good. Once scarring has developed there will be permanent hair loss.

PITYRIASIS VERSICOLOR

Presentation   Pityriasis versicolor is mainly seen in young and middle aged adults (Figure 16.16). It is more common in males (Figure 16.17) 3:2. The disease occurs worldwide but is more common in tropical and subtropical climates.

There are two distinct presentations. The first is of reddish-brown, slightly scaly patches on the upper trunk (Figure 16.18). The second presentation is of hypopigmented areas (Figure 16.19), usually noted in Caucasians after exposure to strong sunlight. The upper trunk is most commonly affected (Figure

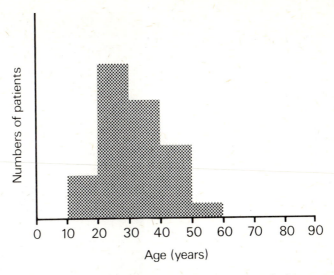

Figure 16.16   Age incidence of pityriasis versicolor

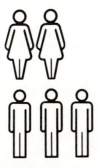

Figure 16.17 Pityriasis versicolor is slightly more common in males (3 : 2)

16.20), but occasionally the lesion will involve the neck and upper arms, and very occasionally it will involve the face and legs. If the disorder is long standing the patches may coalesce to form large confluent areas on the trunk. Apart from the cosmetic problem due to altered colour of the skin the only other symptom which is sometimes present is irritation.

Differential diagnosis   The reddish-brown scaly lesions have to be distinguished from seborrhoeic eczema. The latter is usually confined to the centre of the chest and centre of the back, whereas pityriasis versicolor is usually more extensive. In pityriasis rosea the lesions are

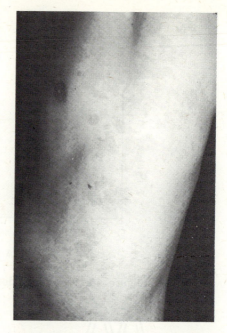

Figure 16.18 Reddish-brown patches of pityriasis versicolor

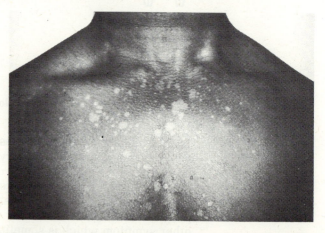

Figure 16.19 Hypopigmented areas due to pityriasis versicolor

redder, oval and have centripetal scaling. In addition the lower trunk is usually affected. Erythrasma is usually a similar colour but the lesions are usually mainly in the axillae.

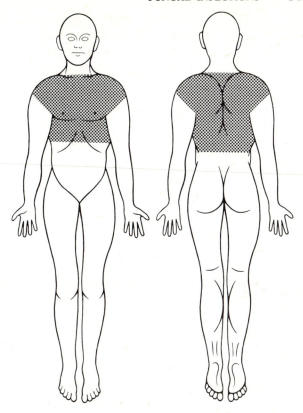

Figure 16.20   Common sites of involvement in pityriasis versicolor

The hypopigmented lesions have to be distinguished from vitiligo, which may be difficult if vitiligo only affects the upper trunk. Demonstration of the fungus is the only certain way of distinguishing between the conditions.

Investigations   The fungus is demonstrated on direct microscopy. In addition to the hyphae it is usual to see numerous spores. The fungus which causes pityriasis versicolor is difficult to culture and therefore this is not attempted for diagnostic purposes.

Aetiology   Pityriasis versicolor is caused by the fungus *Pityrosporum orbiculare*. Moisture and heat encourage growth of the fungus and the disease is common in hot and humid climates. It is not known why the infection tends to be localized to the upper trunk. The loss of pigment that occurs in areas affected by the fungus, particularly after exposure to sunlight, appears to be due to a carboxylic acid which the fungus produces. The acid has the ability to inhibit melanin formation, and thus patients do not tan in the affected areas. The disease is therefore particularly noticeable after a holiday sunbathing in a warm country.

Treatment *Pityrosporum orbiculare* is a fungus which is not sensitive to griseofulvin. Thus treatment is with topical preparations. Half strength Whitfield's ointment (benzoic acid 3%, salicylic acid 1.5%), clotrimazole and miconazole are all effective. If patients do not like creams and ointments, 20% sodium thiosulphate solution may be used. All these preparations should be applied every night to the whole of the trunk, for a month. Success has also been claimed for 2.5% selenium sulphide suspension (Selsun) left on overnight. If the presenting feature is hypopigmented areas, the treatment is the same, but the pigment may not return for a few months. There is no specific treatment to increase the rate of repigmentation.

Prognosis *Pityriasis versicolor* is easy to clear, but there is a relatively high incidence of reinfection. It seems that certain individuals are prone to the infection whilst others have a resistance to it and are not affected despite repeated exposure.

MYCETOMA (MADURA FOOT)

Presentation A mycetoma is a localized chronic infection of the skin, subcutaneous tissues and bones due to various species of fungi or actinomycetes.

The disease is most commonly seen in adult males, but any age or sex may be affected. The earliest lesion is a firm, painless nodule. This is followed by further nodules which produce an irregular surface. Some of the nodules may break down discharging pus containing grains. Gross thickening of the subcutaneous tissues occurs. Extension of the lesion to the bones gives rise to arthritis, periostitis and finally osteomyelitis. Eventually severe deformity is produced as a result of destruction of the tissues. There are numerous sinus tracts with a purulent or seropurulent discharge.

Differential diagnosis   Chronic osteomyelitis may resemble mycetoma in the early stages. Laboratory tests will distinguish between the causative organisms.

Investigations   Examination of the pus by microscopy and culture. If no pus is present a biopsy should be performed. Histology shows a chronic granulomatous reaction. There is destruction of tissue with necrosis.

Aetiology   Mycetoma may be caused by a number of different fungi and actinomycetes which occur as saprophytes in soil or vegetable matter. The organisms gain entry into the tissues following a penetrating injury. The disease occurs most commonly in tropical and subtropical climates in persons who go barefoot. The organisms which cause a mycetoma are not found in temperate climates. The disease is not contagious.

Treatment   The infection is not always cleared by antibiotics although the fungi are sensitive to the drugs *in vitro*. The drugs which are selected for treatment will depend to a certain extent on which organism is found to be the causative agent. Systemic amphotericin B and griseofulvin are effective in some infections, whilst broad spectrum antibiotics, particularly co-trimoxale are effective on others.

Surgery both simple and radical has to be considered if medical treatment fails.

Prognosis   If untreated the disorder is slowly progressive leading to severe deformity and chronic secondary bacterial infection. In the early stages appropriate long term antibiotics may clear the infection.

CANDIDIASIS (MONILIASIS)

Candidiasis is caused by the fungus *Candida albicans*. *Candida albicans* is the fungus most likely to become pathogenic although it is found in the gastro-intestinal tract in a large proportion of individuals without causing any disease. Why *Candida albicans* gives rise to pathological lesions in some individuals and not in the majority, considering how common it is in the environment, is not known. It is considered by some to be an opportunist organism in that it will only cause disease in previously damaged skin or mucosa.

ORAL CANDIDIASIS (THRUSH)

Presentation Oral candidiasis is common in young infants. It may occur however in individuals of any age, particularly in those with previous oral pathology. There is no sex predilection in infants, but oral candidiasis in the adult is more common in women.

The typical lesions are creamy white soft plaques on the oral mucosa. If this material is removed it reveals a red base. Occasionally the condition progresses to ulceration of the mucosa. In adults oral candidiasis may present as a red sore mouth. The infection may spread from the mouth to involve the oesophagus and trachea.

Chronic hyperplastic oral candidiasis is a disease of middle aged adults and presents with white plaques. In these individuals no other abnormality is usually found.

Candida albicans infection may also present as angular stomatitis. Fissuring of the skin at the corners of the mouth is very common in otherwise healthy individuals, and this is frequently secondarily infected with *Candida albicans*. *Candida* infection of the lips may also occur in patients with cheilitis, usually that associated with lip sucking. The lips are red and scaly with fissures.

Differential diagnosis In infants the yellowish-white plaques of candidiasis have to be distinguished from curds of milk. The hyperplastic oral candidiasis is similar to leukoplakia and specimens taken for myocological examination should establish the correct diagnosis. The red mouth has to be distinguished from an allergic reaction to dentures. Other causes of erosions will have to be considered, such as pemphigus, Behcet's disease and aphthous ulceration.

Investigations   Swabs should be taken for microscopy and culture.

Aetiology   Infants seem to be particularly prone to oral candidiasis. The source of the infection may be the birth canal of the mother. Antibiotic therapy predisposes to oral thrush. There is a higher incidence of oral thrush in adults in those who wear dentures, and this seems to be a contributory factor. The problem is generally common in debilitated individuals.

Treatment   Oral nystatin suspension or amphotericin B are effective in clearing *Candida albicans*. For angular stomatitis and cheilitis, creams or ointments containing nystatin should be used. If patients wear dentures these should be soaked in solutions containing nystatin overnight, otherwise they may cause reinfections. In adults, sucking nystatin tablets is more effective than oral suspension. If the patient wears dentures these should first be removed.

Prognosis   In infants the prognosis is good and the condition clears rapidly with treatment. Oral candidiasis in adults often recurs after treatment, but this may be due to the factors which predispose to the infection.

INTERTRIGINOUS CANDIDIASIS

Presentation   Apart from seborrhoeic eczema of infancy which may be associated with *Candida albicans*, intertriginous candidiasis is a disorder of adults. The sex incidence depends on the site of the involvement.

The eruption begins as an erythematous area with some slight scaling at the edges and characteristically there are satellite papules and pustules (Figure 16.21). If the eruption is very acute, pustules appear in the confluent, erythematous area. The eruption tends to remain in the intertriginous areas and does not progress to the surrounding skin. The common sites of involvement are the submammary region in females, folds in the abdominal skin in obese subjects, the groins, and the interdigital spaces of the fingers.

Differential diagnosis   The commonest condition to be distinguished from monilial intertrigo is seborrhoeic eczema involving

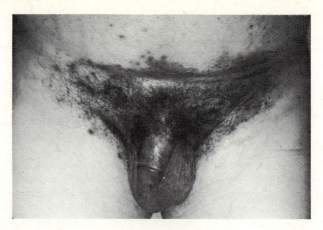

Figure 16.21   Intertrigo with satellite papules suggestive of infection with *Candida albicans*

similar sites. The only way of differentiating the two conditions on clinical grounds is by the presence of satellite pustules. Mycological studies of scrapings of skin or a swab from a pustule will reveal *Candida albicans* if it is present. Ringworm infections of the groins can be distinguished from *Candida* as the former spread out from the intertriginous area and often have a raised scaly edge. Erythrasma does not have satellite pustules and Wood's light examination will show a pink fluorescence. Benign familial pemphigus (Hailey–Hailey disease) is often confined to the intertriginous areas and the distinctive feature is of linear clefts in the area of affected skin.

Aetiology   The warmth and moisture of the intertriginous areas are ideal circumstances for the growth of *Candida albicans*. Conditions which increase warmth and sweating, such as long periods in bed or long plane journeys, predispose towards the condition. It is likely that the eruption begins as simple intertrigo which becomes invaded with *Candida albicans*.

Treatment   Creams containing nystatin, miconazole or clotrimazole are usually effective in clearing the eruption. If the skin is moist and weeping better results are obtained with magenta paint.

Prognosis   Intertrigo caused by *Candida albicans* clears quickly with treatment. However, certain subjects appear prone to the infection and in these persons there is a relatively high incidence of recurrence.

GENITAL CANDIDIASIS: CANDIDAL BALANITIS

Presentation In the uncircumcised individual there is redness and slight moisture of the glans penis and foreskin (Figure 16.22). Small pustules and erosions may be present. If the disorder becomes recurrent fissuring of the foreskin and scarring may develop. *Candida* infections of the penis are relatively rare in the circumcised.

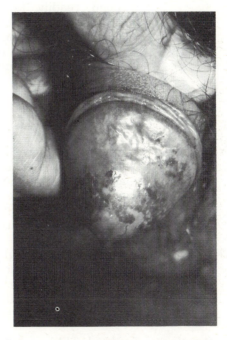

Figure 16.22   Candidal balanitis. Redness and moisture of the glans penis

Differential diagnosis Simple intertrigo occurs in the circumcised and may be difficult to distinguish without mycology tests. Other causes, e.g. balanitis of Zoon, and erythroplasia of Queyrat (intra-epidermal carcinoma) have to be considered.

Investigations A swab should be taken for microscopy and culture, and the urine examined to exclude diabetes mellitus.

Aetiology Certain individuals appear to be prone to the infection and it frequently flares up after intercourse. Occasionally the female partner may be the source of infection, but it also appears that the moisture and trauma of intercourse are factors which precipitate the problem.

Treatment Topical nystatin is effective in clearing the *Candida* infection but the inflammation often remains and a combination of nystatin and hydrocortisone gives better results.

Prognosis Candidal balanitis is often recurrent. Most attacks respond readily to treatment. If the problem becomes chronic with fibrosis of the foreskin, circumcision is usually necessary. Circumcision should also be considered in recurrent infections if the attacks are very frequent.

CANDIDAL VULVO–VAGINITIS

Presentation There is a yellow–white vaginal discharge and white plaques may be seen on the walls of the vagina. The vulva is red and swollen. The infection frequently spreads to the groins and peri-anal skin, presenting with erythema, scaling and satellite pustules. There is usually severe pruritus.

Differential diagnosis Other causes of vaginal discharge and pruritus vulvae must be considered. If the skin is involved simple intertrigo must be considered, but the vaginal discharge and satellite lesions on the skin should distinguish between the two conditions.

Investigations Swabs should be taken for microscopy and culture. The urine must be tested to exclude diabetes mellitus.

Aetiology Diabetes, pregnancy, certain antibiotics (particularly tetracycline) and the contraceptive pill are all factors which increase the susceptibility to *Candida* infection.

Treatment   Nystatin or clotrimazole pessaries should be used, and the vulvitis and skin lesions treated with a combination of nystatin and hydrocortisone cream.

Prognosis   The condition quickly responds to treatment. The predisposing factors should be eliminated if possible to prevent further attacks. Certain individuals appear to be susceptible to recurrent infections, and the reason is not clear.

CANDIDIAL PARONYCHIA

Presentation   Chronic paronychia due to *Candida albicans* is most commonly seen in adults. It may also occur in infants and young children. It is more common in females (Figure 16.23), 9 : 1.

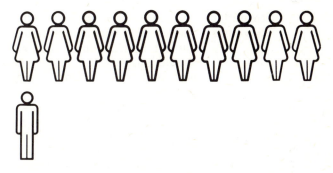

Figure 16.23   Candidal paronychia is mainly a disorder of females

The characteristic features are redness and swelling of the posterior nail folds. The cuticles are lost at early stages. Small quantities of pus may be expressed from under the nail fold. The lateral nail folds may also be involved. There is secondary involvement of the nail plate, beginning at the side of the nail, but eventually all the nail may be affected. There is ridging of the nail plate, and characteristically a brownish green discolouration (Figure 16.24). Initially the infection usually only affects one finger, but eventually others may be involved. It is rare for all the fingers to be affected.

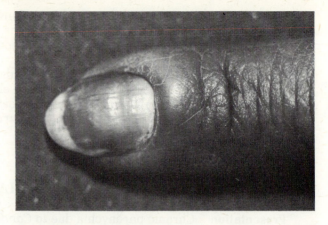

Figure 16.24 Candidal paronychia. Swelling and redness of the posterior nail fold with yellowish-green discolouration of the nail plate

Differential diagnosis The chronicity of the condition and lack of pus should distinguish the condition from an acute bacterial paronychia. The swelling of the nail folds should suggest the diagnosis and distinguish the nail abnormality from ringworm infections and psoriasis.

Investigations As the infection is in the nail bed it is difficult to reach the organisms and infected tissue for examination. Specimens of nail taken for mycological examination may reveal *Candida albicans*.

Aetiology The main predisposing factor appears to be an occupation in which the hands are continually in and out of water. The condition is an occupational hazard in barmaids and fishmongers. The moisture under the nail fold is ideal for growth of the yeasts.

Treatment The most important aspect of treatment is to keep the hands out of water as much as possible. If the patients' occupation is such that they have to have their hands in water, they should wear cotton gloves inside rubber ones. Topical antifungal lotions applied to the junction of the nail fold and nail plate may help slightly. It should be stressed that it may take weeks or even months for the paronychia to clear with treatment.

Prognosis   Candidial paronychia are chronic and unless the hands are kept out of water and detergents the condition will persist for years. Once the problem has cleared it is advisable for the patient still to wear gloves for housework or occupation, otherwise the condition may recur.

CHRONIC MUCOCUTANEOUS CANDIDIASIS

Presentation   The age and sex incidence depends on the type of clinical picture. The clinical presentation may be divided into granulomatous and non-granulomatous. The granulomatous disease is found in children and the sex distribution is equal. The lesions usually commence on the face or scalp. The lesion is localized, raised and has an irregular surface which is red and scaly. Cutaneous horns may develop on the surface. The lesion gradually enlarges and new separate lesions may also develop.

In the non-granulomatous form of chronic candidiasis the mouth and digits are affected. The oral lesions are widespread and paronychia occur on the fingers and toes.

Differential diagnosis   The granulomatous form of the disease has to be distinguished from other granulomas. The differential diagnosis of the oral lesions is that of the conditions mentioned above on oral candidiasis.

Investigations   Mycological tests, and in the case of granulomata, a biopsy is necessary to establish the diagnosis.

Tests for immunological competence should be performed, and these include lymphocyte transformation to *Candida*, immunoglobulins, opsonizing function, and killing of *Candida* by phagocytes.

Endocrine function and serum iron should also be investigated.

Aetiology   There are a number of underlying disorders which may present with chronic candidiasis. Generalized abnormality of endocrine function associated with chronic candidiasis is a rare but well recognized syndrome. Those affected are females.

A number of immunological abnormalities have

been described in this disorder, but not all are present in the same individual. Suffice it to say that in a large proportion there is a demonstrable impairment of normal immunological functions and patients should be investigated to determine which abnormalities may be present.

Iron deficiency is present in some patients, and appears to play some role in the aetiology of the condition, but iron deficiency alone is not the cause of the problem. The iron deficiency appears to be part of a more generalized abnormality which is endocrine or immunological.

Treatment   This depends to a certain extent on which, if any, underlying abnormalities have been found. If possible they should be corrected, particularly a low serum iron. Specific anticandidiasis treatment includes antibiotics given systemically or applied topically. The systemic drugs which have been used are amphotericin B, 5-fluorocytosine and clotrimazole. The topical drugs include those just mentioned and nystatin.

Correction of an opsonization defect with plasma infusion has been helpful in some instances. Transfer factor has also been beneficial in a number of patients.

Prognosis   This again depends on the underlying abnormalities and whether they can be corrected permanently. In the past a number of children with chronic mucocutaneous candidiasis have died, but this has been due to the underlying immunological defects which predispose to infections in general. The prognosis has improved with the newer antibiotics and 'immunological treatments', but there is still a high incidence of morbidity.

17 GENODERMATOSES

NEUROFIBROMATOSIS (VON RECKLINGHAUSEN'S DISEASE)

Presentation A hereditary disease affecting the nervous system, skin, mucous membranes and bones. The incidence is 1 in 3000. It is a worldwide disorder affecting the sexes equally.

One of the characteristic features is the presence of café au lait spots (Figure 17.1). These are sharply defined light brown macular patches. They may be oval or round, usually 2–5 cm. There may also be multiple freckles, mostly in the axillae, on the neck and peri-anal area. Occasionally there is generalized pigmentation.

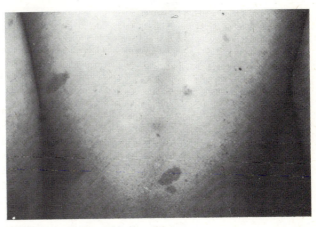

Figure 17.1 Café au lait patches in neurofibromatosis

The neurofibromas, which are visible, vary in their morphology. They may be dome-shaped, pedunculated or plaques (Figure 17.2). They may be skin

159

coloured or pigmented. The numbers of fibromata vary from an occasional lesion to many hundreds. They vary in size from a few mm to a few cm.

Endocrine abnormalities may occur in association with neurofibromatosis and include acromegaly, Addison's disease, cretinism, phaeochromocytoma and sexual precocity. Involvement of the gastro-intestinal tract may give rise to haemorrhage or obstruction. Bone involvement may cause kyphosis, scoliosis, bone cysts and pathological fractures. Malignancy in neurofibromas may occur although the incidence is only 3%, and this change is usually in deeper neurofibromas, rather than in cutaneous or subcutaneous lesions.

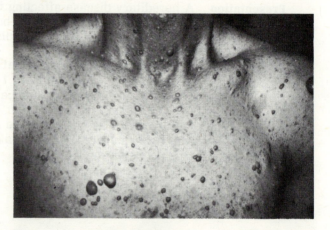

Figure 17.2   Pedunculated and papular neurofibromas

Differential diagnosis

Café au lait spots are common and appear in 15% of the population over the age of five years. Large lesions, i.e. those over 2 cm and more than six in number are suggestive of neurofibromatosis. Café au lait spots also occur in Albright's syndrome; however, they are usually fewer in number and there are no other skin lesions. Café au lait spots may also be present in tuberous sclerosis, but the disorders are easily distinguishable by their other cutaneous features. Plaque-like tumours of the skin have to be differentiated from lepromatous leprosy, and a biopsy may be necessary. Solitary pedun-culated lesions have to be distinguished from simple papilloma and fibro-epithelial polyps.

Investigations This disease is easily diagnosed when the typical skin lesions are present. Only where there is a single feature or internal involvement without skin lesions, is the diagnosis more difficult. A family history, if positive, is helpful.

Biopsy of a neurofibroma shows an increase of loose wavy collagen fibres and cellular proliferation. there is a mucoid degeneration of the stroma. Biopsy of a café au lait spot shows an increase in the number of melanocytes and an increase of melanin in both melanocytes and keratinocytes. Electron microscopy shows giant melanosomes in the melanocytes and keratinocytes of the café au lait spots in neurofibromatosis, but not those of the normal population, or in those with Albright's syndrome.

Aetiology Neurofibromatosis is a hereditary disease due to an autosomal dominant gene. However, it has been estimated that 50% of the cases are due to gene mutation. Neurofibromata are tumours of the peripheral nerve sheaths with proliferation and degeneration of the nerve.

Treatment No specific treatment is available apart from excision of troublesome tumours.

Prognosis At birth the skin is usually clear, but a few café au lait spots may be present, although they usually appear in early childhood. The tumours appear later, usually around puberty. The prognosis in the majority of patients is good, apart from the cosmetic disability. In a small number of patients there may be tumours of the cranial nerves and malignant changes in other lesions.

DARIER'S DISEASE

Presentation An hereditary disorder of abnormal keratinization. It is a rare disease affecting all races, but it is commoner in hot climates. Males and females are equally affected.

The disease is rare in the first years of life and

usually begins between the ages of 8 and 15, and rarely after 40.

The typical clinical lesions are small, firm, brown papules (Figure 17.3), usually associated with the hair follicles. They measure a few mm in diameter and gradually enlarge to become yellowish and covered with greasy scales. The papules may gradually coalesce to form a plaque which covers the area

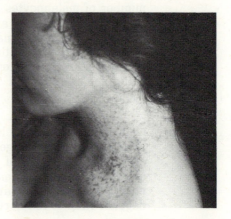

Figure 17.3   Brown papules on the neck in Darier's disease

with gross scaling and crusting. The sites of predilection are the seborrhoeic areas, i.e. the face, neck, behind the ears, mid-chest, back, scalp, buttocks, groins and axillae (Figure 17.4). The lesions are usually symmetrical, but may be localized. On the mucous membrane areas there may be small white umbilicated papules which may coalesce to form patches. There may be punctate keratosis, pits or hyperkeratosis on the palms and soles. The nails become fragile with longitudinal ridges; they are discoloured and there is subungual hyperkeratosis. Internal involvement is rare. Genital hypoplasia, small stature and low intelligence has been reported in some patients with this disease.

Differential diagnosis

Darier's disease may be differentiated from seborrhoeic eczema by its thick warty papules, mucosal involvement and more persistent patches. Acanthosis nigricans involves the flexural areas, with

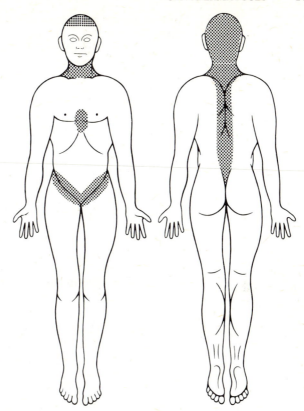

Figure 17.4   Common sites of Darier's disease

hyperkeratotic and hyperpigmented plaques. There may be similar lesions on the palms of the hands.

Benign familial pemphigus also occurs in the flexural areas, but has a history of recurrent vesicles and bullae which cause erosions and crusting. Linear fissures are often present, which are characteristic of benign familial pemphigus.

Localized Darier's disease must be distinguished from warty naevi.

Investigations   A biopsy is helpful. It shows papillomatosis hyper- and parakeratosis, thickening of the epidermis with separation of the cells which lie above the basal layer, causing lacunae. Two specific types of dyskeratotic cells have been described as 'corps rond' and 'grains'. The former have large basophilic masses surrounded by a clear halo. The grains have elongated dark staining nucleus and may be found in the acantholytic cells in the lacunae.

Aetiology   An autosomal dominant hereditary disease with incomplete penetration. The disorder may also be caused by gene mutation. The defect in this disease is one of abnormal synthesis and maturation of keratin.

Treatment   Keratolytic agents such as salicylic acid are of some help. There are reports of topical vitamin A (rectinoic acid) being beneficial. In the past large doses of oral vitamin A (100 000–500 000 IU) daily have been claimed to clear the lesions, but side effects are common with this large dosage. More recently the newer aromatic retinoids given orally have been successful in clearing the lesions in some patients and would now appear to be the treatment of choice in the first instance.

Prognosis   In the initial stages there may be spontaneous clearing of the lesions. However, if the disease becomes extensive it is usually persistent. Heat, humidity, sunlight, and secondary infections may induce new lesions or aggravate those already present.

Secondary infection is common. Kaposi's varicelliform eruptions may occur at the site of the lesions, either due to herpes simplex or vaccinia.

TUBEROUS SCLEROSIS (EPILOIA)

Presentation   A hereditary disease mainly involving the skin and nervous system, with the classical triad of epilepsy, mental retardation and adenoma sebaceum. It has a worldwide distribution. The incidence is 1 in 100 000. There is no sex predilection.

There are usually no skin lesions at birth, but they appear in the first decade of life. There are four characteristic lesions: (1) adenoma sebaceum, which are small discrete pinkish firm papules 1–4 mm, which occur on the naso–labial folds. These subsequently spread to the cheeks, chin and nose (Figure 17.5). (2) periungual fibromas which are present in some of the patients. There are yellowish flesh

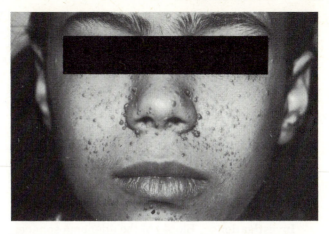

Figure 17.5   Pinkish papules on the face in tuberous sclerosis

coloured, small, firm, smooth tumours emerging from under the nail folds or around the base of the nails. (3) shagreen patches, which are skin coloured plaques, 1–10 cm, occurring in the lumbosacral region. (4) depigmented leaf shaped macules occurring on the trunk or limbs and which vary from a few mm to several cm. The lesions may be solitary or numerous, and this lesion may be present at birth. Other skin lesions which may occur include: café au lait spots, fibro-epithelial polyps and capillary haemangiomas.

The brain is invariably affected with fibrous tumours, causing mental deficiency and epilepsy. The eye is frequently affected, the commonest lesions being a retinal phakoma. There are renal hamartomas in 50% of the patients and 80% have bone abnormalities particularly pseudocysts of the phalanges.

Differential diagnosis   The diagnosis is usually made on the presence of adenoma sebaceum, which is the main diagnostic feature. The lesions must be differentiated from acne, in which comedones and pustules may be present. Epithelioma adenoides cysticum (trichoepitheliomata) are symmetrical, small, translucent nodules around the nose, eyelids and cheeks, and may appear at a similar age. Syringomata (benign sweat gland tumours) which are small, flesh coloured lesions occur mainly around the eyes and not along the nasolabial folds.

The depigmented patches may occur in early childhood and present before the other cutaneous manifestations. If this is so, the lesions have to be distinguished from vitiligo. This can be done by biopsy as in vitiligo; no melanocytes or very few are present, whereas in tuberous sclerosis the melanocytes are present, but show reduced melanin production. Unlike the depigmented patches of leprosy, there is no change in sweating or anaethesia in the lesions. In pityriasis alba, which is mild eczema, there are fine scales on the lesions.

Investigations   Biopsy of the adenoma sebaceum lesions show angiofibromatous proliferation. The sebaceous glands do not show adenomatous changes, and are often atrophic or absent. Biopsy of shagreen patches simply shows fibrous tissue proliferation. The white patches have abnormal melanocytes which show reduced tyrosinase activity and reduced melanin. Wood's light examination helps to demonstrate the white patches. X-ray of the skull may show calcification in the region of the basal ganglion. X-ray of the feet and hands shows cystic changes in the phalanges.

Aetiology   Tuberous sclerosis is a defect of the connective tissue, especially of the skin and nervous system. It is inherited as an autosomal dominant gene with complete penetration. In a large number of patients it is due to a new genetic mutation.

Treatment   The skin tumours may be excised or removed by curettage and cautery, or cryotherapy. Treatment of the internal complications will depend on the nature and severity of the problem.

Prognosis   The skin lesions continue to appear until adolescence and then persist. Morbidity and mortality depend on the degree of internal involvement. If there is minimal involvement, life expectancy is normal. Involvement of the heart and kidney leads to early death. Rhabdomyomata of the heart will usually result in death before the age of five years.

PEUTZ–JEGHER'S SYNDROME

Presentation   Peutz–Jegher's syndrome is a hereditary disorder. The patient is born with mucocutaneous lesions, or they appear soon after birth. The sexes are equally affected.

The clinical presentation is of a blue or dark brown flat patch, oval or round, and a few mm in size. These patches appear over the lips, the buccal mucosa, gums, palate and nose, and a few may be found on the palms and soles. The skin texture is normal. Patients in the second or third decades may have have colicky abdominal pain. This is due to the single or multiple polyps of the intestine. Intussusception is common, and bleeding due to ulceration of the polyps may also occur.

Differential diagnosis   Simple lentigos do not affect the oral cavity. Hyperpigmentation in Addison's disease is usually accompanied by other symptoms, and is not usually confined to the peri-oral region. Freckles on the sun exposed areas occur elsewhere on the face and fade or become paler in the winter. In Cronkhite's syndrome there is pigmentation on the fingers and hands, palms and soles.

Investigations   Radiological investigations show polyps in the small intestine and sometimes in the stomach or large intestine. Occult blood may be present in the stools, and this leads to anaemia. Sigmoidoscopy may show polyps in the colon.

Aetiology   The disease is transmitted by an autosomal dominant gene.

Treatment   Intussusception needs surgical treatment. The skin lesions do not require therapy apart from camouflage.

Prognosis   The lesions are present at birth or appear soon after, becoming more prominent until puberty and may then fade. Malignant transformation of the intestinal polyposes is rare and the prognosis varies from a normal life without symptoms to early death due to repeated attacks of intestinal obstruction.

EHLERS–DANLOS SYNDROME (CUTIS HYPERELASTICA)

Presentation   A hereditary disease with generalized connective tissue defect. It occurs worldwide and is slightly more common in males.

The main clinical features are due to fragility of the tissues and blood vessels; hyperelasticity of the skin (Figure 17.6), and hyperelasticity of the joints. The severity of the condition is variable. The characteristic skin abnormality is that the skin can be 'pulled out' for a few cm and then returned to its original

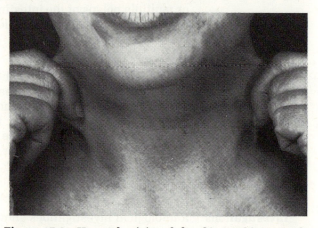

Figure 17.6   Hyperelasticity of the skin in Ehlers–Danlos syndrome

position when released. In later life loose skin folds develop on the hands, elbows, and around the face and eyes. The skin is soft, velvety and fragile. Slight trauma and laceration causes a wide wound which heals slowly with large atrophic umbilicated scarring. A soft dark blue tumour (molluscoid pseudotumours) may develop in the scar. These are more common over joints and prominent bones. Slight trauma to the fragile walls of the blood vessels causes bruising. If large skin vessels rupture, haematomas develop and subcutaneous fat necrosis may occur leading to fibrosis and calcification. Many subcutaneous tumours may be present on the legs, buttocks, and elbows.

Hyperextensibility of the joints may lead to dislocation and ultimately impaired mobility. There may be internal organ defects including cardiac septal defects, gastrointestinal bleeding, spontaneous rupture of the bowel, dissecting aortic aneurysms and pneumothorax. The facies is sometimes characteristic with wide nasal bridge, epicanthic folds and hypertelorism. The eyes may show blue sclera corneal abnormalities, and angioid streaks and ectopic lenses.

Differential diagnosis   The disease must be differentiated from Marfan's syndrome, in which there are loose joints, and ectopic lenses. There may also be striae over the hips and shoulders, but the increase in skin elasticity is slight. In Marfan's syndrome, the pathognomic sign is lengthening of the bones. Ehlers–Danlos syndrome has also to be distinguished from cutis laxa. In this disorder the patient has sagging folds of loose skin on the face and trunk, from the age of two years, but there is no hyperelasticity as in Ehlers–Danlos syndrome.

Investigations   Ehlers–Danlos syndrome with its characteristic features and positive family history can easily be diagnosed. A skin biopsy rather suprisingly does not show any consistent changes in the collagen or elastic tissues. Fibrosis, foreign body, giant cells and calcification may be seen.

An X-ray of subcutaneous tumours may show calcification.

Aetiology   Ehlers–Danlos syndrome has recently been divided into subgroups depending partly on clinical features and partly on biochemical abnormalities. All types are inherited. The majority of cases are due to an autosomal dominant gene, but some are inherited either as an autosomal recessive or X-linked. A number of enzymes concerned with connective tissue have recently been shown to be abnormal and probably account for the abnormalities.

Treatment   There is no specific treatment. Orthopaedic support may be necessary to protect the joints.

Prognosis   The disorder is persistent, there is progressive disability and disfiguration. Internal involvement may lead to premature death.

HEREDITARY HAEMORRHAGIC TELANGIECTASIA (OSLER–RENDU–WEBER DISEASE)

Presentation   An inherited disease with neoangiomatosis of blood vessels throughout the body. The onset of the disease is in childhood, but the majority of lesions appear in early adult life. The characteristic lesions are different types of telangiectasia; punctate, linear and nodular. Lesions of the skin occur most commonly on the lips, face, ears, lower arms, palms and toes (Figure 17.7). The mucosal surfaces always affected are the nasal septum and tongue. Other mucosal surfaces which are usually involved are the conjunctiva, oesophagus, bronchial tree, stomach, intestine,

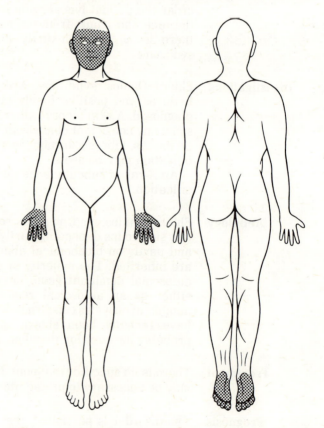

Figure 17.7   Distribution of lesions in hereditary telangiectasia

vagina and rectum. Pulmonary and hepatic arterio-venous fistulas may develop, the latter giving rise to hepatic fibrosis. The commonest presentation is epistaxis, but haemorrhage may occur from any of the abnormal blood vessels.

Differential diagnosis Ataxia telangiectasia must be differentiated from hereditary haemorrhagic telangiectasia. In the former the patient also has telangiectasia on the face and neck in childhood. However, in this disease other features develop, notably partial atrophy of the subcutaneous fat, cutaneous atrophy, ataxia and recurrent infections due to immune deficiency. In generalized essential telangiectasia the lesions are linear and may present in patches. Haemorrhage into the skin and mucous membrane may occur. In Bloom's disease the telangiectasia appear in infancy mostly on the butterfly area of the face and are associated with photosensitivity and stunted growth. In the Rothmund–Thomson syndrome there is photo-sensitivity and reticulate pigmentation of the face with linear telangiectasia. The eyebrows and scalp hair are sparse. The CRST syndrome occurs in adults, in which there is macular telangiectasia of the face, associated with cutaneous calcinosis, Raynaud's phenomenon and sclerodactyly.

Aetiology The disease is transmitted by an autosomal dominant gene.

Treatment The important complication is gastro-intestinal hae-morrhage which requires appropriate treatment. Iron deficiency anaemia may occur. The skin lesions can be treated by cautery.

Prognosis Death may occur prematurely from internal haemor-rhage, but the majority of patients survive to old age.

18 GRANULOMA ANNULARE

Presentation   The disorder may occur at any age but is most common in children and early adult life. The sexes are equally affected. The typical lesion is an annular, raised lesion with normal overlying epidermis, so the surface is smooth (Figure 18.1). The colour of the lesion varies; it may be white, red or violaceous. The size varies from approximately 1 cm to 10 cm. The

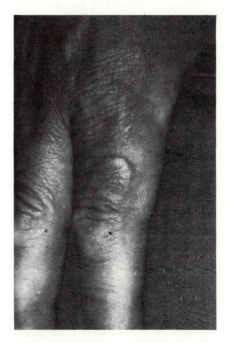

Figure 18.1   Annular lesion on the dorsum of a finger in granuloma annulare

lesions may be multiple or solitary. Occasionally the lesions present as small papules or nodules. The size of this type of lesion is usually less than 1 cm. Very occasionally granuloma annulare may present as a plaque up to 10 cm in diameter. The commonest sites to be involved are the backs of the hands, backs and sides of the fingers, the extensor surfaces of limbs, particularly over the body prominences (Figure 18.2).

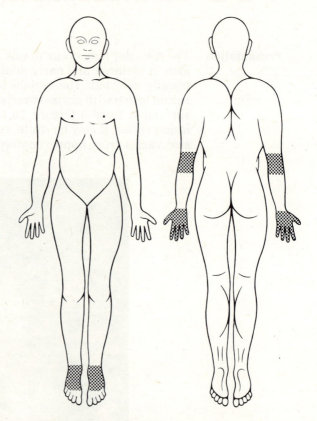

Figure 18.2   Common sites for granuloma annulare

Generalized granuloma annulare   This is a rare form of the disease with numerous lesions on the trunk and limbs. This variety of the disease is seen mainly in adults.

Differential diagnosis   The annular lesions on the limbs have to be distinguished from fungal infections, but the latter are invariably scaly unless treated with topical steroids.

On the fingers the papular lesions have to be distinguished from viral warts; the latter have a roughened clefted surface, and black dots representing thrombosed capillaries may be present. The nodular lesions may be confused with rheumatoid nodules. If the lesions are over the knuckles, they have to be distinguished from knuckle pads. The generalized form of the disease may be confused with lichen planus, other forms of granulomas, and reticulosis.

Investigations   In instances where the diagnosis is in doubt a biopsy should be performed. In the generalized form the urine should be examined for glucose, and a glucose tolerance test carried out if there is no glycosuria.

Aetiology   The cause of granuloma annulare is not known. In the generalized form there appears to be an association with diabetes mellitus.

Treatment   The only worthwhile treatment is intralesional corticosteroids. There is some suggestion that any traumatic procedure such as a biopsy will cause involution of the lesion.

Natural history and prognosis   It has been estimated that 50% of lesions will disappear within two years of onset. In children the majority of lesions certainly seem to disappear in this time. Apart from the association of diabetes mellitus in some patients with the generalized form, the disease is harmless and only a cosmetic disability.

19 HAIR

ALOPECIA AREATA

Presentation Alopecia areata affects all races. It is a common dis-order accounting for 2% of new cases in UK skin clinics. Males and females are equally affected. The disease may occur at any age, but it is most common between 5 and 40, the highest incidence is under the age of 25 (Figure 19.1).

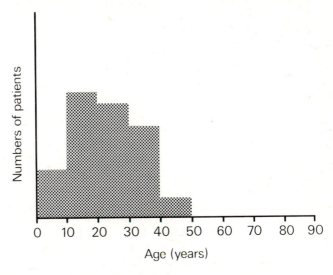

Figure 19.1 Age of onset of alopecia areata

The characteristic presentation is one of several well circumscribed areas of sudden hair loss. The lesions are oval or round (Figure 19.2), usually with normal coloured skin, but occasionally it may be pink. The loss of hair from the affected area may be

177

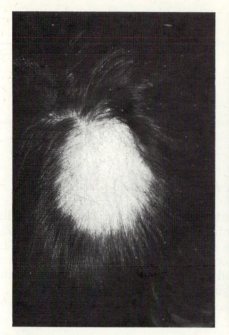 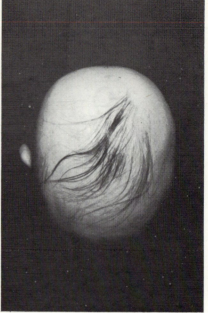

Figure 19.2 Oval bald patch in
alopecia areata

Figure 19.3 Alopecia areata involving nearly all the scalp hair

partial, but is usually total. The hair follicles are visible. On the periphery the pathognomonic exclamation mark hairs may be seen. These are hairs 5 mm in
length, thicker at the distal part, with the shaft
tapering gradually towards the proximal end.

If the lesion is active the hair surrounding the bald
area is easily shed on traction. The lesions may
extend peripherally for a few weeks. Spontaneous
recovery and regrowth usually occurs. First, vellous
and depigmented hairs appear, then normal hair
grows, which may remain grey, but usually repig-
ments. The beard, pubic hair, eyebrows and
eyelashes may also be similarly affected, but the
commonest site is the scalp. Very rarely the hair loss
will involve all the scalp hair (Figure 19.3), and even
all the body hair.

Nail changes usually occur when the hair loss is
extensive and take the form of fine pitting and
ridging and ultimately dystrophy.

Occasionally, a diffuse loss of hair occurs from
the scalp with no bald patches, and does not lead to
baldness, so-called diffuse alopecia areata.

Differential diagnosis   In children, alopecia areata must be distinguished from fungal infections. In the latter the hairs are present, but broken close to the surface of the scalp and the skin is scaly. Alopecia areata is distinguished from syphilitic alopecia by the fact that the latter shows a moth-eaten pattern of multiple and irregular patches, which are not completely devoid of hair.

Trichotillomania is non-scarring, patchy, but shows incomplete hair loss, the hairs being broken at different lengths. The other patchy alopecias, such as lichen planus, discoid lupus erythematosus and pyodermas show changes in the skin.

Total loss of hair from the scalp in alopecia areata has to be distinguished from hair loss due to anti-mitotic drugs. The diffuse type of alopecia areata without total hair loss has to be distinguished from telogen effluvium and drug induced alopecia.

Investigations   Examination of a plucked hair from the active margin may show an exclamation mark hair.

Biopsy of a lesion shows small and immature hair follicles. The follicles are surrounded by mononuclear inflammatory cells.

Aetiology   There is family history of alopecia areata in about 20% of patients. The mode of inheritance is not known. It has been postulated that the disease is an anagen effluvium, and that an acute onset of alopecia occurs when there is a halt in the anagen phase. Auto-immunity has been implicated, but there is no firm evidence to support this at present.

Treatment   Topical steroids are often prescribed, but do not appear to be helpful. Intra-lesional and systemic steroids will certainly result in regrowth of hair, but if the disease process is still active, the new hair will fall out again, when the effect of the steroid wears off. There is no place for the case of long term systemic steroids because of the side effects. Dinitrochlorobenzene (DNCB) sensitization, topical use of other irritants and ultraviolet light, including PUVA (psoralens and long-wave ultraviolet light), have been used, but the results are variable.

Prognosis   It is difficult to predict the course and prognosis. Usually however, if the lesions are not widespread, regrowth occurs within a few months; 90% of the patients can expect regrowth. Occasionally the hair does not repigment in the affected area. Poor prognostic features are involvement of back and sides of the scalp, above the ears, extensive involvement and repeated episodes. Once the disease progresses to total loss of hair from the scalp the prognosis is poor, and it is rare for the hair to regrow.

TELOGEN EFFLUVIUM (TELOGEN ALOPECIA)

Presentation   Telogen effluvium may be defined as excessive hair loss. It may occur at any age, but it is commonest in young adults. Both sexes are affected, but it is more common in females (Figure 19.4). The characteristic feature of this disorder is the latent period of 2–4

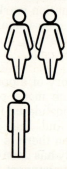

Figure 19.4 Telogen effluvium is more common in females (2:1)

months between the trigger factor and the onset of the hair loss. The patient loses 100–1000 hairs per day depending on the severity of the disease. Characteristically the hair loss is diffuse, but if there is underlying male pattern alopecia this becomes more apparent. The skin of the scalp is normal.

Differential diagnosis   Other causes of diffuse hair loss must be kept in mind, such as hypothyroidism, anaemia or drugs. The diagnosis is based on the history, e.g. pregnancy or serious febrile illness, 2–4 months before onset. Shed hairs are normal microscopically. Plucking the scalp hair and counting the hairs in anagen and telogen will show the number of telogen hairs is much higher than normal.

Aetiology   In normal hair growth each hair has an active growing period. During the telogen phase the hair goes through a rest period which lasts 2–4 months, and then sheds. A new hair then grows in place of the shed one. Nearly 10% of the hair follicles are in the resting phase and loss of up to 100 hairs per day is normal. In telogen effluvium many more hairs go into the telogen phase, and the known precipitating factors include acute febrile disease, haemorrhage, child birth, and stopping the contraceptive pill.

Course and prognosis   The duration of telogen effluvium is variable. It usually lasts 3–6 months, occasionally longer. The eventual prognosis is good, the hair regrowing to its former state.

Treatment   There is no effective treatment to shorten the course of the disorder.

MALE PATTERN ALOPECIA

Presentation   Male pattern alopecia is a gradual thinning and loss of terminal hair from the scalp affecting adults. It is very common throughout the world, and is considered as a normal hair pattern. However, it is less prevalent in the Chinese. The incidence gradually increases between the ages of 20 and 60. The first signs may appear in the late teens.

The hair loss begins with recession of the fronto–temporal hair line and progresses to gradual thinning of the hair over the vertex, especially posteriorly (Figure 19.5). If progressive the balding areas coalesce resulting in loss of hair over the vertex. In severe cases hair only remains on the lower sides and back of the scalp. The scalp never becomes completely bald. The skin is normal and smooth, and there may be vellous hairs.

Differential diagnosis   The main condition from which male pattern alopecia should be distinguished is telogen effluvium, which is an episode of generalized excessive hair loss 3–4 months following certain types of stress.

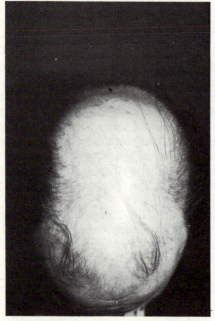

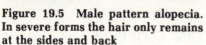

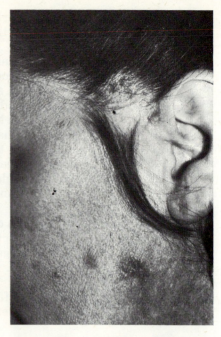

Figure 19.5   Male pattern alopecia. In severe forms the hair only remains at the sides and back

Figure 19.6   Scarring alopecia in discoid lupus erythematosus

Other causes of chronic diffuse hair loss should be considered, such as hypothyroidism and chemical agents applied to the scalp.

Investigations   None are necessary.

Aetiology   The disorder is most probably inherited as a dominant gene. Normal amounts of circulating androgens are necessary for this pattern of hair loss.

Treatment   No effective treatment is available.

SCARRING ALOPECIA

Any cutaneous disorder which results in destruction of the hair follicles will cause scarring alopecia. In this type of alopecia the hair never regrows and the alopecia is permanent. The skin is usually atrophic or scarred, and there are no signs of hair follicles.

There are numerous disorders which cause scarring alopecia such as congenital and hereditary disorders, burns, radio-dermatitis, trauma, neoplasms, infections such as carbuncles, or furuncles, fungal infections such as favus or severe kerions. A number of specific skin disorders may also cause scarring alopecia.

Discoid lupus erythematosus Scalp lesions may occur with or without other manifestations. The lesion is a hairless, red, indurated, scaly plaque (Figure 19.6) and follicular plugging is present. A biopsy for histology and immunofluorescent studies confirms the diagnosis.

Lichen planus This presents as small patches of white atrophic skin, with areas of follicular plugging. Without the typical mucocutaneous or cutaneous lesions it is difficult to diagnose.

Pseudopelade This is an uncommon form of scarring alopecia seen mostly in adults. The aetiology is unknown. It is characterized by oval or irregular patches of cutaneous atrophy. There are white, waxy, depressed areas, without skin inflammation, which gradually progress to destroy the hair follicles. There is no treatment available.

Localized scleroderma (morphoea) This may cause scarring alopecia. The characteristic of the lesion is that of morphoea elsewhere on the body.

TRICHOTILLOMANIA

Presentation Trichotillomania is self-induced alopecia, caused by pulling, twisting, rubbing, or breaking the hair, consciously or unconsciously. Both sexes are affected, but it is more common in women (Figure 19.7). The commonest age of onset is in the 5–10 year age group and young adults (Figure 19.8). The predisposing factors are emotional stress and tension. Patients may show other signs of self-mutilation. The site of predilection is usually the scalp, but it may be seen in the eyebrows, eyelashes and in the pubic hair.

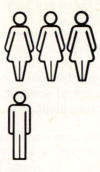

Figure 19.7   Trichotillomania is more common in females (3 : 1)

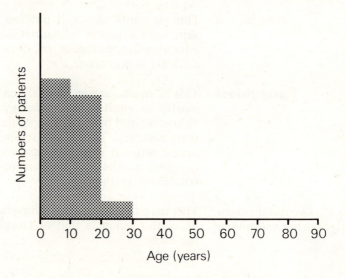

Figure 19.8   Age incidence of trichotillomania

The clinical picture is of a solitary or few patches of hair loss, with an ill-defined edge. The skin is normal or slightly scaly. Careful examination shows different lengths of hair.

Differential diagnosis Alopecia areata has well-defined patches of complete hair loss and normal skin. Tinea capitis shows scaling and sometimes inflammatory changes of the affected skin with broken hairs, and mycology confirms the diagnosis. In secondary syphilis there are moth-eaten patches of only partial alopecia and other signs of secondary syphilis are usually present. The diagnosis is confirmed by positive serology.

Investigations None are usually necessary. If the diagnosis is in doubt, specimens should be taken for mycology.

Treatment Any method of preventing trauma to the hair may be helpful, such as occlusive bandages on the scalp for a few weeks, wearing gloves or shaving the hair until the patient breaks the habit. Sedation and psychotherapy are sometimes required.

Course and prognosis Most children grow out of this habit, and the condition is self-limiting.

ALOPECIA DUE TO DRUGS

Chemicals and drugs can alter and influence the hair growth and loss cycle. The pattern, severity, and course of hair loss depends on the nature and the amount of the drug used.

Antimitotic agents may cause rapid, severe alopecia by arresting the hair growth in the active phase, which causes diffuse rapid shedding of the hair. If the dose is small the drug may simply cause narrowing of the shaft of the active hair. Spontaneous regrowth will occur.

Anticoagulants, e.g. heparin and warfarin, in accidental poisoning or in therapeutic doses increase normal hair loss which is trivial in most instances.

TRACTION ALOPECIA

This disorder is caused by prolonged traction of the hair, which gradually causes thinning in areas where the hairs are pulled. The disease primarily occurs in girls and young women as a result of hairstyles such as plaiting. The clinical appearance of this form of hair loss depends on the area, direction and tension at which the hair is pulled. Usually it is characterized by oval or linear areas of hair loss at the margins of the hair lines.

In traction alopecia the region may be erythematous with papules, scaling and broken hairs. The hair may be surrounded by a small keratin ring. In the earlier stages, if traction ceases the condition is reversible but continued traction will cause permanent alopecia.

HIRSUTISM

Presentation

Hirsutism may be defined as a change of vellous hair to terminal hairs in female subjects. The common sites are the upper lip, chin, midline below the umbilicus, on the abdomen, centre of the chest, around the nipples, legs, thighs and back.

Hirsutism depending on the cause may or may not be accompanied by virilism. Virilism consists of hypertrophy of the clitoris, oiliness of the skin, muscularity, husky voice, enlargement of the thyroid cartilage and recession of the fronto–temporal hairline.

Aetiology

Hirsutism is usually divided into primary and secondary. In primary hirsutism the hair follicles have an increased sensitivity to androgens. In secondary hirsutism there is an increase in circulating androgens. The sources of androgens in females are the ovaries and adrenals.

Primary hirsutism

The commonest form of primary hirsutism is racial. The condition is most common in races from the Middle East, and common in persons from the Indian subcontinent and the southern Mediterranean. The condition usually begins around puberty and is fully established by the age of 25.

Idiopathic hirsutism is so called because it occurs in persons with no genetic predisposition, and no recognized endocrine abnormality, although plasma testosterone is sometimes slightly elevated.

Secondary hirsutism
Polycystic ovaries or Stein–Leventhal syndrome

In this syndrome there are irregular menstrual periods and infertility. The plasma testosterone and androstenedione are raised, but the urinary 17-oxosteroids may be normal or moderately elevated.

Arrhenoblastoma

This is an ovarian tumour with testicular cells. It produces testosterone which results in hirsutism and other signs of virilism. The onset of hirsutism is usually between the ages of 20 and 30. Plasma testosterone is high, and urinary 17-oxosteroids are slightly raised.

Adrenal rest tumour
There is hirsutism, virilism, and Cushing's syndrome. The tumour is situated in the ovary and secretes androgens and cortisol. The plasma testosterone is elevated and the urinary 17-oxosteroids are also raised.

Congenital adrenogenital syndrome (Congenital adrenal hyperplasia)
This is due to an enzyme defect which results in an impairment of the adrenal to synthesize cortisol. The low cortisol levels result in increased production of ACTH and subsequent adrenal hyperplasia. There are raised levels of androgens resulting in virilism and hirsutism, prior to puberty. In addition to the raised androgens there are raised urinary 17-oxosteroids.

Iatrogenic hirsutism
A number of drugs may cause hirsutism and these include anabolic steroids and progesterones derived from nortestosterone.

Cushing's syndrome
Hirsutism is only significant in approximately a third of patients. This is because in the majority of patients cortisol is the principal hormone which is raised and androgens are raised only in proportion. Other symptoms of Cushing's syndrome are present which should establish the diagnosis clinically.

Investigations
In patients with irregular or absent periods, signs of virilism, or Cushing's disease, full endocrinological investigations are necessary, but these are best supervised by an endocrinologist.

Treatment
If the cause is a secondary one then obviously this should be treated accordingly, although even if successful this does not always result in the regression of the hirsutism.

In primary hirsutism, or if the hair persists after treatment of the cause in secondary hirsutism, the hair may be removed by electrolysis, waxing or shaving. Only electrolysis offers the chance of permanent removal of hair. Bleaching of the hair is also helpful from the cosmetic point of view.

Recent success in the treatment of hirsutism has

been claimed with the anti-androgen cyproterone acetate. This is only effective when taken orally and must be combined with oestrogens.

Prognosis   Once established hirsutism tends to persist, and this is often the case with secondary hirsutism even after successful treatment of the underlying endocrine abnormality.

20 HERPES GESTATIONIS

Presentation Herpes gestationis is a distinctive eruption which occurs during pregnancy or the puerperium. It most commonly presents in the third trimester and there is no particular age incidence. The initial lesions usually occur on the abdomen around the umbilicus (Figure 20.1), and soon spread to involve the abdomen and subsequently the rest of the trunk. The

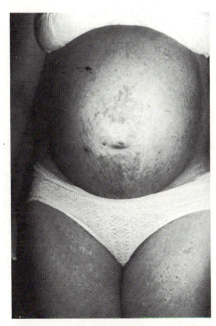

Figure 20.1 Erythematous urticarial eruption around the umbilicus in the early stages of herpes gestationis

limbs are affected a few days later. The first lesions to appear are erythematous, urticarial patches. Subsequently blisters appear. The blisters are more common on the limbs than on the trunk. The blisters vary in size from a few mm to a few cm, are tense and do not rupture easily. The eruption is associated with severe irritation, which sometimes precedes the lesions.

Differential diagnosis   Pruritus is not an uncommon symptom in pregnancy and often occurs without any rash. In herpes gestationis the initial pruritus is subsequently followed by a rash. Erythema multiforme when predominantly urticarial, bullous and widespread may be difficult to distinguish from herpes gestationis. However, so-called target lesions which may be present in erythema multiforme are not found in herpes gestationis. Erythema multiforme is self-limiting and will clear irrespective of the pregnancy. Dermatitis herpetiformis usually begins on the elbows and although intensely irritating, the disease is not usually as widespread as herpes gestationis. Dermatitis herpetiformis usually persists after pregnancy, although it also may be aggravated by pregnancy and improve subsequently. Apart from herpes gestationis there is another eruption associated with pregnancy which is also very irritating, but blisters are not present, and the predominant lesions are papules. It is sometimes referred to as the papular eruption of pregnancy.

Investigations   Skin biopsy shows a subepidermal blister with inflammatory changes in the upper dermis. Immunological tests show the deposition of C_3 complement along the line of the basement membrane. In a small proportion of patients IgG is also found at the same site as the complement. In the serum it is possible to show that a factor (termed the 'herpes gestationis factor') is present which is capable of binding complement to the basement membrane.

Aetiology   The current theory is that herpes gestationis is an immunological disorder. In relation to the foetus an antibody is produced by the mother 'the herpes gestationis factor' which is directed against the basement of the skin, and this results in complement activation and tissue damage. Soon after birth the herpes gestationis factor disappears from the serum and the disease clears.

Treatment In the initial stages or if the disease is not severe, symptomatic treatment with oral antihistamines may relieve the irritation, but does not influence the course of the disease. The only drugs which are effective in suppressing the eruption are oral corticosteroids. Fortunately the dose required is relatively low, being approximately 20 mg per day. Once the rash has cleared a smaller maintenance dose may suffice to suppress the rash until spontaneous remission occurs.

Prognosis Herpes gestationis is self-limiting and clears soon after parturition. In some patients it may clear in a few weeks, whilst in those in whom it begins in the puerperium the eruption may persist for two or three months. It is usual for the disorder to recur in subsequent pregnancies. The foetus is not at serious risk from the disorder. There is no increased incidence of congenital abnormality. There have been a few reports of the child being born with skin lesions similar to those of the mother.

21 HYPERHIDROSIS

Presentation   Hyperhidrosis is excessive sweating when no apparent cause is found, i.e. the usual stimuli of a hot climate, exercise and emotional stress are absent, and is sometimes referred to as essential hyperhidrosis. Essential hyperhidrosis may take two forms, the generalized but rare form, and a more common,

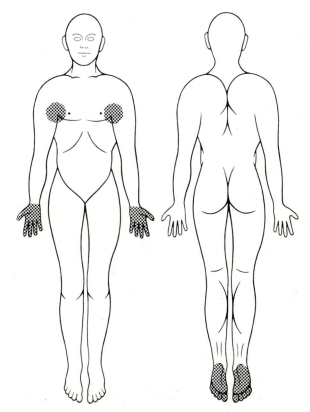

Figure 21.1   Common sites of essential hyperhidrosis

localized one limited to one or more of the emotional sweat areas, the palms, soles and axillae (Figure 21.1). It is even doubtful whether essential generalized hyperhidrosis occurs at all, as a pathological cause is frequently found on investigation.

Essential hyperhidrosis occurs with equal frequency in both sexes, but it is more common on the soles in males, and axillae and palms in females. The condition is invariably symmetrical even if it is only the palms, soles or axillae which are affected. The condition usually begins around adolescence (Figure 21.2). The affected area is continuously moist, but may be worse in the summer; the condition is unaffected by emotional stress as the sweat glands seem to be switched on to maximum all the time. Females often complain of ruining their clothes as a result of axillary hyperhidrosis, and if it affects the hands, it is difficult for the individual to perform a job which necessitates handling paper.

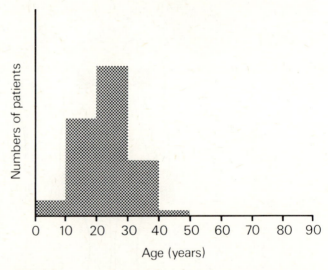

Figure 21.2   Age incidence of essential hyperhidrosis

Differential diagnosis   Essential hyperhidrosis has to be distinguished from pathological causes of sweating, such as hyperthyroidism, pheochromocytoma, malaria, tuberculosis, brucellosis, anxiety state, and central nervous system disease affecting the hypothalamus. Most of these conditions will cause generalized sweating, apart from an anxiety state where the disease does tend to affect only the emotional sweat areas. Localized sweating may occur elsewhere on the body, and this is usually due to an abnormality of the nervous system. Gustatory sweating usually occurs on the lips, forehead and nose after eating hot, spicy foods.

Investigations If there is any doubt as to whether the condition is essential hyperhidrosis, then the patient must be investigated to see if any of the above pathological conditions are present.

Aetiology The cause of essential hyperhidrosis is unknown. The fact that it is often limited to the axillae or palms, or soles, argues the possibility that it is due to an underlying anxiety state, but other symptoms of anxiety are usually absent. The condition may simply be an end organ effect with overproduction of sweat in response to normal stimuli.

Treatment Recently the treatment for essential hyperhidrosis has improved considerably. Sweating is stopped in the majority of patients by a 25% solution of aluminium chloride. The aluminium chloride may be dissolved in water, but it has been claimed that better results are obtained using an alcoholic solution; however, it does take about 3 weeks to dissolve the aluminium chloride in alcohol. The solution should be applied to the affected area 2 or 3 times a week, and left to dry on the skin. It is best applied at night and contact with night clothing should be avoided until the solution has dried. This frequency of application of aluminium chloride is usually sufficient to stop sweating, but it can be used more frequently if necessary. Once control of sweating has been achieved the frequency of using the aluminium chloride can be gradually decreased, and it is often sufficient to use the solution once a week or even every two weeks. If it is found necessary to use it daily or on alternate days it may cause inflammation, particularly in the axillae, but this can be controlled with 1% hydrocortisone cream.

Because of the success of aluminium chloride most of the older remedies need no longer be considered. Local excision of the axillary skin was successful for axillary hyperhidrosis. Sympathectomy is mentioned in many texts but in the author's opinion it should not be used. Most systemic drugs which have been tried are ineffective or have a high incidence of side effects.

Natural history and prognosis   Untreated essential hyperhidrosis may persist for many years. It is rare after middle age, so it can be assumed that the condition does burn itself out eventually. There is some suggestion that continual use of aluminium chloride over a few months results in a long, permanent remission.

22 ICHTHYOSIS

Ichthyosis is a disorder of abnormal keratinization. Clinically the skin appears dry, scaly and cracked. There are many different clinical forms of ichthyosis. Ichthyosis is most commonly hereditary, but may also be acquired. Hereditary ichthyosis is subdivided into distinct entities by the clinical features and mode of genetic transmission.

ICHTHYOSIS VULGARIS

Presentation

This is the most common form of ichthyosis and affects all races. In England it has been estimated that 4 in 1000 are affected, males and females equally. The disorder is not present at birth. The peak age of onset is between 1 and 4 years, and rarely occurs before 3 months of age. It is more prevalent in dry and cold climates and less so in warm and humid ones. The clinical features are dryness and scaling (Figure 22.1), with sparing of the flexures of the limbs, keratosis pilaris on the upper arms and hyperkeratosis of the knees and elbows. The face is often affected in childhood, but not later in life. The disorder is usually symptomless, but there may be irritation.

Differential diagnosis

These include other forms of ichthyosis, dry skin associated with atopic eczema and acquired ichthyosis which occurs in later life.

Investigations

Diagnosis of the disorder can usually be made on clinical grounds. A biopsy shows hyperkeratosis with an absent or poorly formed granular layer. There may be follicular plugging and the sebaceous glands are smaller than normal.

197

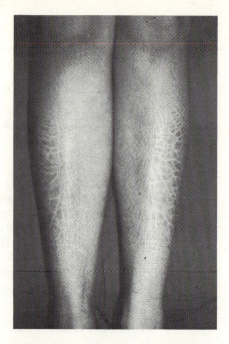

Figure 22.1   Dry skin with superficial cracking in ichthyosis vulgaris

Aetiology This is a hereditary disease with an autosomal dominant gene. The disease may be associated with atopy.

Treatment Ten per cent urea cream applied daily is the most effective treatment at present. Recent success has been claimed with both lactic acid and mandelic acid. These preparations are used at a concentration of 5% in a cream base.

Prognosis The prognosis is good in that the condition improves with age and many clear in adulthood.

X-LINKED ICHTHYOSIS

Presentation A type of ichthyosis seen only in males (Figure 22.2); the rate of incidence in the UK has been reported as 1 in 6000. Clinically the disorder is characterized by the onset of the disease in the first three months of life or it may be present at birth. The scales are

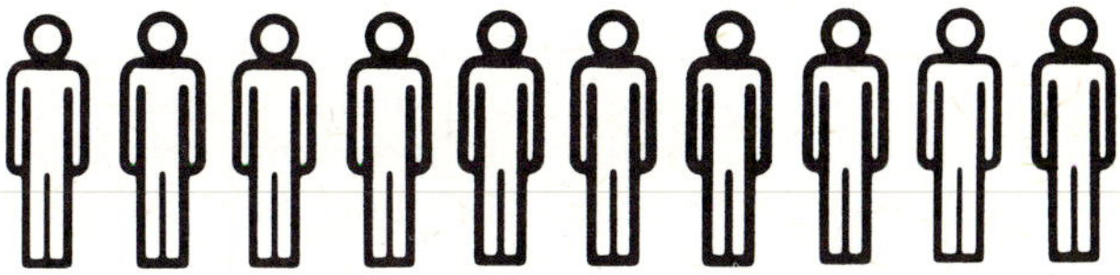

Figure 22.2   X-linked ichthyosis occurs in males

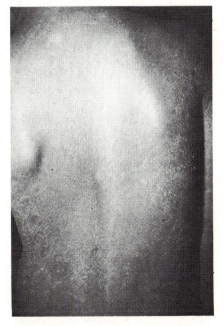

Figure 22.3   Extensive ichthyosis in
the X-linked variety

large and brown, and usually the whole body surface is involved (Figure 22.3), except the palms and
soles. It is more severe on the trunk, face, front of
neck, and scalp. In adults the most involved areas
are the abdomen, lower legs, and politeal fossae.
There is no follicular keratosis. There may be deep
corneal opacity.

Differential diagnosis   X-linked ichthyosis must be distinguished from ichthyosis vulgaris. X-linked ichthyosis has an earlier onset, and only males are affected. There is no involvement of the palms and soles, and there is no keratosis pilaris. There is, however, flexural involvement, and the scales are large and dark brown.

Investigations   The diagnosis is usually made on clinical grounds. A biopsy shows hyperkeratosis, a normal granular layer, and mild dermal inflammatory changes. Unlike ichthyosis vulgaris the sebaceous glands are normal and there is no follicular plugging.

Aetiology   This disorder is inherited by a sex-linked recessive gene, hence its manifestation in males only. Females are carriers. (A deficiency of the enzyme aryl sulphatase has been reported.)

Treatment   Ten per cent topical urea cream is helpful. It must be applied indefinitely as the disease relapses on cessation of treatment. Five per cent lactic acid in a cream base is also beneficial.

Prognosis   This type of ichthyosis is persistent and may become more severe in adult life.

LAMELLAR ICHTHYOSIS (NON-BULLOUS ICHTHYOSIFORM ERYTHRODERMA)

Presentation   A rare congenital disease which affects all races. Males and females are equally affected. The disease is usually present at birth, otherwise it appears within three months of birth. The severity of the disease varies considerably. It may be present as a simple generalized erythema. The skin then becomes thick and scaly (Figure 22.4). The scaling is more prominent in the flexures and persists throughout life. There is moderate hyperkeratosis of the palms and soles, and ectropion is common. In more severe cases the child may be stillborn, or born as a harlequin foetus or a collodion baby (see below, p. 203). Cortical cataracts may occur in lamellar ichthyosis.

Differential diagnosis   In infants the disorder must be distinguished from Leiner's disease. The latter is not usually present at birth and the disorder may be limited to the face and

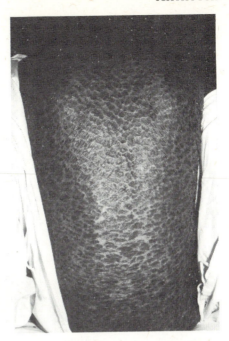

Figure 22.4   Thick scales in lamellar ichthyosis

scalp. There are greasy scales on the scalp, eyebrows and seborrhoeic areas, and there may be lymphadenopathy and diarrhoea. Another cause of infantile erythroderma is epidermal necrolysis, which has a sudden onset of erythema and peeling. Generalized eczema and psoriasis may also be present as erythroderma, although this cause of erythroderma in infants is rare. Finally, it must be distinguished from other types of ichthyosis, particularly bullous ichthyosiform erythroderma.

Investigations   A biopsy shows thickening of the epidermis. The granular layer may be thickened and there is gross hyperkeratosis and perivascular infiltration.

Aetiology   It is transmitted by autosomal recessive gene.

Treatment   Keratolytics such as 5% salicylic acid in propylene glycol lessens the scaling. Hydroxy acids (citric and lactic) have been claimed to be helpful, as have oral aromatic retinoids.

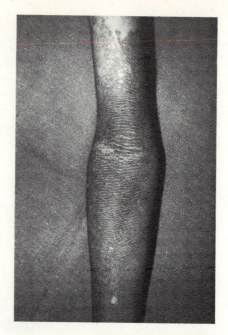

Figure 22.5   Grossly thickened skin with ridging in ichthyosiform erythroderma

Prognosis   In severe cases the child may be stillborn. There is often difficulty in moving and joint mobility. Although this type of ichthyosis improves in childhood, the disorder is persistent throughout life.

BULLOUS ICHTHYOSIFORM ERYTHRODERMA

Presentation   A rare congenital disease affecting all races, males and females equally. Babies are usually normal at birth, but are occasionally born as collodion babies. The onset of the disease is from birth to six months of age. The infant develops repeated attacks of redness, scaling and widespread bullae ranging from 5 mm to several cm, which occasionally cause extensive erosion of the skin and secondary infection. The bullae most commonly occur on the lower legs, and they become less frequent with age. The eruption may remain generalized or be localized to the flexural regions or occur as irregular linear lesions. Lesions may also persist on the lower face, neck, and back of hands and feet. The skin in the affected areas is grossly thickened and often shows deep ridging (Figure 22.5). The skin is a light brown colour. The palms and soles may be involved, but the hair and nails are normal.

Differential diagnosis Other bullous diseases of childhood must be considered, particularly the dystrophic variety of epidermolysis bullosa. In the latter the mucous membranes are involved. Bullous impetigo of infancy and bullous papular urticaria are not generalized and lack hyperkeratosis.

Investigations Biopsy of a lesion shows marked hyperkeratosis, a prominent granular layer, thickening of the epidermis with vacuolization of the epidermal cells, with large keratohyaline granules.

Aetiology This is a hereditary disease with autosomal dominant gene.

Treatment Topical keratolytics will decrease the hyperkeratosis. Oral aromatic retinoids are the best treatment available at present.

Prognosis In the period of widespread bullae and secondary infection the morbidity is high. The condition often improves with age, the life expectancy is normal.

COLLODION BABY (LAMELLAR EXFOLIATION OF THE NEWBORN)

Presentation Collodion baby is not a diagnosis of a particular type of ichthyosis, but may be due to X-linked ichthyosis, lamellar ichthyosis or bullous ichthyosis erythroderma. The condition is rare. It affects both sexes. Babies are born prematurely with erythema and translucent shiny skin which feels hard and rigid. There is ectropion and a cellophane like membrane, and distortion of the face. Several days later the membrane sheds in large scales. The skin may then become normal or take the form of the underlying ichthyosis.

Differential diagnosis   Harlequin babies are similar, but more severely affected.

Aetiology   This is due to the forms of ichthyosis mentioned above.

Treatment   All that is required is simple lubrication of the skin with an ointment such as soft paraffin, and prevention of secondary infection is advisable.

Prognosis   If the baby survives premature birth and subsequent difficulty in feeding, the skin peels after several days and the prognosis is then that of the underlying disease.

ICHTHYOSIS LINEARIS CIRCUMFLEXA

Presentation   Babies are red and scaly at birth or become so in the first few months. Later they develop numerous red, hyperkeratotic scaly lesions with polycyclic or serpiginous configuration and raised borders. These lesions are migratory. There is hyperkeratosis of the flexural areas such as the popliteal and antecubital fossae. The palms and soles are normal, but later develop hyperhidrosis. There is often an abnormality of the hair.

Differential diagnosis   This is mainly from lamellar ichthyosis and bullous ichthyosiform erythroderma.

Investigations   A biopsy shows parakeratosis and acanthosis. The granular layer may be accentuated and there is a mild perivascular infiltrate.

Aetiology   The disease is transmitted as an autosomal recessive.

Treatment   Mild keratolytic ointments may give some symptomatic relief. Oral aromatic retinoids have been reported to be helpful.

Prognosis   The skin lesions may improve at puberty, but do not clear completely.

ACQUIRED ICHTHYOSIS

A type of ichthyosis which occurs due to certain underlying diseases or drugs. It affects either sex and may develop at any age, although it is more likely later in life, after early childhood.

Presentation The clinical manifestation of the disease is similar to ichthyosis vulgaris. The skin is dry with cracking and hyperkeratosis of the palms and soles.

Differential diagnosis It may be distinguished from ichthyosis vulgaris by its later onset, lack of family history and underlying disease. Patients suspected of acquired ichthyosis must be thoroughly examined and investigated to determine the cause, which may be as follows:

Malignant disease In Hodgkin's disease, ichthyosis may appear after the disease is established, or as the first symptom. Ichthyosis may also appear in other reticuloses, carcinoma and mycosis fungoides;

Metabolic and internal diseases e.g. malnutrition, liver damage and malabsorption;

Drugs e.g. drugs which cause malabsorption and nicotinic acid;

Infection Leprosy.

Treatment Treatment is that of the underlying disorder. Ten per cent topical urea cream gives symptomatic relief.

23 LICHEN PLANUS

Presentation Lichen planus affects all races. It accounts for nearly 1% of new cases in UK skin clinics. It occurs at any age, but is rare in childhood and the peak incidence is in the young and middle aged adults (Figure 23.1). Males and females are equally affected.

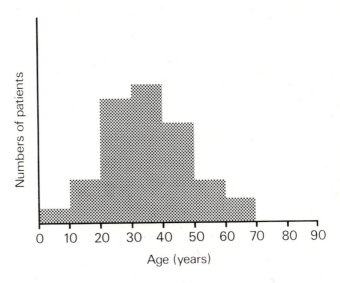

Figure 23.1   Age incidence of lichen planus

The typical skin lesions are characterized by small symmetrical shiny flat-topped violaceous papules (Figure 23.2), which are usually discrete, but may become confluent and form plaques. Occasionally there are white streaks over the papules (Wickham's striae) and there may be a central depression on the surface. The commonest sites of

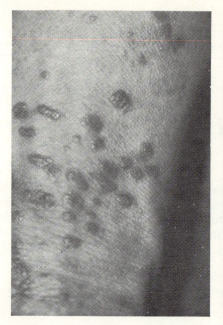

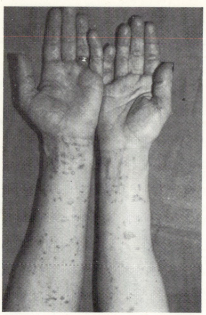

Figure 23.2 Shiny topped flat papules on the wrist in lichen planus

Figure 23.3 Lichen planus papules on a common site of involvement, the wrists and flexor surface of the forearms

predilection are the flexor aspects of the wrists and forearms (Figure 23.3), lumbar region and ankles. However any part of the body can be affected, including the scalp, nails, and mucous membranes. Lichen planus is usually associated with irritation.

Lichen planus may arise at the sites of trauma, e.g. excoriations, where the lesions have a linear configuration (the Koebner phenomenon). On the palms and soles the disorder is often confluent and presents as hyperkeratotic plaques. On the legs the lesions are larger than the papules elsewhere, and have a hyperkeratotic surface. This type of lesion is sometimes referred to as hypertrophic lichen planus, and varies from a few mm to a few cm, and the lesions may be solitary.

Nail involvement is uncommon, but when present takes the form of longitudinal ridging and in severe forms the nails are destroyed by pterygium formation. On the scalp lichen planus causes scarring alopecia due to destruction of the hair follicles. The

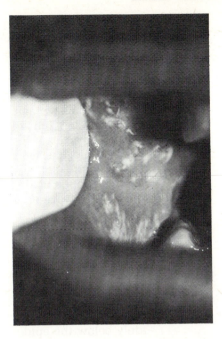

Figure 23.4 White papules and streaks on the buccal mucosa in lichen planus

skin of the scalp eventually has a smooth atrophic appearance and no follicles are visible.

Mucous membrane involvement is common and the lesions have a characteristic appearance. On the buccal mucosa, tongue, lips, vulva and vagina the lesions present as white streaks or papules (Figure 23.4) and there may be erosions. On the glans penis the lesions have an annular configuration. Mucous membrane involvement may occur without cutaneous lesions.

Occasionally lichen planus lesions may give rise to bullae. A rare form of lichen planus is seen when the disease is limited to the hair follicles, giving rise to a follicular eruption.

Differential diagnosis Hypertrophic lichen planus must be distinguished from lichenified eczema on the legs, and unless there are features of lichen planus elsewhere it may be difficult to distinguish between the two disorders.

Lichenoid drug eruptions often have a similar

appearance to lichen planus and the correct diagnosis is made by obtaining a history of taking a drug which causes a lichenoid eruption. Psoriasis, particularly the guttate variety, may mimic widespread lichen planus, but psoriasis is more erythematous in colour and silvery scales are usually present.

The papulo-squamous type of rash in secondary syphilis is non-itchy and shows a predilection for the palms and soles. If there is any doubt about the diagnosis serological tests must be performed.

The white streaks on the buccal mucosa and tongue must be distinguished from *Candida albicans* infection. Severe erosions may mimic pemphigus.

Investigations The diagnosis is usually made on the typical lesions of lichen planus but if there is doubt a biopsy should be performed. This shows mild hyperkeratosis, slight thickening of the granular layer, increase of the prickle cell layer with a saw tooth arrangement of the rete pegs, basal cell liquefaction degeneration and band-like mononuclear cell infiltration immediately below the epidermis.

Aetiology The cause of the disease is unknown; viruses, bacteria, and other infective organisms have been postulated but not proven. An auto-immune aetiology of the disease has also been suggested.

Certain drugs may provoke lichen planus-type lesions, e.g. antimalarial drugs, particularly mepacrine or the antituberculosis drugs, p-amino salicylic acid and isoniazid, and heavy metals, e.g. gold and organic arsenic.

Treatment In very mild cases no treatment is required. When there is irritation potent topical steroids are helpful. In hypertrophic and resistant patches potent topical steroid ointments under polythene occlusion at night can be used for 2–3 weeks.

Intralesional steroids (e.g. triamcinolone) are very effective in hypertrophic lesions. If the condition is widespread systemic steroids, in the form of prednisone, 30 mg daily for two weeks, clear the lesions. However, the recurrence rate after withdrawal of the steroids is high, and a maintenance dose may be required until the disease goes into remission. Mucosal lesions which do not give rise to symptoms do not require treatment. Topical steroids in orabase and ß-methasone, 17-valerate mouth pellets or aerosols are helpful. If the lesions are severe and ulcerated, systemic steroids will control the lesions.

Prognosis   The course is variable. In most patients the rash clears spontaneously without scarring, but there may be residual post inflammatory hyperpigmentation which takes some months to disappear. Involvement of the scalp produces scarring alopecia which is permanent. If nail involvement is severe there is permanent nail loss. The mucous membrane lesions if persistent may rarely progress to leukoplakia and carcinoma.

The average duration for spontaneous recovery is approximately six months, although the hypertrophic lesions may last for a few years. It is rare for lichen planus to recur after it has cleared.

24 LICHEN SCLEROSIS AND ATROPHICUS

Lichen sclerosis and atrophicus is a rare condition. Sometimes it is found in association with morphoea (see Chapter 28).

Presentation Although it can commence at any age, it does so in prepubertal girls, or, most commonly, women around the menopause (40–60 years) (Figure 24.1). Women are chiefly affected, the female : male ratio is 10 : 1 (Figure 24.2). All races are affected, but it is less common in negroes.

The lesions may be predominantly extragenital or anogenital in location. The latter are more common.

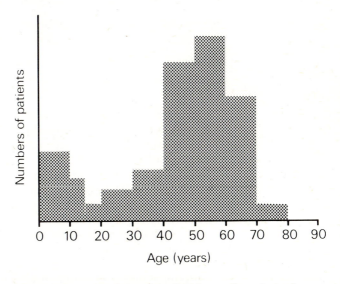

Figure 24.1 Age of onset of lichen sclerosis and atrophicus

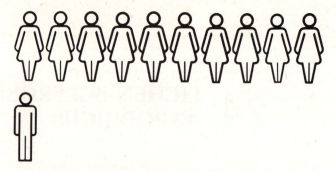

Figure 24.2   Sex ratio in lichen sclerosis and atrophicus is 10 female : 1 male

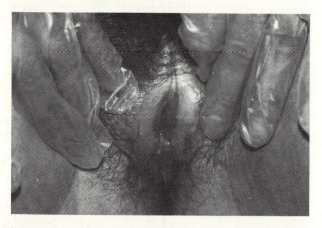

Figure 24.3   Lichen sclerosis and atrophicus of the vulva showing the typical shiny white appearance with a red margin

Extragenital lesions are most common on the upper trunk and wrists. Anogenital lesions surround the anus and involve the vulva (Figure 24.3), often in a figure of eight distribution; penile lesions are rare and are usually confined to the glans and prepuce, and cause phimosis. Extragenital lesions accompany the anogenital lesions in 30% of cases. The mouth is rarely involved.

There have been some familial cases.

The extragenital lesions commence as shiny white papules with follicular plugging, often with telangiectasis, purpura and a red margin. They may be bullae. Later they become white, atrophied and depressed (Figure 24.4). In dark people these

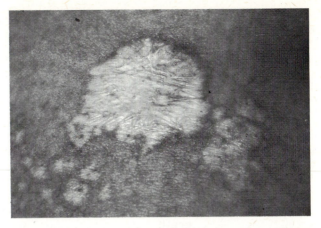

Figure 24.4 Extragenital lichen sclerosis and atrophicus, the lesions are white and atrophied with a red margin

may give rise to numerous small guttate depigmented areas.

The genital lesions are white and shiny with a red border (Figure 24.3). Telangiectasia, purpura and erosions from bullae are seen. The normal structures become atrophied and obliterated. There is dyspareunia and intense pruritus. Squamous carcinomas develop in 5% of patients with vulval lesions, and thickened white or ulcerated areas must be viewed with suspicion and biopsied.

There is an increased incidence of auto-immune disease in patients with lichen sclerosis and atrophicus, and in their families.

Differential diagnosis The presence of follicular plugging differentiates it from morphoea. In vitiligo the skin though white is otherwise normal. Genital lesions may cause confusion with *primary atrophy*, which lacks the shiny white appearance, and atrophic lichen planus; the presence of typical lesions elsewhere distinguishes the latter.

Diagnosis and investigations Skin biopsy will confirm the diagnosis, and in the vulva area must be performed on suspicious areas so that the pre-malignant and malignant change is detected early.

Aetiology The cause is unknown; local factors are important as transplanted skin takes on the character of the local skin. Hormonal factors are important as shown by its relationship to the menarche and menopause; oestrogens and progesterones seem to protect. An increased incidence of auto-immune disease suggests that disordered immunity may be involved.

Treatment   There is no effective treatment. Potent topical steroids alleviate the pruritus of genital lichen sclerosis and atrophicus. It is hoped that by reducing scratching and trauma the incidence of squamous carcinoma may be reduced. Close supervision for early detection of carcinoma is essential. Vulvectomy is necessary if squamous carcinoma develops. The lichen sclerosis and atrophicus often recurs in the graft.

Natural history and prognosis   The childhood cases often remit with puberty, but about one third persist throughout life. Most adult cases do not remit. The extragenital lesions cause purely cosmetic problems, but the vulval lesions have a poorer prognosis because of the development of carcinoma.

25 LUPUS ERYTHEMATOSUS

The term lupus erythematosus encompasses a wide spectrum of diseases. They range from the localized purely cutaneous discoid lupus erythematosus (discoid LE) to systemic lupus erythematosus (SLE) with multi-system involvement. The relationship between the two is not clear. Some patients have a transitional clinical picture.

DISCOID LUPUS ERYTHEMATOSUS

This is the cutaneous form.

Presentation   Discoid lupus erythematosus usually presents in adults; any age can be affected, but most present in

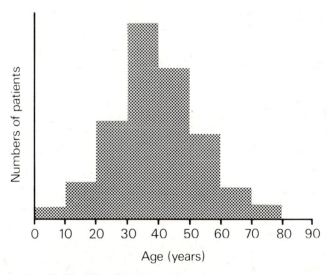

Figure 25.1   Age of onset of discoid LE

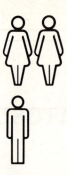

Figure 25.2   Sex ratio of discoid LE

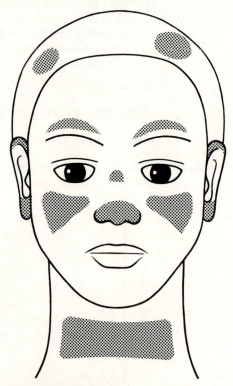

Figure 25.3   Distribution of discoid LE on the face

their late thirties (Figure 25.1). Females outnumber males 2 : 1 (Figure 25.2). It occurs in all races.

It is located chiefly on the light exposed areas. The face is most often involved, particularly the

cheeks, and there may be a butterfly distribution
(Figure 25.3). The nose, ears, scalp, the backs of the
fingers and hands and arms are also typical sites.
The V of the neck is the commonest site on the trunk
(Figure 25.4). Occasionally there are lesions in the
mouth and vagina.

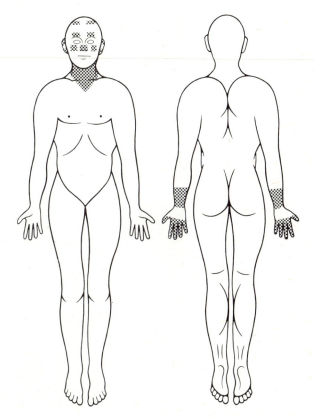

Figure 25.4   Distribution of discoid LE on the body

The lesions can be single or multiple. They vary in
size from one to many centimetres.

The early lesion is a raised red plaque. There may
be a brownish scale. Follicular plugging with keratin
is a prominent feature (Figure 25.5). The lesions
heal from the centre. There is a red advancing edge.
The centre is atrophied, with telangiectasia and thin
skin; it is usually hypopigmented (Figures 25.5, 25.6
and 25.7), although there may also be hyperpigmentation particularly in negroes (Figure 25.7).

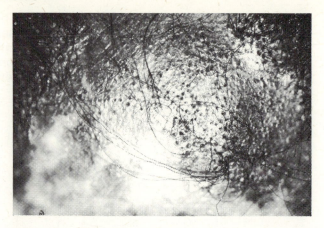

Figure 25.5   Discoid LE on the scalp: there is marked follicular plugging, hypopigmentation and scarring alopecia

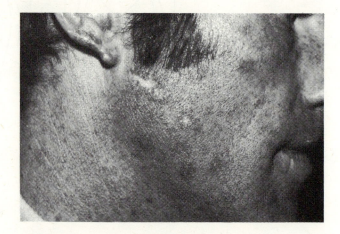

Figure 25.6   Discoid LE on the ear and cheek: the centre of the lesion is white and atrophic with telangiectasia; there is a red scaly advancing edge

Depressed scars may be formed. The scalp lesions heal with scarring and permanent hair loss (Figure 25.5). The mucous membrane lesions are well defined red erosions.

The lesions may itch. Sunlight may precipitate or exacerbate discoid lupus erythematosus. Premenstrual flares occur.

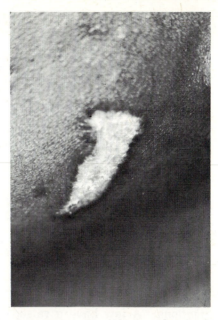

Figure 25.7   Discoid LE on the cheek of a negro: erythema, atrophy and hypopigmentation are prominent. The border is hyperpigmented and there is adjacent hyperpigmentation from a lesion that has resolved

Differential diagnosis

The early plaques closely resemble sarcoid, or other granulomata, and scaly lesions may resemble solar keratoses.

Discoid lupus erythematosus may closely resemble systemic lupus erythematosus (SLE).

The cicatrical alopecia may be difficult to distinguish from lichen planus.

Diagnosis and investigation
Skin biopsy

A skin biopsy from the lesions is necessary to confirm the diagnosis. The histology is characteristic. There is liquefaction of the basal layer of the epidermis, thickening of the basement membrane, a lymphocytic dermal infiltrate and follicular plugging.

Direct immunofluorescence of the lesion shows immunoglobulin and C_3 deposits in a lumpy band at the dermo–epidermal junction (the LE pattern) (Figure 25.8). IgG, IgM and IgA may all be found. IgM is the most common. There are no deposits in the uninvolved skin.

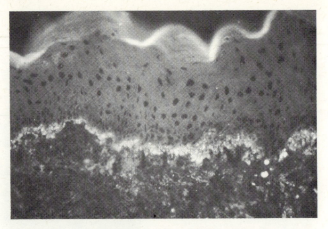

Figure 25.8 'LE band': immunofluorescent demonstration of IgM at the basement membrane region

Haematological investigations   Most patients have no abnormalities in their serum. A few have a raised ESR (20 mm/h), anaemia and leukopenia. The ANF may be positive (diffuse pattern), as may LE cells, WR and RA latex. DNA antibodies are not elevated.

Aetiology   It is thought that discoid lupus erythematosus represents an altered immune response to some unknown antigen.

A small proportion (5%) may develop SLE, and the two diseases may have the same aetiology, the host response determining the different features. However, this small group may be SLE, with DNA antibodies, from the start and there may be no crossover.

Treatment   Steroids are effective. The very potent topical steroids speed resolution and reduce scarring. Intralesional steroids are helpful. Small doses of systemic steroids (prednisone 5–10 mg daily) may suppress the lesions, but the necessity for very long term therapy restricts their use.

Antimalarials will completely suppress discoid lupus erythematosus. Chloroquine must be given for short periods only and with careful ophthalmic supervision as it can induce irreversible retinopathy. Mepacrine is not toxic to the eyes but some patients find the yellowing of the skin unacceptable.

Sunlight should be avoided (see Chapter 33: Photosensitivity).

Natural history and prognosis   The early lesions may resolve rapidly. Most are chronic, persisting for years, healing centrally and slowly advancing. The atrophy and pigmentary change can be very disfiguring.

Modern treatment has altered the prognosis considerably.

Squamous cell carcinoma develops in longstanding scars.

Five per cent develop manifestations of SLE. This group may have always been different from the onset.

GENERALIZED DISCOID LUPUS ERYTHEMATOSUS

Presentation   A small number of patients, mostly women, have generalized discoid lupus erythematosus.

The lesions are symmetrical on light exposed areas, with extension to covered areas. The face, upper chest, backs of hands and arms (Figure 25.9) are most commonly affected. The palms and soles more rarely. The scalp is often affected.

The skin is erythematous, atrophied and telangiectatic (Figure 25.9). Nail fold telangiectasia occur. Scalp involvement causes a diffuse or localized scarring alopecia.

Systemic symptoms of arthralgia and Raynaud's phenomenon may be present.

Differential diagnosis   SLE may be very difficult to distinguish clinically.

Diagnosis and investigations
Skin biopsy   This will show the characteristic histology of LE (see above). Direct immunofluorescence on the involved skin shows the 'LE pattern' (Figure 25.8). IgM predominates. The uninvolved skin may show the same pattern.

Blood tests   A moderately raised ESR (30–50 mm/h), anaemia, leukopenia, positive ANF (diffuse pattern) may be found. LE cells may be found. DNA antibodies are *negative*. Renal function is normal.

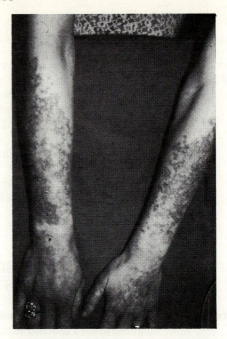

Figure 25.9   Generalized discoid LE: atrophy, erythema and scaling on the backs of the hands and arms

Treatment   Low dose systemic steroids, or the antimalarial Mepacrine, suppress the rash (see above, p. 223). Mepacrine is the drug of choice because of less serious side effects.

LUPUS PROFUNDUS

This is a rare variant of discoid lupus erythematosus.

Presentation   It occurs in young adults, and is more prevalent in women.

The cheeks, upper arms and trunk are mainly affected. The lesions consist of firm mobile nodules, typical skin changes of discoid lupus erythematosus may overlie them. They are tender. They resolve with scarring and atrophy of the dermis. The depressed scars are very disfiguring.

Differential diagnosis	The nodules require biopsy to distinguish them from panniculitis or sarcoid. The scars may resemble those from insulin injection atrophy.
Diagnosis and investigations *Biopsy*	A biopsy shows the histology of LE.
Investigations	The serological findings are similar to discoid lupus erythematosus.
Treatment	Intralesional or systemic steroids, or antimalarials may reduce activity of the disease.
Natural history and prognosis	This condition is persistent. It is very mutilating.

CHILBLAIN LUPUS ERYTHEMATOSUS

This is a rare subgroup of discoid lupus erythematosus.

Presentation	The patients are usually young women, with a history of poor circulation, chilblains and often discoid lupus erythematosus elsewhere.
	The fingers, toes, heels and calves are affected and rarely the nose and ears. The lesions are raised, and purple; there may be scaling and fissuring (Figure 25.10). They persist into warm weather. Occasionally an erythema multiforme like rash may be present.
Differential diagnosis	They are often dismissed by both patient and doctor as 'ordinary chilblains'. They are sometimes confused with lupus pernio of sarcoid.
Diagnosis and investigations *Skin biopsy*	A biopsy may show LE histology. Immunofluorescence of the lesions shows the LE pattern of immunoglobulins, especially IgM deposits (Figure 25.8).
Blood tests	The same abnormalities occur as in DLE; however the ANF is usually of the speckled pattern.
Therapy	There is a poor response to treatment. Systemic steroids and antimalarials help a few patients. Warmth is the most important factor.

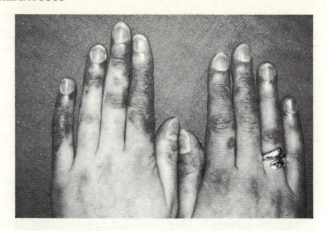

Figure 25.10 Chilblain lupus: persistent chilblains, erythema, scaling and discoid LE on the fingers

Natural history and prognosis

The chilblains persist indefinitely, despite remission of associated discoid lupus erythematosus lesions.

It is thought that a higher proportion progress to SLE than in uncomplicated discoid lupus erythematosus.

SYSTEMIC LUPUS ERYTHEMATOSUS (SLE)

This disease may affect all organs and systems.

Presentation

It can occur at any age but is commonest from the ages of 20–50. Females outnumber males 9 : 1

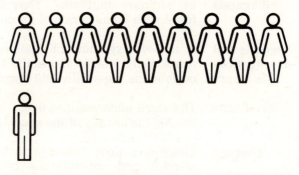

Figure 25.11   Sex ratio in SLE

(Figure 25.11). It occurs in all races but the incidence is highest in American negroes and West Indians, in whom as many as 1 in 250 may be affected.

Cutaneous manifestations   There may be marked photosensitivity. The rash may be confined to light exposed areas and precipitated or exacerbated by sunlight. Excessive sun exposure may also worsen systemic involvement.

The face   The skin of the face is often involved with erythema, induration, scaling and telangiectasia. This occurs on the bridge of the nose and cheeks forming the classical butterfly rash (Figure 25.12). Rarely discoid LE like lesions may occur.

The hands   The hands are affected in many ways. Erythema, telangiectasia and scaling may occur on the backs of the hands and thenar eminences. There may be periungual and knuckle erythema (Figure 25.13). Nail fold telangiectasia, infarcts (Figure 25.13) and splinter haemorrhages occur.

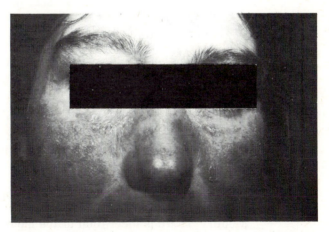

Figure 25.12   SLE: typical butterfly rash with erythema, scaling and telangiectasia

The fingers may be shiny and tapered. The finger pulps may show small infarcts from vasculitis or severe Raynaud's phenomenon.

The feet   The changes are similar to the hands.

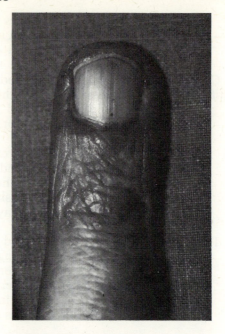

Figure 25.13 SLE: periungual and knuckle erythema and nail fold infarcts

The arms	Erythema and scaling occur on the elbows. Panniculitis, with deep red nodules that ulcerate, affects the upper arms.
The legs	A scaly erythema can affect the knees. Vasculitis causes leg ulceration, and livedo reticularis or purpura may occur. Panniculitis often involves the fat of the legs.
Scalp	Dry brittle hair and diffuse alopecia are common.
Mouth	There is ulceration of the mouth.
Urticaria	The transient itchy weals of urticaria affect 15% of SLE patients.
General manifestations	Lassitude, malaise and fever are common. Splenomegaly and lymphadenopathy may be found.
Musculo-skeletal	Arthralgia and arthritis are frequent presenting symptoms. Deformities and erosions are rare. Myal-

gia, with severe pain, and myositis are common. It is said that 'the bark of SLE is worse than its bite', i.e. the pain is very severe but little structural damage occurs. Tendon contractures, particularly of the flexor tendons of the hands, are common. Avascular necrosis of bone occurs.

Renal
Fifty per cent of patients have renal involvement. This ranges from mild haematuria or proteinuria, to nephrotic syndrome, nephritis, hypertension or renal failure. Severe renal involvement is a major cause of death. Subclinical renal involvement may occur in the others.

Chest
Pleurisy is common. Diffusion defects are often demonstrable but asymptomatic. Chest X-ray may show basal atelectasis or raised diaphragms (the shrinking lung).

Central nervous system
The CNS manifestations are common and may be mild or life threatening. They include migrainous headache, nerve palsies, aseptic meningitis, fits and strokes. Psychiatric disturbances range from mild depression to psychosis.

Cardiovascular system
Pericarditis, myocarditis and the rare Libmann–Sachs endocarditis occur. Raynaud's phenomenon is a frequent symptom.

Haematological system
Anaemia is common; it may be due to bone marrow suppression by the disease or to auto-immune haemolysis. Leukopenia, lymphopenia and thrombocytopenia also occur.

Gastro-intestinal involvement
Gastro-intestinal involvement is rare. Ascites occurs and hepatitis may be induced by salicylates.

Pregnancy
There is a high rate of spontaneous abortion.

Drug induced lupus erythematosus
Certain drugs can cause a systemic lupus erythematosus-like syndrome: including hydralazine, procaine amide, griseofulvin, penicillin, reserpine, phenylbutazone and some oral contraceptives. This syndrome is very like true lupus, but renal and central nervous system involvement is rare. DNA antibodies are absent.

Penicillin and sulphonamides may precipitate or exacerbate true SLE.

Differential diagnosis

The butterfly rash may be confused with other photosensitive eruptions, rosacea and seborrhoeic eczema.

Generalized discoid LE may cause confusion.

Diagnosis and investigations

Skin biopsy

Histology of the rash may be helpful. Immunofluorescence of the involved skin and the uninvolved shows IgG and/or IgM, rarely IgA or C_3 deposits in a lumpy linear LE pattern (Figure 25.8).

Renal biopsy

This is often diagnostic. Electron microscopy may show immunoglobulin deposits.

Blood tests

A raised ESR, anaemia, and leukopenia are common. Coombs' test may be positive. LE cells are positive, ANF is positive in high titre, and DNA antibodies are postive. C_3 may be low, and this indicates renal damage. Lymphocytotoxic antibodies may be present.

Renal function tests

Should be performed.

Pulmonary function tests

Should be performed.

Aetiology

Family studies suggest a genetically determined predisposition to auto-immune disease. Animal studies suggest an abnormal reaction by an immunologically defective host to a slow virus.

Many of the symptoms and signs are explicable in terms of immune complex deposition and a vasculitis. The lymphocytotoxic antibodies cross react with brain and placental cells, and may be involved in central nervous system disease and the spontaneous abortions.

Treatment

Precipitating and exacerbating factors, e.g. sunlight, oral contraceptives, and certain antibiotics, can be identified in some patients and must be avoided.

Treatment should be conservative. Analgesics,

anti-inflammatory drugs, and antimalarials may be very helpful. Salicylates must be used cautiously because hepatitis can be induced. Steroids may be required for severe relapses, in combination with azathioprine or cyclophosphamide for renal disease. Low dose maintenance steroids may be required.

Natural history and prognosis   Ninety per cent survive five years. Those that do die, do so from fulminating renal or central nervous system disease.

It is characterized by relapses and long periods of remission. Many survive for decades.

26 METABOLIC DISORDERS AND THE SKIN

The cutaneous effects of the following metabolic disorders are discussed: amyloid (see page 17), diabetes mellitus, gout, hyperlipidaemias and porphyrias (see page 289).

DIABETES MELLITUS

Diabetes mellitus has several cutaneous manifestations and associations, and in addition renders the skin more susceptible to certain disorders. The most striking and common are listed below:

Infections *Staphylococcus aureus* skin infections (see page 345) and nasal carriage are common in diabetics. Pyogenic skin infections are a presentation of diabetics, and diabetes should always be sought in those with recurrent skin infections.

Candida infections (see page 149) are frequent in diabetics. Candidal vulvovaginitis and associated pruritus vulvae, or balanitis may be presenting symptoms of diabetes. Oral and intertriginous candida are less common. Chronic candida paronychia reflect the vascular damage of diabetes, and are common in both non-diabetics and diabetics.

Vascular disease The severe vascular disease of diabetics has cutaneous signs.

Chronic ischaemia causes changes in the skin of the feet, lower legs and nails. The skin becomes thin and hairless and has poor healing; the nails become brittle, ridged and discoloured. Acute ischaemia causes arterial ulcers on the legs, ischaemic infarction and gangrene of the toes.

Neurotrophic ulcers Diabetic peripheral neuropathy causes neurotrophic ulcers on the soles of the feet from unperceived and neglected trauma. The susceptibility to infection and ischaemia further compound the problem.

Diabetic dermopathy The small blood vessel disease of diabetes is thought to be the cause of diabetic dermopathy. The lower shins are the site of this eruption. Small red papules form and resolve leaving brown atrophic scars.

Necrobiosis lipoidica Necrobiosis lipoidica (Figure 26.1) occurs in less than 1% of diabetics. It may precede the diabetes by many years, or the diabetes may be detected only by

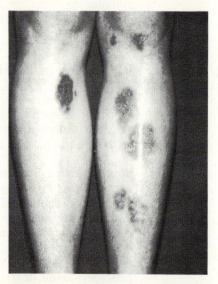

Figure 26.1 Necrobiosis lipoidica: shiny yellow telangiectatic plaques on the front of the shins

a glucose tolerance test with carbohydrate or steroid provocation. There is no relation of extent of necrobiosis to duration, severity or control of diabetes.

Small vessel disease has been suggested as the cause.

Granuloma annulare Granuloma annulare, particularly if generalized, may be associated with diabetes (Figure 26.2).

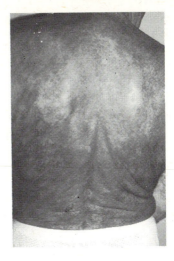

Figure 26.2   Generalized granuloma annulare in a diabetic

Bullous disease of diabetics   Large, tense bullae are occasionally found on the hands and feet of diabetics. The blisters are subepidermal.

Xanthomata   The hypertriglyceridaemia and chylomicronaemia that may arise in diabetes can cause eruptive xanthoma (Figure 26.3).

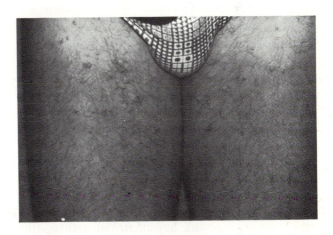

Figure 26.3   Eruptive xanthomata

Acanthosis nigricans Diabetes that is symptomatic of pituitary or adrenal dysfunction may be accompanied by acanthosis nigricans (see page 1). The obesity that is often seen in diabetics may cause pseudo-acanthosis nigricans (see page 2).

Lipo-atrophy There is a rare form of familial diabetes associated with generalized lipo-atrophy.

Lipo-atrophy at the site of insulin injections is common.

GOUT (HYPERURICAEMIA)

Gout is the clinical disease associated with hyperuricaemia; there are joint, skin and renal manifestations.

Presentation Men present between 30 and 60, women later, after the menopause. Men more commonly have clinical disease. It is inherited as a dominant gene, but can also be secondary to other diseases or therapy: genetic, thiazide diuretics, starvation and myeloproliferative disorders.

Cutaneous signs The ears, hands and extensor surfaces of the hand and limb joints are involved, the nodules are related to peri-articular structures, e.g. bursa and tendon sheaths. The lesions are large nodules, with tight, shiny skin overlying and fixed to them (Figure 26.4). Occasionally they ulcerate and discharge.

Gouty tophi are rare in the absence of arthritis, and usually appear only in chronic gout with many recurrent attacks of arthritis. Tophi usually indicate renal involvement.

Hyperuricaemia is often associated with hyperlipidaemia, and xanthomata may be present.

Arthritis Gout usually affects one joint at a time, and causes an asymmetrical arthropathy. The big toe is most frequently involved.

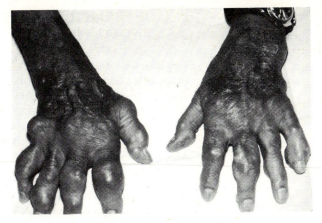

Figure 26.4   Gouty tophi on the hands

Renal disease   Hyperuricaemia causes nephropathy by deposition of uric acid in kidney. This causes proteinuria and renal failure.

High concentrations of uric acid in urine may form renal calculi. Renal colic can be a presenting symptom.

Differential diagnosis   Gouty tophi and arthritis may be confused with rheumatoid arthritis, or osteoarthritis with Heberden's nodes. The asymmetry of gout, and the location of the tophi, are diagnostic.

Diagnosis and investigations
Blood tests   Serum uric acid *must* be measured. Renal function should be assessed. A full blood count and film eliminate myeloproliferative disorders.

X-rays   Reveal characteristic joint changes.

Microscopy   Joint aspirate discharge from tophi show characteristic crystals.

Aetiology   Hyperuricaemia results from over production or accumulation of uric acid; these may be primary or secondary.

Treatment   Allopurinol lowers uric acid. Secondary hyperuricaemia should be treated by treating the cause.

Natural history   The renal problems of gout cause death from renal failure in a few patients.

THE HYPERLIPIDAEMIAS
(XANTHOMATOSIS)

The hyperlipidaemias are a group of serious systemic disorders that may present to the dermatologist with xanthomata. The hyperlipidaemias have been classified into six types on the basis of biochemical abnormality, and electrophoretic and ultracentrifugation analysis (see Table 26.1). There is a good but *not* absolute association between the types and the various kinds of xanthomata (Table 26.2). The types are not absolute; patients may change from one type to another, and more than one type may be present within a family.

Table 26.1   The types of hyperlipidaemias

Type	Biochemical abnormality	Electrophoretic abnormality	Ultracentrifugational abnormality	Cutaneous signs
I	Chylomicra	Chylomicra	Chylomicra	Eruptive xanthoma
II A	Cholesterol	ß-lipoprotein ↑	LDL ↑	Xanthelasma
II B	Cholesterol and triglycerides	ß-lipoprotein and pre-ß-lipoprotein ↑	LDL and VLDL ↑ }	Tuberous and tendinous xanthoma Corneal arcus
III	Abnormal triglycerides	Broad 'B' band	IDL ↑	Xanthoma palmaris Tuberous and tendinous xanthoma
IV	Triglycerides	Pre-ß-lipoprotein ↑	VLDL ↑	Eruptive xanthoma
V	Triglycerides and chylomicra	Pre-ß-lipoprotein and chylomicra ↑	VLDL ↑	Eruptive xanthoma

Key: LDL – low density lipoprotein
VLDL – very low density lipoprotein
IDL – intermediate density lipoprotein

Table 26.2   Xanthomata and their underlying types of lipidaemia

Xanthomata	Type
Eruptive xanthoma	I, IV or V
Xanthelasma	II
Palmar xanthomata	III
Tuberous and tendinous xanthomata	II or III

Presentation
Type I

This is the rarest of the hyperlipidaemias. It presents in the first 10 years of life. Both sexes are affected. The inheritance is an autosomal recessive. The biochemical abnormality is an excess of circulating chylomicra.

Skin lesions

Eruptive xanthomata are characteristic of this condition. They may be found anywhere on the skin and mucous membranes, but are usually found on the buttocks and extensor surfaces of the limbs. The xanthomata are small yellow papules, often with an erythematous base (Figure 26.3).

Visceral lesions

Abdominal pain and acute pancreatitis are common. Hepatosplenomegaly occurs.

Cardiovascular system

There is no increased incidence of cardiovascular disease.

This hyperlipidaemia is due to a lack of lipoprotein lipase.

Type II

There are two subgroups of Type II; Type II A characterized by increased cholesterol and Type II B in which cholesterol and triglycerides are raised. Many cases are familial and genetically determined. Some are secondary; causes of secondary hyperlipidaemias include alcoholism, diabetes mellitus, dysproteinaemias, hyperuricaemia, hypothyroidism and renal disease.

Homozygous cases present in childhood, the others in middle life. Men and women are both affected but men usually present earlier.

Skin lesions

Xanthelasma, symmetrical and affecting the upper and lower eyelids, are common. They are flat yellow plaques (Figure 26.5).

Tendinous xanthomata are soft yellow nodules overlying tendons.

Tuberous xanthomata are yellow nodules or polypoid lesions (Figure 26.6), commonly situated on knees, elbows, buttocks and heels. A corneal arcus may be present.

Cardiovascular system

There is a marked increase in coronary heart disease in patients with this disorder. Homozygotes usually die before 30. Xanthelasma are found in patients with normal lipids.

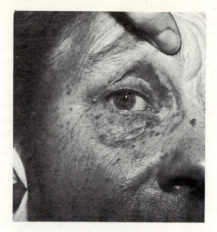

Figure 26.5   Xanthelasma

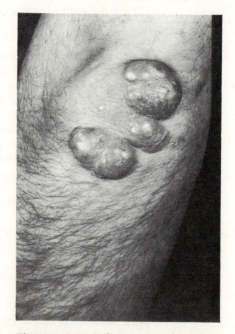

Figure 26.6   Tuberous xanthomata

Type III   This is a rare genetically determined hyperlipidaemia. There is an abnormal lipoprotein giving a broad
'B' band on electrophoresis.
    It presents in adult life, both sexes are affected.

Skin lesions	Palmar xanthomata are characteristic; there are linear yellow xanthomata in the palmar creases. Tuberous and tendinous xanthomata (Figure 26.6) may also be present.
Cardiovascular system	There is a high incidence of peripheral vascular disease.

Type IV   This is a common hyperlipidaemia. There is excess triglyceride in the blood. It is often a secondary phenomenom, as in Type II.
It usually presents in middle age.

Skin lesions	Eruptive xanthomata (Figure 26.3) are the characteristic skin lesions.
Cardiovascular system	Coronary heart disease and peripheral vascular disease are both common.

Type V
Skin lesions   Eruptive xanthomata (Figure 26.3) are characteristic.

Visceral lesions   Attacks of acute pancreatitis are common.

Cardiovascular system   Coronary heart disease and peripheral vascular disease are common.

Differential diagnosis   Eruptive xanthomata may be confused with papular sarcoid or lichen planus, but their yellow colour is distinctive.
Tuberous and tendinous xanthomata are differentiated from rheumatoid or sarcoid nodules by their yellow colour.

Diagnosis and investigations   Lipid studies including electrophoretic or ultracentrifugational studies are essential. A glucose tolerance test, protein electrophoresis, urea, urate and thyroid function studies should be performed to discover any cause for the hyperlipidaemia.

Aetiology   The precise enzyme defect is not known in most cases.
Xanthomata are localized deposits of lipids, but the reason for their deposition is not known.

Treatment   Treatment of hyperlipidaemias should be done by an expert. Dietary manipulation often in combination with drugs e.g. clofibrate cholestyramine, nicotinic acid and sex hormones, can return the lipids to normal. Xanthomata respond well to lowering lipids.

Xanthelasma can be destroyed by chemicals or cauterization. Excision is also satisfactory.

Natural history and prognosis All except Type I have a decreased life expectancy from cardiovascular disease.

27 MIXED CONNECTIVE TISSUE DISEASE

Presentation This is an overlap syndrome, with features of SLE, scleroderma and myositis.

It commences between 30 and 40 but usually presents much later. Women are much more commonly affected than men.

Cutaneous manifestations The fingers are usually swollen with tight shiny skin; There may be nail fold and finger pulp infarcts (Figure 27.1). Severe Raynaud's phenomenon is common.

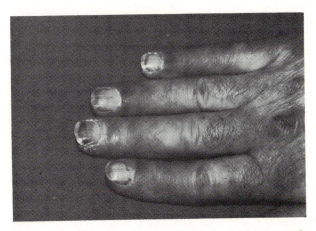

Figure 27.1 Hands of patient with mixed connective tissue disease; the fingers are swollen and there are nail fold infarcts

The skin elsewhere may be thickened and immobile as in scleroderma.

Vasculitis may occur, giving rise to tender red nodules and ulcers.

Other systems	Arthritis and myositis are common. Pulmonary and oesophageal involvement occurs. Renal involvement is rare.
Differential diagnosis	It may be difficult to distinguish this syndrome clinically from SLE or scleroderma.
Diagnosis and investigations *Skin biopsy*	Immunofluorescence may show on LE band of IgM.
Blood tests	ANF is often positive (speckled pattern). ENA antibodies and nRNP (nucleic ribonucleic acid protein) antibodies are positive. DNA antibodies are not raised.
Treatment	There is a good response to systemic steroids.
Natural history and prognosis	This disease is persistent but because of the lack of renal involvement death is rare.

28 MORPHOEA

Morphoea is also known as circumscribed scleroderma, though its relationship, if any, to scleroderma (see Chapter 44) is very poorly defined. There have been occasional reports of patients with morphoea and scleroderma. Lichen sclerosis and atrophicus may also coexist with morphoea (see Chapter 24).

Presentation Morphoea presents in early childhood or else chiefly between 20 and 40. It can commence at any age. Females are affected three times more commonly than men (Figure 28.1). It occurs in all races but in contradistinction to scleroderma is less common in Negroes.

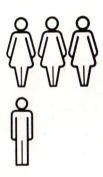

Figure 28.1   Sex ratio

There are four major types:

Plaque morphoea This occurs on the trunk and limbs, the intertriginous areas are usually spared. The lesions are plaques or bands. They may be single or multiple.

They are initially purple in colour, and then cream, thick and shiny (Figure 28.2), often with an active purple halo. The hairs are lost and follicular orifices become prominent. There may be purpura and bullae. The plaques are attached to the deep tissues. They resolve often with residual hyperpigmentation.

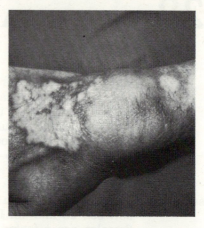

Figure 28.2   Morphoea: the cream plaque is surrounded by a halo

Linear morphoea   Linear morphoea is commonest in childhood. A single limb, particularly a leg, is affected most frequently, sometimes the trunk. The lesion extends along the length of the limb. The lesions are pale and

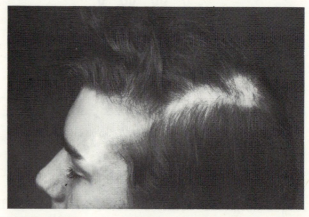

Figure 28.3   En coup de sabre of the forehead and scalp. The skin is pale and there is hair loss.

waxy with a purplish advancing edge. They involve the underlying muscle and bone. Atrophy, severe shortening and contractures may arise. Sometimes amputation is necessary.

'En coup de sabre'   This is the colourful descriptive name given to fronto-parietal morphoea, likening it to a sabre cut. The lesion commences in the scalp and extends down across the forehead (Figure 28.3), and may traverse the cheek and jaw to the neck. The tongue is often involved. The skull may be indented. The first sign is a white hard hairless groove in the scalp, the edges may be hyperpigmented. It extends over the face, and there may be hemiatrophy of the face and tongue.

Generalized morphoea   This form of morphoea commences on the trunk and extends to head and limbs. Large plaques of typical morphoea, sometimes with scaling and brown in colour, appear and coalesce. Bullae may be a troublesome feature. Scarring alopecia occurs. Large plaques over joints result in contractures and flexion deformities. The limbs become atrophied. The patient may become increasingly immobile.

Differential diagnosis   Lichen sclerosis and atrophicus (see page 213) is distinguished by follicular plugging and a red border. The diffuse skin changes of scleroderma do not have a distinct border.

Diagnosis and investigations

Skin biopsy   This shows the changes similar to scleroderma.

Blood tests   ANF is positive in a few cases of generalized mor-phoea.

Aetiology   The cause is unknown.

Treatment   Penicillamine has been reported to be helpful in a few cases particularly in the linear morphoea of childhood.

'En coup de sabre' morphoea may be helped by plastic surgery.

Natural history and prognosis   Plaque morphoea slowly resolves over a period of several years, leaving atrophy or hyperpigmentation in some cases.

'En coup de sabre' does not usually resolve.

Some cases of generalized morphoea progress inexorably until the patient is very disabled.

29 NECROBIOSIS LIPOIDICA

This was at one time thought to be a manifestation of diabetes, but this is not so in all cases.

Presentation Young and middle aged adults are chiefly affected; those patients without diabetes tend to be older. Women outnumber men 3 : 1 (Figure 29.1).

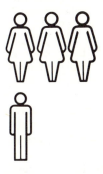

Figure 29.1   Sex ratio in necrobiosis lipoidica

The lesions are located chiefly on the front of the shins (Figure 29.2), but sometimes elsewhere on the legs; lesions may also be present elsewhere on the body. They are often symmetrical. The majority of these cases are associated with diabetes, and others will develop it. Atypical necrobiosis lipoidica is situated on the face or scalp and not usually associated with diabetes. It is usually a single plaque.

The lesions are plaques with a raised red margin and a shiny, yellow, atrophied centre, often with telangiectasia (Figure 29.2). The lesions can ulcerate. The facial lesions are less atrophic.

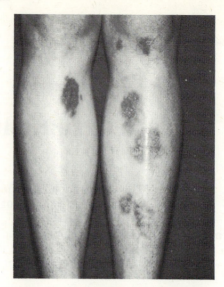

**Figure 29.2 Necrobiosis lipoidica:
the shiny yellow telangiectatic plaques
on the fronts of the shins are typical**

Differential diagnosis Granuloma annulare and annular sarcoid may cause confusion, but necrobiosis is distinguished by yellow atrophied centre and telangiectasia.

Diagnosis and investigations Skin biopsy confirms the diagnosis.
  Glycosuria should be sought, and a glucose tolerance test performed if there is evidence of diabetes.

Aetiology It is thought that the microvascular changes of diabetes may be important in initiating necrobiosis.

Treatment Intralesional steroids are rarely helpful. Skin grafting may be necessary for ulcerated lesions.
  Good control of the diabetes makes no difference.

Natural history and prognosis The lesions usually slowly enlarge. Sometimes they remit.

30 PARASITOPHOBIA (DELUSIONS OF PARASITOSIS)

Presentation The condition is a delusion of infestation of the skin by parasites. The condition is three times more common in women (Figure 30.1). It is a disorder of the middle aged and elderly (Figure 30.2). The patient

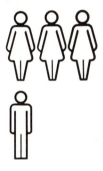

Figure 30.1 Delusions of parasitosis are three times as common in females

does not complain of irritation but of insects biting and crawling into the skin. The patient will bring with them scales from the skin which they claim are fragments of insects they have in or on the skin. Frequently excoriations are found on the skin but otherwise no other skin lesions are present. The history suggests the diagnosis.

Diagnosis The most obvious differential diagnosis is the patient who is genuinely being bitten by insects. However, in this instance papular urticarial lesions are usually seen, and the patient does not bring a collection of scales to the doctor.

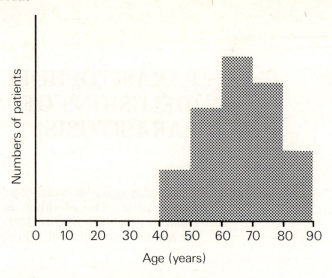

Figure 30.2   Age incidence of parasitosis

Investigations   The patient's delusions are sometimes due to organic disease or a deficiency state, and a full blood count, and if necessary serum B12 levels, performed. Vitamin B12 deficiency in the elderly may present as a delusional state.

Aetiology   The disorder is either a psychiatric one or occasionally due to a deficiency state or toxic confusional state.

Treatment   A full medical examination and screening tests for deficiency states should be carried out. If no abnormality is found, psychiatric assessment is necessary.

Natural history and prognosis   Often despite psychiatric help the condition persists for many years.

31 PEMPHIGOID

Presentation Pemphigoid is a disease of the elderly, the majority of patients being over the age of 60 (Figure 31.1). Females are more commonly affected than males, the ratio being approximately 2 : 1 (Figure 31.2).

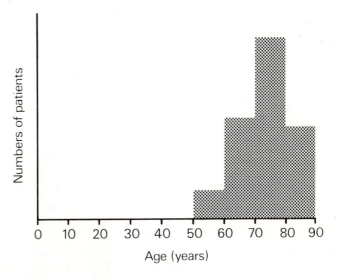

Figure 31.1 Age of onset of pemphigoid

Pemphigoid frequently begins on the limbs, but the trunk is invariably affected after a few days. In the majority of patients the disease is widespread and symmetrical, but occasionally the disease is localized to small areas such as the lower legs. The face and scalp are not commonly affected, nor are the mucous membranes.

Pemphigoid is one of the so-called bullous disorders, but prior to the blisters the rash may present

253

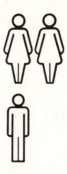

Figure 31.2 Pemphigoid is more common in women (2 : 1)

as urticarial or red, scaly lesions and there is often quite severe irritation. Blisters usually appear within a few days or weeks. The blisters tend to be large (1–2 cm in diameter), and tense, and do not rupture easily, and therefore tend to be persistent. When the blisters appear they are usually on an urticarial base and large plaques of urticaria may be present (Figure 31.3).

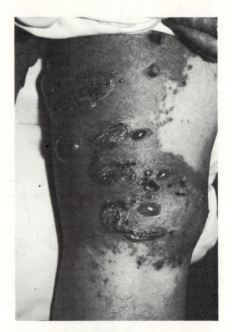

Figure 31.3 Blisters on an erythematous urticarial base in pemphigoid

Differential diagnosis Pemphigoid has to be distinguished from other diseases which may present with blisters. In pemphigus, the blisters are more superficial and rupture easily, and are not found on an urticarial base, but the surrounding skin has a normal appearance. Oral lesions are common in pemphigus, but rare in pemphigoid. Erythema multiforme in the elderly may be difficult to distinguish from pemphigoid. Erythema multiforme is usually less extensive than pemphigoid, and is frequently localized to the distal part of the limbs. Target lesions may be present in erythema multiforme but not in pemphigoid. Occasionally dermatitis herpetiformis becomes generalized and large blisters may be present; in these patients the disease looks like pemphigoid. On clinical features of the eruption it may be impossible to distinguish between the two conditions. However, pemphigoid occurs in the elderly and dermatitis herpetiformis usually begins in early or middle adult life. If doubt exists the diagnosis can only be made by response of the rash to dapsone and immunological findings. Drug eruptions may mimic pemphigoid, but once the drug is stopped the rash usually clears quickly.

Diagnosis and investigations The diagnosis of pemphigoid is confirmed by a skin biopsy and immunological tests which show the binding of antibody to the basement membrane in the skin, and a circulating antibody to basement membrane in the serum.

Skin biopsy Ideally an intact blister should be excised. If no small blisters are present then the biopsy should be taken through the edge of a blister, but biopsy should include the skin surrounding the blister. Histologically the blister in pemphigoid is subepidermal, the primary site of pathology being the basement membrane region.

Immunological studies A biopsy from the edge of a blister extending into the surrounding urticarial skin should be taken; the actual blister is of no use for these tests. Using immunofluorescence, IgG and C_3 complement are found in the region of the basement membrane (Figure 31.4). In approximately 75% of patients a circulating antibody of IgG class to the basement membrane is detectable in the serum.

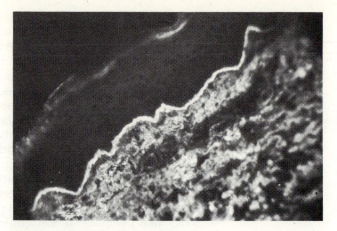

Figure 31.4   IgG deposits along the line of the basement membrane in pemphigoid

Aetiology   Pemphigoid is now considered to be an auto-immune disease, the antibody being directed against the basement membrane of the skin. However, like a number of other auto-immune disorders, there is some argument whether the antibodies are of primary significance or secondary to tissue damage.

Treatment   The treatment of pemphigoid is with oral cortico-steroids. The initial dose is equivalent to 80 mg of prednisone daily. Once the disease is under control and no new lesions are appearing, the dose of pred-nisone is gradually reduced. Most patients will require a maintenance dose of prednisone which usually varies from 5 to 20 mg daily. There is now reasonable evidence that a lower dose of cortico-steroid can be obtained for maintenance treatment by using other immunosuppressive drugs in addition to corticosteroids. The drug most widely used is aza-thioprine in a dose of 100–200 mg daily. Patients will be required to be followed up in a skin depart-ment, and the dose of their drugs altered according to the state of the disease.

Prognosis   Prior to corticosteroids the prognosis of pemphigoid was very much better than that of pemphigus; only in one-third of patients could death be attributed to the disease. Untreated pemphigoid is a chronic disease, but even before corticosteroids, spontan-eous remissions were reported, but usually only after two years. The incidence of complete remission (not requiring maintenance treatment) is now approximately one-third, and this remission may occur after a few months or a few years. Most other patients have the disease easily controlled with small doses of corticosteroids and azathioprine. A small proportion will die from the side effects of corticosteroids and immunosuppression.

BENIGN MUCOUS MEMBRANE PEMPHIGOID

This disease is so called because firstly it does not severely affect general health, and even before the days of corticosteroids did not prove fatal, and mucous membranes or areas of skin close to mucous membranes are affected.

Presentation   Benign mucous membrane pemphigoid is a disease of the elderly: the majority of patients are over 60 years, when the disease first begins (Figure 31.5). The disorder is more common in females, the ratio of female to male being 2 : 1 (Figure 31.6).

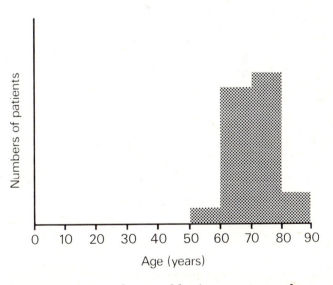

Figure 31.5   Age of onset of benign mucous membrane pemphigoid

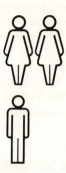

Figure 31.6 Benign mucous membrane pemphigoid is more common in females (2 : 1)

The mucous membranes affected are the conjunctivae, oral cavity, nose, throat, upper oesophagus, genital organs and anus. The mouth and conjunctivae are the commonest mucous membranes to be affected. When the skin is involved it is usually close to mucous membranes, but not necessarily adjacent. The scalp is a common site to be affected.

In approximately half the patients, only the mucous membranes are affected. Very occasionally the skin may be affected without involvement of the mucous membranes. The lesions of mucous membrane pemphigoid, whether involving the mucosae or skin, cause scarring of the affected tissues.

In the mouth the initial lesions are small blisters, which eventually rupture and give rise to superficial ulcers. These ulcers are slow to heal, but usually are not painful. Healing eventually does occur and is often associated with scarring. In the mouth the scars are usually of no significance, but in the oesophagus strictures may form. Conjunctival involvement usually begins as a mild conjuctivitis which in itself is of little trouble. However, scarring will eventually occur, although the process is slow and may take a number of years. The commonest lesions are adhesions between the bulbar and palpebral conjunctiva (Figure 31.7). In the more severe forms the cornea is involved and scarring at this site will lead to impairment of vision.

The skin lesions may appear as blisters which are tense and usually 1–2 cm in diameter. The second type of skin lesion is red plaques which show superficial ulceration and eventually scarring. If this

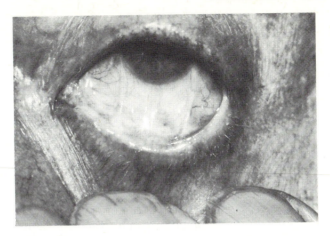

Figure 31.7   Scarring of the conjunctiva in mucous membrane pemphigoid

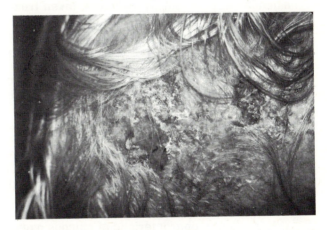

Figure 31.8   Erosion and hair loss due to scarring in mucous membrane pemphigoid

occurs in the scalp it will lead to permanent hair loss (Figure 31.8).

Differential diagnosis   The oral lesions have to be distinguished from other causes of chronic mouth ulceration, such as pemphigus, erosive lichen planus, severe and recurrent aphthous ulcers and Behcet's disease. In pemphigus the lesions are usually more painful, and there is no scarring when the ulcers heal. In lichen planus the white streaks characteristic of the disease may be seen elsewhere in the mouth. Chronic aphthous ulcers in the early stages usually have a yellow base. Behcet's disease usually occurs in younger persons and is characteristically associated with genital ulceration and iritis and uveitis. The skin lesions may sometimes resemble pemphigoid, but are usually less extensive.

Investigations Biopsies from the skin or mucosal lesions for routine histology and immunological studies should be performed to establish the diagnosis.

Biopsy Skin or mucous membrane should be biopsied. Ideally a blister should be excised for routine histological examination. Histology shows a subepidermal blister with inflammatory cells in the upper dermis.

Immunological studies A biopsy should be taken from the perilesional and involved skin or mucous membrane. Immunoglobulin deposits of IgA and IgG class are found in the region of the basement membrane. C_3 complement is also present. Unlike pemphigoid, the incidence of circulating antibodies to the basement membrane is low, being found only in 25% of patients.

Aetiology Benign mucous membrane disease is classified as an auto-immune disorder. The antibody is directed against the basement membrane region, and in that respect is similar to pemphigoid. However, the nature of the antigen would appear to be different to pemphigoid, for in the latter disease, the mucous membranes are only rarely involved, whilst it is a characteristic of mucous membrane pemphigoid.

Treatment Treatment is symptomatic and is not always required. If the skin lesions are present and extensive systemic steroids are required, the dose is considerably lower than in pemphigoid. The initial dose for control of the eruption is 30–40 mg prednisone daily. The dose is reduced as soon as skin lesions clear and a maintenance dose may be required until spontaneous remission occurs. In the localized plaque form of the disease potent topical steroids such as clobetasol propionate may heal the lesions.

The oral lesions if troublesome can be controlled by systemic steroids, often with relatively small doses; e.g. prednisone 5–10 mg daily. Local steroids in the form of betamethasone 17-valerate mouth pellets are helpful. However, if lesions are not particularly troublesome, no treatment is required. The ocular lesions should be treated by an ophthalmologist.

Prognosis   Benign mucous membrane pemphigoid is a chronic disease, lasting many years. There is often spontaneous remission of oral and skin lesions, but further bouts of activity of the disease may follow. The most serious complication is blindness from severe eye involvement but fortunately this is rare, occurring in less than 20% of patients. The only other complications which are serious, although rare, are oesophageal stricture and squamous cell carcinoma developing in the chronic oral lesions.

32 PEMPHIGUS AND HAILEY–HAILEY DISEASE

PEMPHIGUS

Presentation Pemphigus is a disease of adults; the commonest age of onset is in the fifth and sixth decades, but it may occur in younger and older age groups (Figure 32.1). There is a slightly higher incidence in females.

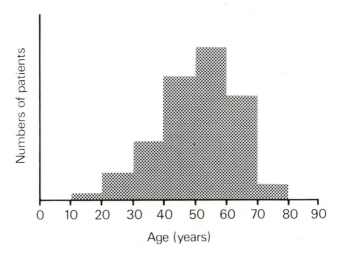

Figure 32.1 Age of onset of pemphigus

The skin lesions vary in pemphigus. The disease may present as red scaly patches, crusts, superficial erosions or blisters. It should be stressed that although pemphigus is often classed as one of the so-called bullous diseases, blisters are often not seen in pemphigus (Figure 32.2) and this leads to delay in the diagnosis. The lesions of pemphigus may occur on any part of the body and there is no particular site of predilection. In some patients there are only a few

263

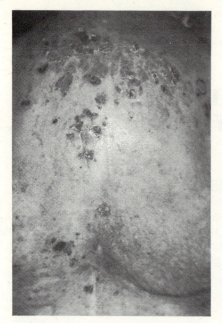

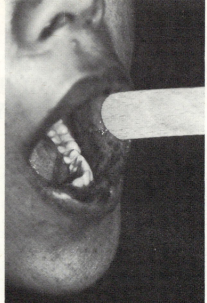

Figure 32.2 Erosions in pemphigus, the commonest type of lesion

Figure 32.3 Erosions in the mouth in pemphigus

lesions, whilst in others large areas of skin are affected by the disease.

Pemphigus affects mucous membranes as well as the skin. The commonest membrane affected is the oral cavity, and in one third the mouth is affected prior to the skin. Occasionally the disease may be confined to the oral cavity for a number of years and this may give rise to difficulty in diagnosis. On the mucous membranes the lesions present as painful erosions with a red base (Figure 32.3). They may vary from a few mm to large areas of a few cm, with total loss of the upper epithelial surface.

Differential diagnosis   Eczema may present as widespread, red, scaly patches. In eczema, however, patients usually complain of irritation. When blisters are present other bullous disorders have to be considered. Pemphigoid usually occurs in the elderly, and the blisters are tense and do not rupture easily as in pemphigus. Dermatitis herpetiformis is very irritating, and lesions occur predominantly on the elbows, knees and buttocks. Erythema multiforme is usually a symmetrical

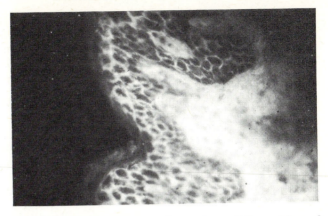

Figure 32.4 IgG bound to the surface of the epidermal cells in pemphigus

disorder, unlike pemphigus which shows no tendency to symmetry, and urticarial and so-called target lesions are usually present. Bullous eruptions due to drugs have also to be considered, but a careful history and stopping the suspected drug should substantiate the correct diagnosis. Severe and widespread impetigo may have similar lesions to pemphigus, i.e. blisters, erosions and crusts and hence the term pemphigus neonatorum is used in the older texts, when infants developed widespread impetigo.

If the lesions are confined to the mouth, then the other disorders that have to be considered are erosive lichen planus, Behcet's disease, and severe and persistent aphthosis.

Investigations The diagnosis of pemphigus is established by skin biopsy and detection of the pemphigus antibody in the skin and serum.

Skin biopsy Ideally a small, intact blister should be excised for histological examination. If none is present then an early lesion whatever its morphology should be taken. Histology will show an *intra-epidermal* blister, and so-called acantholysis, in which the epidermal cells drift apart from each other, and the space between them becomes filled with fluid.

Immunological studies A skin biopsy from the edge of a lesion should be taken and examined for the presence of IgG (by immunofluorescent techniques). The IgG in pemphigus is found bound to the surface of the epidermal cells (Figure 32.4). The pemphigus antibody is present in the serum in over 80% of patients, and is detected by indirect immunofluorescent techniques.

Aetiology Pemphigus is now considered to be an auto-immune disease. The auto-antibody is directed against the surface of the epidermal cells derived from the ectoderm. This results in loss of attachment of the cells from each other, and the cells drift apart and the architecture of the epidermis is destroyed. Pemphigus is sometimes associated with other auto-immune disorders.

Treatment The treatment of pemphigus is with systemic steroids. Unfortunately large doses of steroids, i.e. 100 mg of prednisone daily, are required in the initial stages. As soon as the disease shows signs of remission the dose of prednisone is gradually reduced. Most patients will require maintenance therapy to keep the disease process suppressed. The dose of steroid for maintenance varies from 5 to 40 mg daily.

Other immunosuppressive drugs, particularly methotrexate and azathioprine, have been used in the management of pemphigus, but their value has not been proven.

Prognosis Before the advent of corticosteroids, pemphigus was invariably fatal. The speed with which the disease killed the patient depended on the severity of the disease. The mortality is now below 25% and death is often due to complications of steroid therapy or the other immunosuppressive drugs used in the management of the disease. There is a high morbidity from steroid therapy, and this is directly related to the dose required for maintenance. In a number of patients the disease eventually goes into remission and all treatment can be stopped. In those patients who do go into complete remission it is usually later than two years after the onset of the disease.

HAILEY–HAILEY DISEASE (BENIGN FAMILIAL CHRONIC PEMPHIGUS)

This disease is not a variety of pemphigus, but is a rare, distinct clinical entity.

Presentation   The disease usually presents in early or middle adult life, and both sexes are equally affected. The common sites of involvement are the intertriginous areas, namely groins, axillae and under the breasts. A non-intertriginous area that may be affected is the neck (Figure 32.5). Small blisters may be present in the early stages but these soon break, giving rise to red, eroded areas, and crusts soon form. A typical feature is small linear cracks in the affected skin (Figure 32.6).

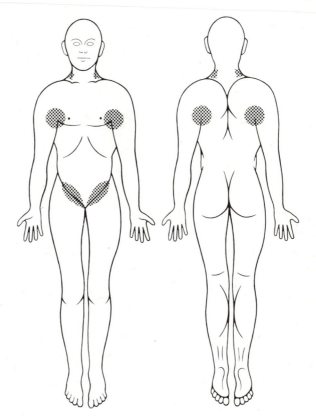

Figure 32.5   Common sites of Hailey–Hailey disease

Differential diagnosis   Other disorders which affect intertriginous areas have to be considered. These include seborrhoeic eczema, psoriasis, fungal and monilial infections. These infective disorders can be distinguished by the appropriate investigations, and psoriasis and seborrhoeic eczema respond well to treatment.

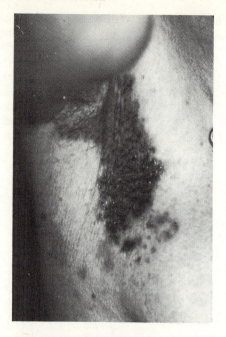

Figure 32.6 Erythematous eroded area in the axilla, with linear fissures in Hailey–Hailey disease

Investigations   A skin biopsy shows an intra-epidermal blister as seen in pemphigus. However, it is not so severe as in pemphigus. Acantholytic cells are also present. These are protrusions into the blisters by villi lined with a single layer of cells. Intercellular bridges are still present to some degree and some cell contact is frequently maintained. The tono filaments show abnormal configuration and this leads to abnormal keratinization. Pemphigus antibodies are not present. Bacteriological studies usually show staphylococci to be present.

Aetiology   The disorder is considered to be a genetic epidermal defect. However, although the gene responsible for the disease is thought to be dominant, only just over half the patients have a positive family history. The high incidence of bacteria and *Candida albicans* in the lesions has led to the suggestion that these organisms may in some way precipitate the lesions in susceptible individuals.

Treatment   This is directed against secondary bacterial infection and towards keeping the area as dry as possible. Astringent lotions such as magenta paint, or lint soaked in potassium permanganate solution 1 : 8000 are helpful. Topical antibiotic preparations containing neomycin should be used if the above lotions do not control the problem. If there is secondary infection with *Candida albicans* this should be treated with topical nystatin. There is some evidence that potent topical steroids may be helpful in addition to antibiotics.

If the condition is very troublesome and not responding to treatment the area may be excised and grafted.

Natural history and prognosis   The disease tends to be persistent, but long remissions may be induced by simple measures. The disorder tends to burn itself out and is less troublesome in old people.

33 PHOTOSENSITIVITY

An eruption on light exposed areas evoked by ultra violet radiation is termed a photosensitive eruption or photodermatosis. All human skin is sensitive to ultra violet radiation (UV), but in certain individuals or under certain conditions it becomes abnormally sensitive, being affected by low doses of radiation or wavelengths that are usually inactive.

The wavelengths evoking photosensitivity lie between 280 and 400 nm. The shorter wavelengths (280–320 nm) are termed UVB, and cause sunburn and carcinogenesis. Longer wavelengths (320–400 nm) are called UVA, and have little effect on normal skin, but are active on photosensitized skin. UVA passes through glass and light clothing. UVA and UVB are not perceived by the human eye. Visible light (wavelengths 400–800 nm) causes problems only in the very severely photosensitized.

The effects of sunlight on normal skin

UVA and UVB radiation have both acute and chronic effects on the epidermis, particularly the dividing cells and the blood vessels and connective tissue of the dermis. The extent of the effect depends on the amount of sunlight, determined by duration of exposure, latitude, season and time of day, and the degree of protective pigmentation of the individual.

The major effects of sunlight are described below:

Acute effects
Erythema

Sunlight causes an initial flushing or erythema that soon subsides. Several hours later there is a second prolonged erythema, due to vasodilation associated with blood vessel damage and inflammation secondary to cell damage and death.

Sunburn

Results from severe damage due to large doses of UVB in sunlight. There is cell death and damage in the epidermis, and blood vessel damage in the dermis. The delayed erythema is intensified and there is oedema and blistering. The skin is very painful. The dead cells are shed and the skin peels several days later. Topical steroids give symptomatic relief in severe cases of sunburn. Prostaglandins have been implicated as mediators of sunburn, and their inhibitors e.g. indomethacin should in theory ameliorate sunburn.

Thickening

Sunlight stimulates the epidermal cells to divide; this causes thickening of the epidermis, and provides a protective filtering of UV irradiation. This persists for several weeks. In people who do not tan this is the main form of protection from sunlight.

Tanning
Immediate
tanning

UVA causes immediate darkening of preformed melanin precursors; this results in tanning within minutes, the peak occurring within an hour and the colour slowly declining thereafter. UVA solariums cause this kind of tan.

Late tanning

UVB radiation causes late tanning. The melanocytes are stimulated to produce melanin, which is distributed to the epidermal cells. This commences about ten hours after exposure, and persists for weeks.

Immediate and late tanning both protect the skin from damage by sunlight, by filtering and scattering UV radiation. A deep tan reduces the amount reaching the basal epidermis by 90%.

Chronic effects of
sunlight

Chronic exposure to sunlight causes changes in the skin. These are more pronounced the greater and more prolonged the exposure, and the more fair skinned the individual. They give to the skin an 'aged' appearance, and there is usually a marked contrast between the exposed and covered skin in people exposed to excess sun.

The changes are most marked in:

Epidermis

There is thinning of the epidermis and loss of the pattern of the dermal papillae.

Dermal
connective tissue

The connective tissue fibres, both collagen and elastic, are altered and become degenerate. This change when severe is termed *solar elastosis* and produces yellowing of the skin.

The lack of supporting fibres causes loss of skin resilience, with wrinkling and furrowing (Figure 33.1) and fragility; loss of connective tissue around blood vessels causes easy bruising, telangiectasia and dilated blood vessels.

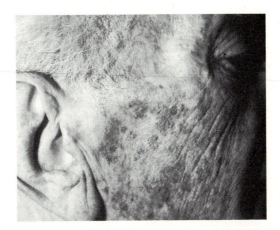

Figure 33.1   The effects of chronic sun exposure: the skin is wrinkled and there is hypo- and hyperpigmentation

Sebaceous glands   These often become atrophied leading to a dry skin. The atrophic cavity may dilate causing a senile comedone.

Melanocytes   Chronic sunlight damages and inactivates melanocytes producing areas of hypopigmentation (Figure 33.1). Some enlarge and become giant melanocytes, these produce excess pigment and form actinic lentigos (Figure 33.1).

Carcinogenesis   The chronic damage to the DNA of the cells of epidermis by UVL can result after a long latent period in carcinogenesis. The incidence of skin cancers and melanomas increases in the fair skinned with their proximity to the equator. Solar keratoses which may be premalignant, squamous cell carcinomas and basal cell carcinomas (Chapter 47) are all attributed to the chronic effects of sunlight. This effect is greatly accelerated in patients with xeroderma pigmentosum, who cannot repair UV induced damage to their DNA.

Protection of the skin from sunlight

Protection of skin from exposure to sunlight is necessary for the very fair skinned living in the tropics, or those suffering from a photosensitive eruption. There are several methods of reducing exposure, and they should be combined.

Reduction in exposure

Sunlight passes through the atmosphere which filters out the UVB and UVA. The shorter the distance travelled through the atmosphere the less UV is absorbed. UV radiation passes through cloud. The atmosphere also scatters the UV, so that much is present in shadow. Brightness is not a measure of the amount of UV radiation.

UV radiation is greatest between 10.00 and 14.00 hours (this may be different in different areas), greater in summer than winter, nearer the equator, and at high altitude.

The photosensitive patient should live in cold temperate areas, keep inside at midday, and avoid skiing, mountaineering and sunbathing holidays.

Natural protective mechanism

Thickening of the epidermis is the major protection in the very fair skinned. It gives a four-fold reduction in the amount of light reaching the basal layer.

In pigmented people or those who tan, pigmentation is a very valuable method of screening out sunlight. It is more efficient than artificial sunscreens.

The increased skin thickness and pigmentation that occur during the summer partially explain the improvement of some photosensitive rashes as the summer progresses.

Clothing

Light clothing reduces but allows some transmission of UVA. Large brimmed hats, and thick, covering clothing all protect the skin. Hairstyles can modify the amount of light reaching the face, ears and neck.

Sunscreens

Sunscreens are applied to the skin, and act by absorbing or reflecting sunlight. Para-aminobenzoic acid (PABA) absorbs UVB radiation and is widely prescribed by dermatologists. The high protection commercial products are more effective. Titanium dioxide reflects light, but is much less cosmetically acceptable, and it does *not* screen out all UV and visible radiation. A deep tan is the most effective sunscreen.

PHOTOSENSITIVE ERUPTIONS

Photosensitive eruptions result from either endogenous or exogenous photosensitizers. The differentiation is important as the avoidance of an external photosensitizer results in cure.

EXOGENOUS PHOTOSENSITIVE ERUPTIONS

Exogenous photosensitizers are widely distributed in plants and plant extracts, cosmetics, antibacterials, industrial processes and drugs. Psoralens are found in certain plants and in oil of bergamot which is used in perfumes and many cosmetic preparations, and are used therapeutically to photosensitize the skin to UVA in the PUVA (psoralen and UVA) treatment for psoriasis.

Presentation Any age can be affected but because exposure to photosensitizers is much more frequent in adult life, exogenous photosensitive eruptions are most commonly seen in adults. Men and women are equally susceptible. The distribution of the rash is determined by the mode and sites to which the photosensitizer is applied, and the areas exposed to sun-

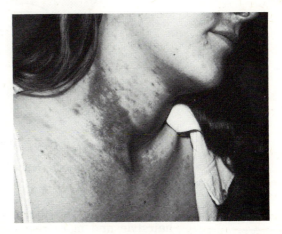

Figure 33.2 Acute photosensitive reaction to perfume and resulting hyperpigmatition (Berloque dermatitis)

light. Topical photosensitizers affect only the areas in contact, e.g. Berloque dermatitis, characterized by hyperpigmentation at the site of perfume application (usually the sides of the neck) (Figure 33.2). Blisters appear at sites where plants containing photosensitizers have brushed against the skin. Systemic photosensitizers give the typical picture of a photosensitive eruption, i.e. face (with sparing of upper eyelids), tips of ears, neck (except under the chin) (Figure 32.3), upper trunk especially the V of the neck, and backs of the hands (Figures

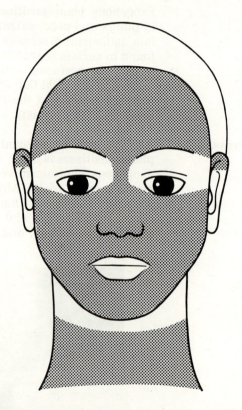

Figure 33.3 Characteristic distribution of photosensitive eruption on face

33.4 and 33.5). The distribution will be modified by hairstyle and more revealing clothing. There is a sharp cut off at the edges of clothing (Figures 33.5 and 33.6)

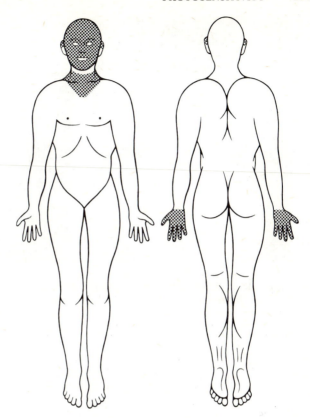

Figure 33.4   Characteristic distribution of photosensitive eruption on the body

The eruption may be painful, burning and pruritic. The first sign is erythema and oedema (Figure 33.5). In severe cases there are vesicles and blisters, and later scaling (Figure 33.5). There may be hyperpigmentation Figure 33.2).

There is a history of exposure to a topical or systemic photosensitizer, though this may be very difficult to identify. A full history of contact with plants, soaps or cosmetics, and a detailed occupational history and complete drug history must be taken.

Photo-onycholysis   An unusual form of exogenous photosensitization affects the finger nails. This is called photo-

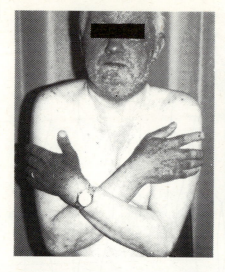

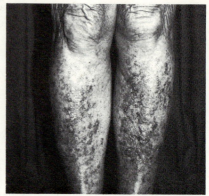

Figure 33.5 Photosensitive eruption due to thiazide diuretic. There is erythema, oedema and scaling. There is a sharp cut off at the edge of the clothes

Figure 33.6 Drug induced photodermatosis: there is erythema and scaling on the lower leg, the thighs and knees were protected by a skirt

onycholysis. There is pain in the finger tips and this is followed by onycholysis, separation of the distal finger or toe nail from nail bed (Figure 33.7). It is usually caused by tetracyclines and appears several weeks after commencing them. It may also occur during PUVA therapy.

Differential diagnosis

This history of a photosensitizer differentiates exogenous from endogenous photosensitivity. It may be impossible clinically to distinguish from airborne contact eczema.

The endogenous photodermatoses are differentiated by history and appearance. The inherited porphyrias commence early in life. Polymorphic light eruption and Hutchinson's summer prurigo are distinguished by the presence of papules on normal skin. Lupus erythematosus is characterized by atrophy and telangiectasia. Photosensitive eczema is insidious in onset.

Diagnosis and investigations

Photo-patch tests and ordinary patch tests are necessary to confirm the source of topical photosensitizers and to exclude airborne allergens.

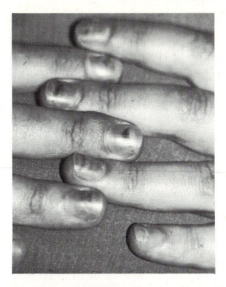

Figure 33.7   Photo-nycholysis due to tetracycline. The distal portion of the nail plate has separated from the nail bed

Table 33.1   The common photosensitizers

Systemic photosensitizers

Therapeutic	Nalidixic acid
	Phenothiazines
	Protryptiline
	Psoralens (PUVA therapy)
	Sulphonamides
	Tetracyclines
	Thiazides
Endogenous	Porphyrins

Topical photosensitizers

Cosmetic	Psoralens in perfumes
	scented preparations
	suntan preparations
	Antibacterials in soaps
Occupational	Dyes
	Pitch
	Tars
Accidental	Plants

Aetiology The most common photosensitizers are shown in Table 33.1.

Two mechanisms are involved in causing photosensitivity; they are phototoxicity and photoallergy.

Phototoxicity This occurs when a substance sensitizes cells to UV light. This may be by combination with DNA, proteins or membranes. The substance must reach a critical concentration before it does this. This occurs within two hours with psoralens, or may take days or weeks, e.g. with tetracyclines. The effect is dose related.

Photoallergy This is a much rarer idiosyncratic response. The compound present in the skin is modified by UV light and an allergic response is elicited. There is a latent period of at least a week on first exposure and the response is not dose related.

Many compounds can act by either mechanism, and it is often impossible to differentiate them.

PUVA therapy uses the phototoxic effect of oral or topical psoralens in combination with UVA irradiation. It is known to have interactions with the bases in DNA and to form cross links.

Therapy The cause must be identified and removed. The patient must be instructed in protection of the skin from sunlight (page 274).

Topical potent steroids or moderate dose systemic steroids may be helpful in severe cases.

Natural history and prognosis Once the skin is photosensitized it takes weeks or months to return to normal. The rate of inactivation and removal of the photosensitizer determines this. Photosensitivity due to nalidixic acid may persist for many months. Eventually recovery occurs.

ENDOGENOUS PHOTOSENSITIVE ERUPTIONS

There are two groups of endogenous photosensitive eruptions; those where the cause of the photosensitization is unknown (these are termed idiopathic), and those in which a metabolic cause for the photosensitization has been identified (see Table 33.2).

Table 33.2 Classification of endogenous photodermatoses

Idiopathic	Polymorphic light eruption
	Hutchinson's summer prurigo
	Solar urticaria
	Actinic reticuloid − photosensitive eczema
Metabolic	The porphyrias
	Xeroderma pigmentosum

There are also a number of dermatoses that are precipitated or exacerbated in certain patients by sunlight (see Table 33.3), and may present as a photosensitive eruption.

Table 33.3 Dermatoses which may be aggravated by sunlight

Atopic eczema
Discoid lupus erythematosus
Systemic lupus erythematosus
Psoriasis
Rosacea

POLYMORPHIC LIGHT ERUPTION

This is the most common photodermatosis. It is becoming more widely recognized with the increased exposure to the sun.

Presentation The disease can begin at any age, from infancy to late middle age, but the teens and twenties are most common (Figure 33.8). Women are affected more commonly than men. The female to male ratio is 4 : 1 (Figure 33.9). It is found in all races, but is rare in Australia.

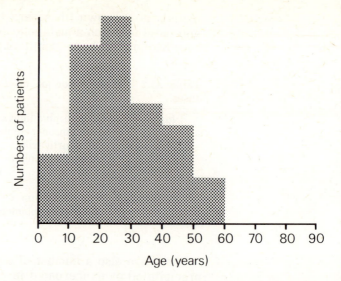

Figure 33.8   Age of onset of polymorphic light eruption

The distribution is usually that of a typical photosensitive rash, the face, neck, and backs of hands being affected (Figures 33.3, 33.4 and 33.10). Other areas, e.g. legs and upper trunk which are uncovered or covered only by light clothing, may also be affected. The face is occasionally spared.

The rash commences within 2–48 hours of exposure to the sun, and if there is no further exposure, remits within a few days. There is great variation in the intensity and duration necessary to evoke it. Some people are affected in temperate winter, others only in tropical summer. The lesions consist of erythema and papules. They are very itchy and may be excoriated (Figure 33.10).

It often becomes milder as the summer progresses.

There may be associated solar urticaria (see below, page 286).

Many patients have a personal or family history of atopy. A family history of photosensitivity is also common.

A familial form has been described in North American Indians.

Differential diagnosis   Other photosensitive eruptions are differentiated by age of onset and history. In children it is important to differentiate if from the porphyrias. In young

women the possibility of systemic lupus erythematosus should be considered, but the morphology and
persistence of the lesions in lupus should distinguish
them.

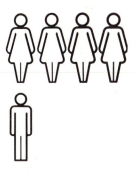

Figure 33.9   Sex ratio of polymorphic light eruption

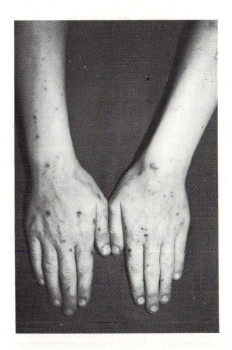

Figure 33.10   Polymorphic light eruption: red excoriated
papules on the backs of the hands

Diagnosis and investigations
Skin biopsy

Biopsy is rarely helpful.

Blood tests

Porphyria should be excluded and the ANF and DNA binding checked.

Monochromator tests

Testing with narrow wavelengths of light is useful in confirming the diagnosis by eliciting the rash, and for advice on sunscreens.

Aetiology

The cause is unknown.

Therapy
General

Exposure to sunlight should be minimized by choice of holiday, clothing and keeping inside at midday. Protective clothing and sunscreens are helpful (see above, page 274). The thickening and pigmentation of the skin as summer progresses often permits longer exposure to sun.

Systemic therapy

ß-carotene, antimalarials and thalidomide are all of benefit to some patients. Chloroquine and thalidomide must be used with great caution because of ocular and teratogenic effects.

Systemic steroids will often suppress the eruption and may be justified for 2–3 weeks each year.

Natural history and prognosis

Once manifest, polymorphic light eruption usually persists for many years, but it is less troublesome in old age. The severity may fluctuate. Gradual exposure to sunlight may reduce the sensitivity, presumably because of increased pigmentation and thickness of the skin.

HUTCHINSON'S SUMMER PRURIGO

Hutchinson's summer prurigo is a rare photodermatosis. In the past it was often confused with polymorphic light eruption. Some dermatologists do not consider it to be a distinct entity.

Presentation

Most cases commence before the age of 10. Females outnumber males 3 : 1 (Figure 33.11). There is often a family history of the disease.

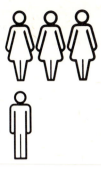

Figure 33.11   Sex ratio of Hutchinson's summer prurigo

Familial cases occur in certain racial groups in South and North America.

The light exposed areas are affected, particularly the cheeks, tip of the nose (Figure 33.12) and backs of hands, but covered areas e.g. the buttocks may also be affected. The lesions comprise itchy red papules (Figure 33.12) which may become lichenified. Occasionally they heal with scarring.

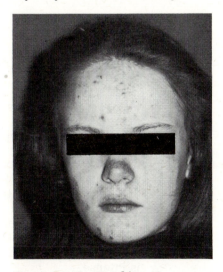

Figure 33.12   Hutchinson's summer prurigo: red papules on the tip of the nose, cheek, chin and forehead

The eruption is worse in summer, and exacerbation after exposure to strong sunlight is common. It persists for months and often through the winter.

Differential diagnosis Erythrohepatopoietic protoporphyria is distinguished by the early onset, and acute diffuse erythema on exposure to sunlight.

Polymorphic light eruption is distinguished by the shorter time course.

Diagnosis and investigations Blood, urinary and faecal porphyrins should be looked for.

Aetiology The cause is unknown.

Therapy General measures to avoid the sun and the use of sunscreens (see page 274) are usually disappointing.

Thalidomide has been used successfully by some workers. Short courses of systemic steroids may be given for summer holidays.

Natural history and prognosis Some cases improve or remit completely at puberty. Others persist indefinitely.

SOLAR URTICARIA

Solar urticaria is one of the rarest of the urticarias. Fifty per cent of cases are associated with polymorphic light eruption, a few with systemic lupus erythematosus or the porphyrias.

Presentation Solar urticaria affects all age groups and both sexes; however, young women predominate because of the association with polymorphic light eruption.

Any area exposed to light is affected. It commences within minutes of exposure to sunlight, and resolves within an hour of leaving sunlight. There is initially erythema and later confluent weal. Pruritus is intense.

Differential The rapid onset and resolution distinguish solar urticaria from the other photodermatoses. The distribution and history exclude the other urticarias.

Diagnosis and investigations UV irradiation of skin confirms the diagnosis by inducing urticaria. Associated polymorphic light eruption, porphyria and systemic lupus erythematosus should be excluded.

Aetiology An immunological reaction involving antibody and antigen and UV radiation is inferred from the passive transfer by serum to normal skin of the urticarial response to irradiation. It is assumed that a cytophilic antibody has been transferred.

Therapy Avoidance of the sun (see page 274) is the only successful method of preventing solar urticaria. Gradually increasing exposures to sun lessen the severity of succeeding attacks.

Antihistamines are not helpful.

Natural history and prognosis It persists indefinitely.

ACTINIC RETICULOID-PHOTOSENSITIVE ECZEMA

Actinic reticuloid and photosensitive eczema were originally thought to be two separate diseases, but are now considered to be probably two ends of a spectrum. Patients have been observed to transform from one to the other. Photosensitive eczema is a much milder disease than actinic reticuloid.

Presentation This is a disease of middle and old age (see Figure 33.13). It affects men exclusively.

There is often a long history of some other previous dermatosis. The light exposed areas are most severely affected (Figures 33.3 and 33.4). Severe cases of actinic reticuloid have a generalized rash, with sparing of intertriginous areas only, and episodes of erythroderma are common.

The rash of photosensitive eczema is red and scaly. Actinic reticuloid often commences similarly but progresses to thick, erythematous lichenified skin (Figure 33.14), often with indurated plaques. Pruritus is severe.

Patients with photosensitive eczema are sensitive to a narrow band of UVB radiation, those with actinic reticuloid to a very wide spectrum of radiation from UVB, to UVA and even visible light. Some

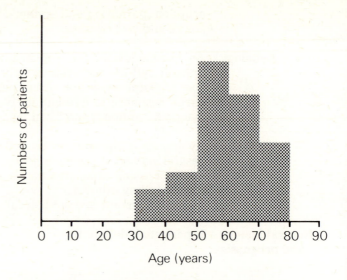

Figure 33.13   Age of onset of actinic reticuloid

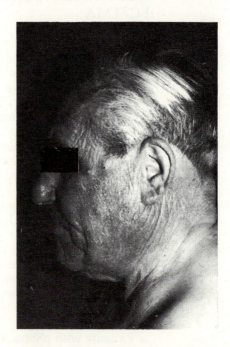

Figure 33.14 Actinic reticuloid: there is erythema and thickening of light exposed skin

unfortunate patients with actinic reticuloid are so light sensitive that they are unable to go out during the day, needing to remain inside with drawn curtains, and unable to tolerate fluorescent lights.

Differential diagnosis Contact dermatitis to an airborne allergen or a photocontact allergy may be very difficult to distinguish, but these rarely become generalized.

Diagnosis and investigation In cases of actinic reticuloid, skin biopsy may suggest a malignant cutaneous lymphoma.

Aetiology There is a high incidence of positive patch tests to oleo resins from plants and potassium dichromate. It is not clear whether these or other allergens are involved in producing the dermatosis. The positive patch tests may reflect an abnormally reactive skin.

Treatment
General The usual methods to reduce exposure to sunlight (see page 274) are essential. Severe cases of actinic reticuloid require a nocturnal existence, while others manage with the use of special windows and reflectant sunscreens.

Topical therapy Very potent topical steroids are helpful.

Systemic therapy Systemic steroids are used in acute episodes of erythroderma. Azathioprine has been reported to induce remission.

Natural history and prognosis Most cases persist for life. The nocturnal life is so depressing that a high proportion of patients commit suicide.

THE PORPHYRIAS

The porphyrias are a group of metabolic disorders in which there is overproduction of porphyrin during the production of haem and cytochromes. The biochemical defect is sited in either red blood cells or liver, depending on the type of porphyria (Table 33.4), and they are classified accordingly. Most are inherited.

Table 33.4   Classification of the porphyries

Erythropoietic	Congenital erythropoietic porphyria
Erythrohepatic	Erythrohepatic protoporphyria
Hepatic	Porphyria variegata
Acquired	Porphyria cutanea tarda

(Acute intermittent porphyria – no cutaneous manifestation)

The porphyrins or their oxidation products fluoresce pink with ultraviolet light. They act as endogenous photosensitizers and cause photosensitivity.

CONGENITAL ERYTHROPOIETIC PORPHYRIA

This is a rare but very striking disorder. It is also known as Gunther's disease.

Presentation It is manifest soon after birth. Both sexes are affected. There is a worldwide distribution. The inheritance is recessive.

All light exposed skin is affected. There is extreme photosensitivity. Blisters form and often become infected. Scarring is severe, with sclerosis, hypo- and hyperpigmentation and hirsutes. The nose and fingertips become obliterated. Mutilation is extreme (Figure 33.15).

The eyes are photosensitive and blindness occurs.

Porphyrins in bones and teeth cause fluorescence and fragility.

There is a haemolytic anaemia and associated splenomegaly.

The urine is pink and fluorescent. The red blood cells fluoresce.

It is suggested that these horrific nocturnal children gave rise to the werewolf legends.

Differential diagnosis The full blown picture is characteristic. Early cases may cause confusion with polymorphic light eruption, erythrohepatic protoporphyria and xeroderma pigmentosa, but the blisters and pink urine are diagnostic.

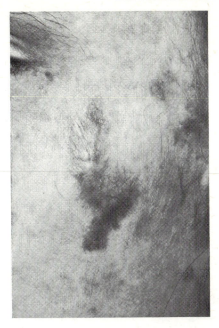

**Figure 33.15   Congenital erythropoi-
etic porphyria showing mutilation,
pigmentary changes and hirsutism**

**Diagnosis and
investigations**
Wood's light

Examination of teeth, blood and urine reveals the characteristic pink fluorescence.

Blood tests

Excess porphyrins are present in red cells, also in urine and faeces.

A full blood count and reticulocyte count are essential to assess the extent of the haemolytic anaemia.

Aetiology

There is a specific biochemical defect in the red cells leading to an excess of Type 1 prophyrins.

Treatment

Rigorous avoidance of the sun (see page 274) with protection of the eyes is essential to minimize scarring and ocular damage.

**Natural history
and prognosis**

Progressive mutilation is the rule. The haemolytic anaemia often causes premature death.

ERYTHROHEPATIC PROTOPORPHYRIA

This is much more common than congenital erythro-poietic porphyria and less devastating in its effects.

Presentation   Most cases present in early childhood, both sexes are equally affected. The inheritance is dominant, but some cases are never manifest. It is found world-wide.

The light exposed skin is affected (Figures 33.3 and 33.4). There is marked photosensitivity, present-ing as an intense burning sensation in sunlight, which may be accompanied by erythema, oedema and rarely solar urticaria (see page 286). Scarring is linear.

Gall stones due to excess biliary excretion of the porphyrins occur.

Liver failure due to cirrhosis is sometimes a late but fatal event.

Differential diagnosis   Differentiation from the other childhood photoder-matoses is made on clinical and biochemical grounds.

Diagnosis and investigations

Skin biopsy   Shows characteristic staining with PAS.

Biochemical   Excess protoporphyrin is present in faeces and in red cells which fluoresce. The urine is normal.

Aetiology   There is a specific metabolic defect in liver and red cells causing excess protoporphyrin production.

Treatment
General   Sunlight exposure must be minimized (see page 274).

Systemic therapy   Orally administered ß-carotene gives symptomatic improvement.

Natural history and prognosis   This condition is persistent.

PORPHYRIA VARIEGATA

Presentation   This inherited porphyria does not usually present until adult life. The sex ratio is equal but men have predominantly cutaneous manifestations and women acute attacks of porphyria. The inheritance is

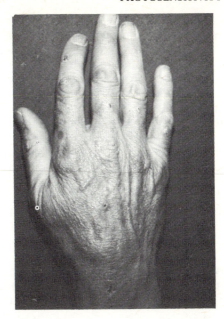

Figure 33.16 Porphyria variegata: premature ageing and erosions on the backs of the hands

dominant. It is particularly common in the Afrikaaners of South Africa.

Cutaneous lesions are usually confined to the face and hands. There is increased sun sensitivity and blisters and crusted erosions are seen (Figure 33.16). There is scarring with hypo- and hyperpigmentation and hirsutism. The skin is very fragile and prematurely aged (see page 272 and Figure 33.16).

The systemic symptoms of the acute attack are abdominal pain, neurological and psychiatric disease.

Oestrogens exacerbate the disease; acute attacks are precipitated by pregnancy, menstruation and the oral contraceptive.

Many drugs can precipitate an attack (see Table 33.5).

Table 33.5   Chief drugs exacerbating porphyria variegata

Oestrogens
Barbiturates
Griseofulvin
Sulphonamides

Differential diagnosis   The cutaneous lesions distinguish this from acute intermittent porphyria. Porphyria cutanea tarda and exogenous photosensitive eruptions are distinguished by history, and the latter by the absence of 'aged' skin.

Diagnosis and investigations   Excess porphyrins are always present in the faeces. Urinary porphyrins are detectable during an acute attack.

Aetiology   A metabolic defect allows overproduction of porphyrins by the liver.

Treatment   Exposure to sunlight must be minimized (see page 274). All drugs precipitating attacks must be scrupulously avoided.

Natural history and prognosis   Death may result from neurological or psychiatric disease. The prognosis is improved by careful avoidance of all exacerbating drugs.

PORPHYRIA CUTANEA TARDA

This is the only porphyria that is not inherited. It is also called symptomatic hepatic porphyria.

Presentation   It usually presents in middle or old age. It is much more common in men. It is very common among the Bantu. Epidemics have occurred after accidental ingestion of hepatotoxins. The most common association is with alcoholic liver disease.

All light exposed areas (Figure 33.3 and 33.4) are photosensitive, with blistering, scarring and pigmentary changes. There are no systemic features.

Chloroquine worsens the disease and may cause abdominal symptoms (but paradoxically is used in treatment). Oestrogens have an adverse effect on it.

There are often associated signs of hepatomegaly, liver failure and alcoholism.

Differential diagnosis   Porphyria variegata and other photodermatoses are distinguished by the absence of liver disease.

Diagnosis and investigations   Excess porphyrins are present in the urine. Blood and faecal porphyrins are normal.

Serum iron is often raised.

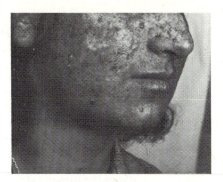

Figure 33.17 Xeroderma pigment-osum: showing typical scarring hyper-and hypopigmentation

Aetiology   Liver damage causes the abnormal hepatic porphy-rin metabolism. A genetic susceptibility has been postulated.

Alcoholic liver damage is the chief cause.

Treatment   General measures are avoidance of sunlight (see page 274), and cessation of drinking or treatment of any remediable liver disease.

Venesection relieves the photosensitivity for many months. Cautious chloroquine administration causes eventual symptomatic improvement.

Natural history and prognosis   The prognosis depends on the patient; improvement occurs if drinking is discontinued. Persistent alco-holism leads to worsening of the photosensitivity and hepatic failure.

XERODERMA PIGMENTOSUM

Presentation   Xeroderma pigmentosum is a rare hereditary disease characterized by photosensitivity and the develop-ment of skin malignancies at an early age. All races are affected, males and females equally. The skin is normal at birth. The age of onset varies according to the degree of exposure to sunlight, but is usually around 2–3 years of age.

The characteristic feature is photosensitivity manifested by intense erythema of the exposed areas after exposure to sunlight. There may be vesiculation and oedema, and conjunctivitis and blepharitis in more severe cases. At an early age irregular macular pigmented areas appear on the exposed areas and at a later stage in the non-exposed areas (Figure 33.17). The skin becomes atrophic, dry, and wrinkled, and telangiectasia appears. In early childhood, benign tumours such as keratosis, keratoacanthomas and cutaneous horns develop. These are followed by malignant tumours, which include basal cell carcinomata, squamous cell carcinomata, malignant melanomas and various sarcomas. In most cases the tumour stage is reached before adolescence. The eyes are usually affected in the early stages with photophobia, conjunctivitis, and excessive lacrimation. Pigmentation of the conjunctiva, opacity of the cornea, ectropion and malignant tumours of the eyes may appear. In some patients there is microcephaly, hypogonadism, and mental retardation.

Differential diagnosis

In the early stage of xeroderma pigmentosum, poikiloderma has to be considered, but this is usually patchy and not confined to the exposed areas, and although there is atrophy and telangiectasia the macular pigmentation is not present.

Radiodermatitis may give similar changes to xeroderma pigmentosum, but it is unlikely to occur at such an early age.

Erythropoietic protoporphyria appears in the same age group and presents as acute photosensitivity. The disease does not progress to pigmentary changes. Photosensitive eczema is rare in children, but may well resemble the early stages of xeroderma pigmentosum. Photophobia and conjunctivitis do not usually occur in eczema.

Investigations

The diagnosis is established by studies on cultured skin fibroblasts. These cells show reduced ability to repair ultraviolet light damaged DNA. Culture of amniotic fluid of pregnant carriers shows a similar defect and is an indication for termination of a pregnancy.

Skin biopsy of a lesion shows atrophy and changes associated with damage due to UV light. Tests with a monochromator show an increased susceptibility to light with a wavelength of 280–310 nm.

Aetiology Xeroderma pigmentosum is a hereditary disorder and the mode of inheritance is autosomal recessive. The patient's skin and eyes show an increased sensitivity to all light with a wavelength 280–310 nm. Initially this is manifested by acute erythema after exposure and subsequently by atrophic changes of the skin, and tumours. In xeroderma pigmentosum there is abnormal repair of damaged DNA following exposure to UV light, and this is thought to be due to reduction of the enzyme endonuclease. However, more recent studies have shown a number of abnormalities in DNA repair, and these appear to be deficiencies of more than one enzyme.

Treatment Patients must be rigorously protected from exposure to sunlight with clothing and avoidance of sunlight. Topical sun screen preparations should be used.

Various drugs such as antimalarials and vitamin A derivations have been used in an attempt to decrease the photosensitivity.

5-Fluorouracil cream should be used in the early stages of skin changes in an attempt to destroy the abnormal cells. Once malignant tumours form they should be treated by surgery or currettage and cautery. If grafts are necessary these should be from a non-exposed area.

Prenatal diagnosis is now possible.

Course and prognosis Xeroderma pigmentosum is a progressive disease with irreversible skin damage. The course depends on the severity of the disease. The majority of patients die before the age of 20 due to skin malignancies. When the onset of the disease is later in life the prognosis is better.

34 PIGMENTARY DISORDERS

VITILIGO

Presentation A common disorder of skin pigmentation more pronounced in darker individuals. The sexes are affected equally. The common age of onset is in young adults, but it presents at any age (Figure 34.1).

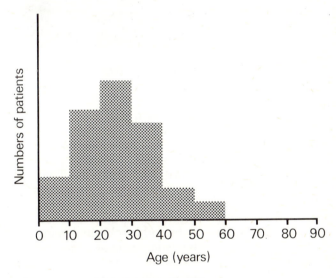

Figure 34.1   Age of onset of vitiligo

The skin lesions are characterized by sharply defined, white, flat patches with oval or irregular configuration (Figure 34.2). The lesions vary from a few mm to several cm, and they may extend peripherally. The involved skin has a normal texture. The overlying hair may be white or grey, and there may be a hyperpigmented border surrounding the depigmented skin. The lesions may be a few or cover the

299

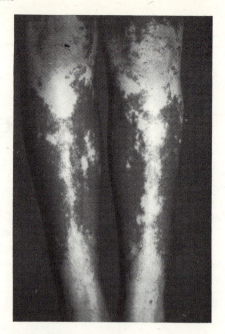

Figure 34.2   Depigmented areas in vitiligo

whole skin surface. They are usually symmetrical and multiple, but may rarely be single or unilateral. The sites of predilection are the face, backs of hands and wrists, flexures, particularly the axillae and groins, and genitalia. The lesions are symptomless apart from being sensitive to sunlight.

Differential diagnosis   Pityriasis versicolor is usually confined to upper limbs and trunk with hypopigmented patches and not depigmented ones as in vitiligo. The lesions have fine scales and may irritate. Scrapings of the skin taken for mycology will demonstrate the fungus.

In post-inflammatory hypopigmentation there is usually, but not always, a history of inflammation of the skin, and the skin is hypopigmented and not depigmented.

Pityriasis alba is hypopigmentation with slightly scaly areas, usually on the face, and is due to mild eczema.

Albinism, partial or generalized, is present at birth and is not progressive. There is an abnormal iris and usually a white forelock.

Hypopigmented patches of leprosy have no hair, and do not perspire and are anaesthetic. The diagnosis can be confirmed by biopsy.

Lichen sclerosis and atrophicus, and morphea, may present as hypopigmented areas, but they have an abnormal skin texture.

Investigations A biopsy shows the absence of dopa-positive melanocytes. There may be organ specific antibodies in a small proportion of patients.

Aetiology It has been suggested that vitiligo may be auto-immune, on the basis of a slightly higher incidence of organ specific auto-immune disorders such as Addison's disease, thyrotoxicosis, pernicious anaemia and diabetes.

Treatment A very small percentage may respond to topical steroid therapy. A more effective treatment is psoralens and ultraviolet light. The best results are obtained with oral psoralens. The treatment is time consuming and may have to be continued for up to 2 years. Asians and negroes respond better to treatment than Caucasians.

If the disease is causing cosmetic embarrassment, suitable camouflage will help. Occasionally when the disease is very extensive it may be advisable to depigment the few remaining pigmented areas with topical hydroquinones to give a uniform colour to the skin.

Prognosis The course of the disease is variable. The onset may be sudden or gradual. The lesions may persist as small patches or gradually extend with new lesions developing. Very rarely the whole of the body may ultimately be affected. Spontaneous recovery is unusual.

POST-INFLAMMATORY PIGMENTARY CHANGES

After acute or chronic inflammatory diseases of the skin there may be pigmentary changes in the lesions. The sexes are equally affected. It is very common in individuals with dark skin, i.e. Asians and negroes

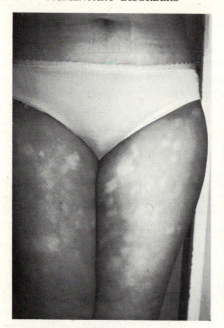

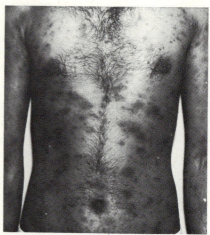

Figure 34.3   Post-inflammatory hypo-pigmentation

Figure 34.4   Post-inflammatory hyper-pigmentation, after eczema

and there may be either an increase or a decrease in the pigmentation. There are numerous skin disorders which cause localized inflammation. The common causes of post-inflammatory hypopigmentation are: eczema, pityriasis alba, pityriasis versicolor, psoriasis, leprosy, syphilis and yaws. The lesions are paler than the normal skin and confined to the area of inflammation and are hypopigmented rather than depigmented (Figure 34.3).

The pathogenesis of the hypopigmentation is not known, and may differ in different diseases, e.g. it may be due to oedema of keratinocytes in eczema, which cannot accept the normal amount of melanin pigments or a rapid epidermal turnover as in psoriasis and therefore a short duration of contact with melanocytes. The diseases which may cause hyperpigmentation are eczema (Figure 34.4) infections, lichen planus, discoid lupus erythematosus, scleroderma, and pinta. The hyperpigmentation may be due to increased activity or hyperplasia of melanocytes, or a retention of melanin pigments in the upper dermis in macrophages after injury to the basal cell layer and melanocytes.

Treatment   None is usually necessary or effective.

Course and prognosis   Post-inflammatory hypo- and hyperpigmentation usually gradually disappear in a few months but occasionally may persist for longer periods.

MELASMA (CHLOASMA)

Presentation   A common disorder of facial skin pigmentation occurring mainly in women (Figure 34.5). The highest incidence is during the reproductive years (Figure 34.6). It

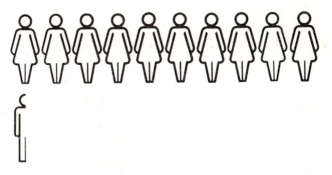

Figure 34.5 Melasma predominantly seen in women

is often precipitated by pregnancy and/or the taking of the contraceptive pill. However, it does occur spontaneously. It is particularly common in persons from the Middle East. The lesions are pale or dark brown, flat patches with an irregular border (Figure 35.7). The sites of predilection are the cheeks, nose, upper lip and forehead.

Differential diagnosis   Hyperpigmentation on the face, after using topical photosensitizing agents in cosmetics or soap, must be considered. Peribuccal pigmentation of Brocq has diffuse pigmentation on the face, mostly around the mouth. In poikiloderma of Civatte, there is reticular hyperpigmentation, atrophy and telangiectasia on the sides of the cheeks and on the neck. Systemic drugs may cause photosensitivity and subsequent

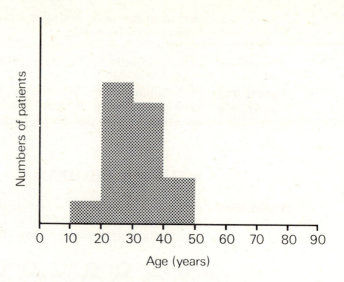

Figure 34.6   Age of incidence of melasma

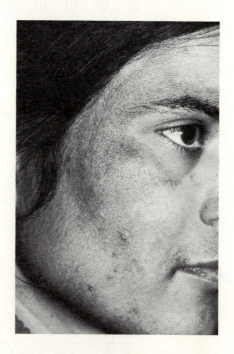

Figure 34.7 Hyperpigmented patches around the eye in melasma

pigmentation; the drugs most likely to produce this effect are chlorpromazine, nalidixic acid and tetracycline. Post-inflammatory hyperpigmentation on the face after various dermatoses may be confused with melasma. In Addison's disease hyperpigmentation usually occurs at other sites.

Investigations Diagnosis is made on clinical features alone.

Aetiology Melasma is due to increased activity of melanocytes in the skin in response to sunlight and/or increased female hormones. Genetic factors may also play some role in the aetiology. It is particularly common in the dark skinned Europeans and Asians living in the Middle East.

Treatment Topical hydroquinones may be helpful but should only be used under strict medical supervision.

Prognosis The lesions become paler during the winter; they may fade slowly after pregnancy or stopping of the contraceptive pill if due to either of these causes. However, they may persist for years, particularly if not directly related to pregnancy or the contraceptive pill.

FRECKLES (EPHELIDES)

Presentation Freckles are a very common disorder of skin pigmentation. There is a racial and hereditary influence and the condition usually affects blonds and redheads. Freckles become more prominent during the summer and the commonest age of onset is 5–7 years. Both males and females are affected.

The characteristic clinical lesion is a light brown macule measuring a few mm. They may be multiple on the sun exposed areas, especially the face, and fade or become paler during the winter.

Differential diagnosis Freckles must be differentiated from lentigines which are more prominent and may be anywhere on the skin. Junctional naevi are permanent, not limited to exposed areas, usually darker and fewer in number. Xeroderma pigmentosum is associated with photophobia, photosensitivity, and skin neoplasms.

Investigations   None are usually necessary. A biopsy of the lesion shows normal numbers of melanocytes, but they are larger than normal and show increased production of melanin granules.

Aetiology   Freckles are considered to be an autosomal dominant disorder. The increased activity of the melanocytes is due to exposure to the sunlight.

Treatment   Topical sunscreen agents during the summer are helpful.

Prognosis   The lesions fade or become paler in the winter, but will recur on further exposure to sunlight.

LENTIGINES

Presentation   A lentigo is a small permanent hyperpigmented lesion on the skin. It is very common especially in Caucasians, and both sexes are affected. Lentigines usually appear in childhood and increase until adult life.

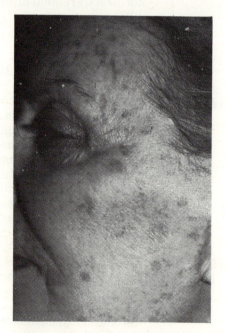

Figure 34.8 Actinic lentigines

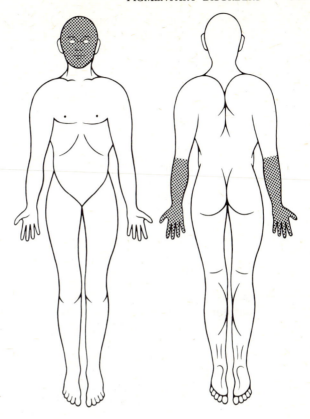

Figure 34.9   Common sites of actinic lentigines

Clinically they are small, flat or slightly raised lesions of a few mm in size, varying from light to dark brown. They may be round or polycyclic and may be slightly scaly. They may be single or multiple and may be present on any part of the skin and muco-cutaneous junctions. Multiple lentigines may occur without other abnormalities, but they may be a sign of other disease such as Peutz−Jegher's syndrome, neurofibromatosis and the Leopard syndrome (cardio-cutaneous syndrome).

Actinic or senile lentigines (Figure 34.8) occur on the exposed areas (Figure 34.9) in middle and late life in Caucasians who have spent a great deal of time in the sun. The stronger the sun the more likely the lesions are to appear.

Differential diagnosis   Careful examination is important to establish whether the lentigines are the only abnormality, or part of a more generalized disorder. Freckles are found on the sun exposed areas, and vary in colour according to the degree of sunlight. Café au lait spots which occur in neurofibromatosis are light brown, and larger, and are always flat and smooth. Junctional naevi are either solitary or few in number.

Investigations   None are necessary. A biopsy of the lesion shows an increased number of melanocytes and melanin granules; there is epidermal thickening and hyper-keratosis. The epidermal rete pegs are elongated and clubbed.

Aetiology   Lentigines are probably due to an inherited defect. It is thought that they are due to autosomal dominant gene. The actinic lentigines are a direct effect of sunlight on the skin.

Treatment   If the lesions are extensive it is difficult to offer treatment. Cryotherapy has been reported to be successful and so has dermabrasion for the facial lesions. Camouflage should be offered for facial lesions.

Prognosis   Some lesions may fade and even disappear after a few years, and others will persist. The actinic lentigines are persistent even if patients are no longer exposed to sunlight.

35 PITYRIASIS ROSEA

Presentation Pityriasis rosea is a mild common inflammatory disorder. It has a worldwide distribution, but it is more common in temperate regions particularly during the autumn and spring. It occurs mainly in young adults (Figure 35.1) and both sexes are equally affected.

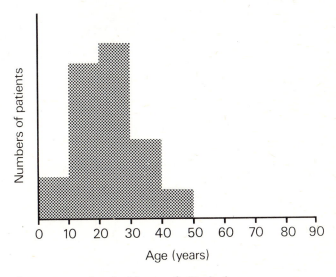

Figure 35.1 **Age incidence of pityriasis rosea**

Characteristically a herald patch first appears, which is solitary and larger than subsequent lesions. The herald patch may be oval, discoid, or annular, is red in colour, slightly raised and has a scaly surface. It usually occurs on the trunk. After an interval of one or two weeks other lesions appear. The sites of predilection are the trunk, upper limbs, neck, groin, and axillae, but it rarely affects the extremities

309

(Figure 35.2). The eruption is usually generalized and symmetrical. These lesions are characteristically oval, dull red discrete patches. Some may coalesce. The long axis of the lesions runs parallel to the lines of the skin cleavage (Figure 35.3). Characteristically there is centripetal scaling (Figure 35.4). Occasionally the eruption is papular rather than the flat oval patches. Irritation is usually minimal.

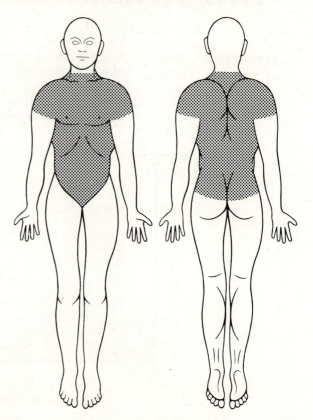

Figure 35.2 Common sites of involvement of pityriasis rosea

Differential diagnosis

The seborrhoeic variety of eczema also occurs on the trunk, but has a slower onset. There is often a previous history of eczema elsewhere. Characteristically seborrhoeic eczema affects the centre of the chest and back.

Guttate psoriasis often has a sudden onset but may also affect the limbs. The silvery scales of

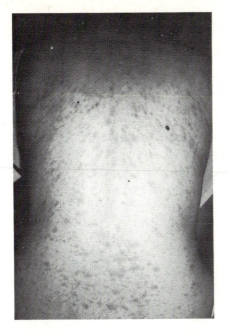

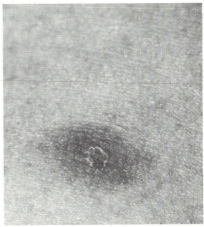

Figure 35.3   Widespread eruption in pityriasis rosea. The long axis of the oval lesion is parallel to the intercostal nerve

Figure 35.4   Scaling in the centre of the lesion (centipetal scaling) in a lesion of pityriasis rosea

psoriasis should also help to distinguish the conditions.

Drug eruptions may mimic pityriasis rosea, but they have a more rapid and generalized onset with irritation. There is usually a history of taking a suspected drug.

Some forms of secondary syphilis have a similar appearance to pityriasis rosea. In syphilis there may be papules on the palms and soles, and oral lesions. If there is any doubt, serological tests for syphilis should be carried out.

The herald patch may be confused with tinea corporis, but vesiculation may be seen in the edge of this type of fungal lesion.

Investigations None are usually necessary. The disorder can be easily diagnosed by the typical lesion, distribution and self-limiting nature as well as the lack of irritation and general upset.

Aetiology   The cause is unknown. An infective agent has been suggested, but not demonstrated.

Treatment   There is usually none required. In patients with irritation systemic antihistamines are helpful at night. Mild topical steroids may shorten the course and lessen the irritation.

Prognosis   Pityriasis rosea is a mild self-limiting disease with spontaneous remission within 6–8 weeks. Further attacks may occur in a small percentage of patients.

36 PRURITUS AND PRURIGO NODULARIS

PRURITUS

Presentation Pruritus is the Latin word for itch. Pruritus is a subjective symptom. Many skin disorders are associated with pruritus, but some patients will complain of pruritus with a particular disease and others will not. In this section the symptom of pruritus *without* any visible skin disease is considered. Pruritus has been described in a number of conditions, and they include the following:

Hepatic disease Obstructive biliary disease, where it is thought that the elevated bile salts in the skin are responsible for the pruritus. Pruritus may be the presenting feature of primary biliary cirrhosis, and precedes other symptoms of the disease by 1–2 years.

Endocrine Pruritus has been reported to occur in both hypo- and hyperthyroidism. A small proportion of patients with diabetes mellitus may have generalized pruritus as opposed to pruritus vulvae which is common.

Pregnancy and the contraceptive pill Pruritus is not an uncommon symptom in pregnancy. It usually occurs late in pregnancy and disappears after birth of the child. These subjects usually develop pruritus in subsequent pregnancies or if they take the contraceptive pill.

Renal disease Pruritis occurs during the end stages of chronic renal failure. It does not occur in acute renal failure. The problem is seen less nowadays because of renal dialysis.

Reticulosis Hodgkin's disease may present with pruritus and precede other symptoms or signs of the disease by as long as 2 years. Pruritus has also been described in chronic lymphatic leukaemia and polycythaemia.

Psychogenic Probably the commonest cause of pruritus is psychogenic. However, care must be taken to exclude the other organic diseases which may present with pruritus. There are often other features to suggest that the patient is suffering from a psychoneurosis.

Parasitic Internal parasitic infections, particularly hookworm, *infections* roundworm, onchocerciasis and filariasis may present with pruritus.

Climatic changes Pruritus is often a common symptom in winter or cold climates and presents particularly when the patient removes clothing, and seems to be related to change in weather. It occurs most frequently in subjects who are atopic and it may be associated with a dry skin, but no eczema is present.

Differential Excoriations are often absent in patients with pru-
diagnosis ritus and nothing is seen on examination of the skin. It is important to exclude a dermatosis which may be minimal but cause severe pruritus. Scabies may cause severe nocturnal pruritus and yet only minimal lesions may be visible, and a thorough search for burrows on the hands, and papules on the buttocks and male genitalia should be sought. Pediculosis pubis, as well as corporis, may present with diffuse irritation, particularly in males who have a great deal of body hair, and a search should be made for nits on the hair of the body, legs and axillae in pediculosis pubis.

The possibility of psychogenic pruritus may be suggested on the interview and the past medical history.

Investigations
Haematological Full blood count and ESR.

Biochemical Liver function tests, urine analysis, blood urea.

Stools For ova and cysts.

Immunological Mitochondrial antibodies to detect primary biliary cirrhosis.

Endocrine Thyroid function test, and glucose tolerance test if diabetes is suspected.

Radiological Chest X-ray.

Aetiology The mechanism of the pruritus is known only in a minority of these diseases. In obstructive biliary disease it is the bile salts which are thought to be responsible for the symptom. In pregnancy and the contraceptive pill the cause is hormonal. The biochemical process involved and the trigger factor in the other organic diseases are not understood.

Treatment This will depend on the cause of the disease. Obviously, if possible the treatment is directed against the primary organic disease. If none can be found then treatment is symptomatic with systemic antihistamines. Most topical preparations are not effective or it is not practical to use them to cover the whole surface of the body.

Natural history and prognosis This will depend on the underlying cause and whether treatment is satisfactory.

PRURIGO NODULARIS

Presentation Prurigo is taken to mean an intensely irritating eruption, but one in which the cause of the eruption is not known, or cannot be classified into the existing category of diseases. The term prurigo is rapidly being discarded in dermatology as it was purely descriptive and applied to various forms of well established clinical entities. The word is now only used for a few conditions and one of these is a distinct clinical entity termed prurigo nodularis.

The disease characteristically presents in the middle aged (Figure 36.1), usually females (Figure 36.2). The typical lesion is a hard, scaly nodule which protrudes from the surface of the skin. The size varies from 0.5 to 2.0 cm. The lesions frequently show scabs due to excoriation (Figure 36.3). The lesions tend to heal (usually after months), leaving scars and pigmentation. The nodules tend to occur on the outer aspect of the arms, front of the legs, upper back, chest and abdomen. These sites suggest that excoriations play some role in the production of the lesions.

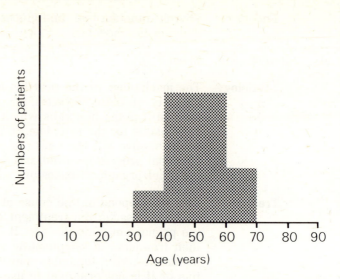

Figure 36.1   Age incidence of prurigo nodularis

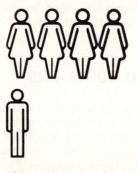

Figure 36.2   Prurigo nodularis is more common in females

Differential diagnosis   The disease may be confused with a reticulosis, but in the latter the lesions are not scaly or excoriated. Hypertrophic lichen planus tends to occur only on legs. Chronic discoid lichenified eczema, or lichenified areas in atopic eczema, must be distinguished from prurigo nodularis; in the eczematous conditions the lesions are often flatter and less nodular, and there may be changes in the surrounding skin, particularly in atopic eczema.

Investigations   If the diagnosis is in doubt then a biopsy should be performed. Screening tests for gluten-sensitive enteropathy should be performed, and if there is any

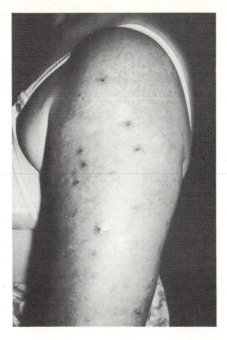

Figure 36.3   Excoriated nodules in prurigo nodularis

suggestion that this may be present, then a small intestinal biopsy should be performed.

Aetiology The cause of the condition is unknown. However, a number of causes or associations with other disease entities have been claimed. There is often said to be an underlying psychological disorder, but this is difficult to define. Prurigo nodularis has been considered to be a variant of atopic eczema because of the thickening of the skin which histologically is similar to that of lichenified eczema. Recently there have been reports of gluten-sensitive enteropathy in this condition and improvement of the skin lesions with a gluten-free diet.

Treatment No satisfactory treatment is known other than a gluten-free diet if it can be established that the patients have a gluten-sensitive enteropathy. Topical steroids may help slightly but the condition soon relapses and new lesions continue to appear. Systemic steroids are not justified, as they have to be given long term, and intralesional steroids are not practical as the lesions are too numerous. Psychiatric treatment has not been shown to be of any help.

Natural history and prognosis   The disorder is persistent and usually lasts for many years. It does seem to lessen in old age.

37 PSORIASIS

Presentation   Psoriasis is a common disorder and it has been estimated that it affects 2% of the population in European
countries. It is more common in Caucasians than in
Asians and negroes. Psoriasis is very rare under the
age of 5, and rare under the age of 10. The
commonest ages for the first appearance of psoriasis are the late teens and early adult life (Figure
37.1). However, psoriasis may present for the first
time at any age. Males and females appear to be
equally affected.

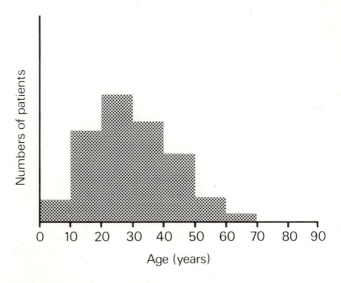

Figure 37.1   Age of onset of psoriasis

The appearances of the lesions of psoriasis vary
depending on the sites affected. In addition there
are a number of different presentations of psoriasis,

319

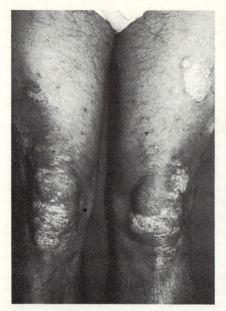

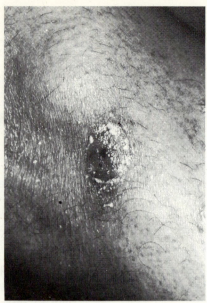

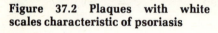

Figure 37.2 Plaques with white scales characteristic of psoriasis

Figure 37.3 Capillary bleeding points after removal of the scales in psoriasis

and these may be related to the activity of the disease process, and factors which are not fully understood at the present time.

The typical lesion of psoriasis is a well demarcated, raised, red patch with white scales (Figure 37.2). If the scales are not present but the disease is suspected, then the lesion should be gently stroked with a wooden spatula, and this will often produce the white silvery scales which are virtually diagnostic of psoriasis. This type of scaling depends on the fact that the keratin layer of the skin is abnormal and the scales are not bound firmly to each other, so that minor trauma produces disruption of the abnormal keratin. If the lesion is rubbed more strongly with the spatula the keratin is easily removed and capillary bleeding points appear which are also typical of the psoriatic lesion (Figure 37.3).

The commonest sites for psoriasis are the extensor surfaces of the elbows and knees (Figures 37.2 and 37.4). The eruption tends to be symmetrical affecting both sides of the body equally. The next

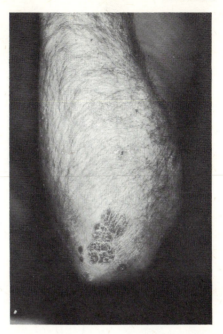

Figure 37.4   One of the commonest sites for psoriasis is the elbow

commonest sites are the scalp and sacral area (Figure 37.5). Psoriasis may be limited to one or two patches, or there may be numerous plaques affecting the whole body (Figure 37.6).

Guttate psoriasis   This is the sudden appearance of small (less than 0.5 cm), red papules of psoriasis on the trunk and limbs (Figure 37.7). The lesions subsequently develop the white silvery scale. The lesions may enlarge to form plaques or they may undergo spontaneous resolution. Guttate psoriasis may be the first presentation of the disease, or it may occur in patients who already have a few plaques of psoriasis. This type of psoriasis usually implies that the disease process is very active.

Koebner phenomenon   This is psoriasis developing at sites of trauma to the skin. Clinically this is seen at recent operation sites, or after a fall. It is possible to induce psoriasis by various physical stimuli such as scratching, but this only occurs if the psoriatic process is active.

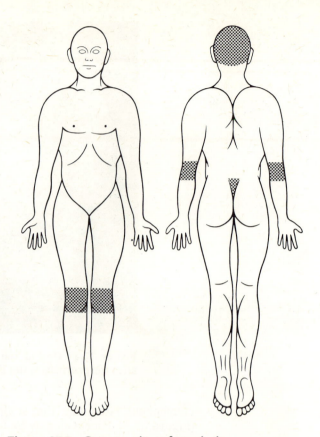

Figure 37.5   Common sites of psoriasis

Scalp   Psoriasis may affect the scalp with lesions elsewhere on the skin, or it may be the only part of the skin affected. There may be only one or a few plaques of psoriasis, or the disease may affect the whole of the scalp, but it usually stops at the hairline. The plaques are usually raised and the scales frequently become adherent to the hair, and are heaped up on each other rather than shed as from hairy parts of the skin. The surface of a psoriatic lesion is often irregular because of the thick scales, and the lesions are easily palpable.

Palms and soles   Because the keratin on the palms and soles is different from the keratin elsewhere on the skin, the features of psoriasis are different when it involves these sites. There are no raised, discrete plaques with silvery scales. Psoriasis presents on the palms

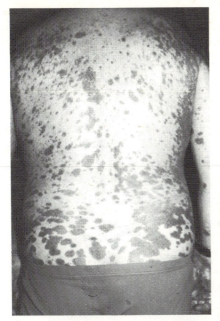

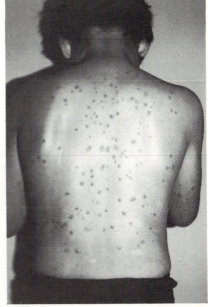

Figure 37.6   Extensive psoriasis

Figure 37.7   Small red scaly papules – guttate psoriasis

and soles as redness and scaling, but the latter is often indistinguishable from that seen in eczema. There may be a few discrete lesions, or the whole of the palm or sole may be affected, often with a sharp line of demarcation from the uninvolved skin on the side of the hand or foot. The line of demarcation occurs where the thick keratin of the palm or sole changes to the less thick keratin.

Occasionally psoriasis only involves the palms or soles and this gives rise to difficulty in establishing the diagnosis.

Flexural psoriasis Psoriasis involving the intertriginous areas, e.g. axillae, groins, peri-anal skin, loses the white dry silvery scales because of the increased moisture in the intertriginous areas. The excess keratin and moisture give rise to white macerated skin. However, like psoriasis elsewhere there is often a sharp line of demarcation between the affected and unaffected skin. Psoriasis is often limited to the intertriginous areas and stops when the skin is no longer occluded by other surface skin. Thus psoriasis in the intertriginous areas presents as a well demarcated red patch with maceration of the keratin. Psoriasis in the intertriginous areas, particularly the posterior natal cleft, often develops fissures which may be painful.

Erythrodermic psoriasis

Psoriasis very rarely may affect the whole of the skin (Figure 37.8). This is termed erythrodermic psoriasis. The skin is red, but unlike the plaques, there are no thick white silvery scales, but much finer

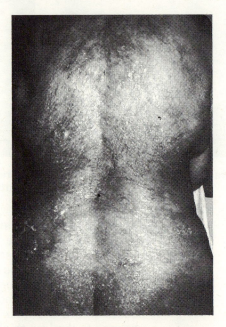

Figure 37.8   Erythrodermic psoriasis

scales. It is thought that erythrodermic psoriasis represents a more acute or active form of the disease, so that the keratin is lost more rapidly. The scales therefore do not accumulate to form a thick mass of keratin.

Patients with erythrodermic psoriasis are often seen to be shivering as there is excessive heat loss from the skin. These patients are at risk from hypothermia. Ankle oedema is also a common feature in erythrodermic psoriasis and is due to the excessive vasodilatation and the fluid collecting in the dependent parts.

Pustular psoriasis There are two types of pustular psoriasis; one is the rare *generalized* form, and the other is the *localized* form, confined to the palms and soles.

In the *generalized form*, the patients have very extensive psoriasis and are often erythrodermic. Numerous small pustules appear in waves on the erythematous skin. There is usually severe constitutional upset with fever. The pustules are sterile.

The *localized form* presents as a discoid, red scaly area on the palms and soles, and small pustules develop in the affected area (Figure 37.9). Pustular

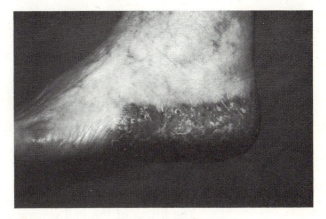

Figure 37.9   Localized pustular psoriasis

psoriasis may remain as one small area, on one palm or sole, or there may be a few discoid lesions. Very occasionally the whole of the palm or sole may be affected. The disorder tends to be persistent and has also been termed persistent pustular eruption of the palms and soles. The pustules are sterile. There is some dispute whether pustular psoriasis of the palms and soles is a manifestation of psoriasis or a separate entity.

Nails Approximately 50% of patients with psoriasis will have involvement of the nails. The commonest abnormality is pitting of the nails (Figure 37.10). These are small depressions in the nail plate approximately 1 mm in diameter. There may be a few or many on each nail, and the abnormality may be seen on a few or several of the nails. The second abnormality of the nails in psoriasis is lifting of the nail plate from

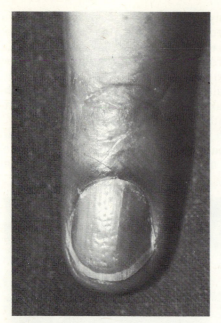
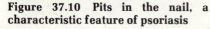
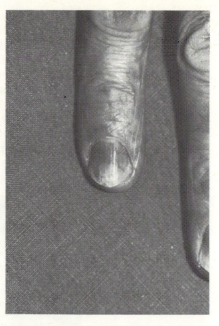

Figure 37.10 Pits in the nail, a characteristic feature of psoriasis

Figure 37.11 Onycholysis. A common abnormality of the nail in psoriasis

the nail bed, so-called onycholysis (Figure 37.11). The lifting of the nail commences distally and may involve the distal two-thirds of the nail plate. The appearance of onycholysis is of a whitish as opposed to a pink nail. This is because the nail is no longer in contact with the underlying nail bed which is reddish-pink. Occasionally there is secondary infection with chromogenic bacteria under the nail plate when it lifts up and this presents as a greenish or black discolouration under the nail. As with pitting of the nail onycholysis may involve one nail or several nails.

Yet another abnormality of the nail in psoriasis is softening and breaking of the nails. This may affect only part of the nail and only a few nails. The opposite may also happen to the nail, and it may in fact become thickened and harder than normal.

Finally, psoriasis of the nail bed causes hyperkeratosis of the nail bed and this lifts up the nail and causes distortion of the nail.

Arthropathy   The incidence of the arthropathy in psoriasis is approximately 5%. Unlike rheumatoid arthritis, which is commoner in females, the sexes are equally affected. The disorder is distinguished from rheumatoid arthritis by the fact that it is sero-negative (the rheumatoid factor is absent in the serum). Psoriatic arthropathy may be present without skin lesions. Nail changes are commoner in patients with joint involvement (about 80%), than in those patients without joint involvement.

Psoriatic arthropathy may present with single joint involvement, but multiple joint involvement is the common presentation. Clinically the distinguishing feature from rheumatoid arthritis is involvement of the distal interphalangeal joints. In other respects the disease is indistinguishable from rheumatoid arthritis. The disease may be mild and only affect a few joints, or it may be severe and progress to severe deformities, particularly of the hands.

Differential diagnosis The differential diagnosis will depend on the sites involved and the extent of the disease. The typical plaques found on the extensor surfaces of the knees and elbows do not usually present any problems. However, if psoriasis is found elsewhere on the trunk and limbs in discoid patches the commonest differential diagnosis will be eczema, usually the discoid variety. However, the lesions of eczema are less well defined and the scaling tends to be different. On the legs, hypertrophic lichen planus has to be considered, but the lesions are usually violaceous rather than red. The acute or guttate variety of psoriasis has to be distinguished from pityriasis rosea, secondary syphilis and eczema. Pityriasis rosea may have a herald patch, and the lesions show centripetal scaling. Secondary syphilis often affects the palms and soles with brown scaly papules, and the oral mucosa, with superficial ulcers.

If psoriasis only affects the scalp it may be difficult to distinguish from seborrhoeic eczema. In psoriasis the surface of the lesions tends to be irregular and on palpation this feels 'rocky'. Both diseases may be patchy but this is more likely to occur with psoriasis. Conversely both diseases may affect the whole of the scalp and stop at the hairline. Signs of both diseases should be looked for elsewhere.

If only the palms and/or soles are involved and the lesions are confluent, it can be difficult and sometimes impossible to distinguish from chronic eczema.

The diagnosis can only be made if lesions elsewhere subsequently appear. A biopsy is not always helpful and as a rule palms and soles should not be biopsied unless it is absolutely necessary. In psoriasis the lesions may be more discrete and smaller. Occasionally lichen planus of the palms and soles may present as hyperkeratotic plaques and mimic psoriasis but more typical lesions of lichen planus are usually present elsewhere.

Flexural psoriasis has to be distinguished from seborrhoeic eczema, fungal infections and erythrasma. If only the intertriginous areas are involved it may be impossible to distinguish between psoriasis and seborrhoeic eczema. In ringworm fungal infections there is usually an advancing scaly edge outside the intertriginous area; if *Candida albicans* is a secondary invader in seborrhoeic eczema, then satellite pustules are usually present. Erythrasma has a slightly more brown colour, and can be distinguished from psoriasis by ultraviolet light examination and microscopy of skin scrapings.

Erythrodermic psoriasis and erythroderma due to eczema have the same appearance. The history of the condition may be helpful in distinguishing between them. Erythroderma may also occur in mycosis fungoides and the Sezary syndrome; in these circumstances a biopsy would be helpful in establishing the diagnosis.

The generalized pustular form of psoriasis has to be differentiated from pemphigus, subcorneal pustular dermatosis, and a very rare condition termed impetigo herpetiformis, although many consider it to be pustular psoriasis. Impetigo herpetiformis however is usually reserved for the condition when it occurs in pregnancy. Biopsies will be helpful in distinguishing pemphigus and subcorneal pustular dermatosis from psoriasis. The localized form of pustular psoriasis on the palms and soles may be confused with secondary infected pompholyx eczema and fungal infections on the soles. Bacteriological and mycological tests will give the correct diagnosis.

If characteristic lesions of psoriasis are present on the skin then nail involvement does not usually present problems in the differential diagnosis. However, the skin lesions may be few or uncharacteristic, and then the nail abnormalities have to be distinguished from those due to other disorders. Pits in the nails also occur in alopecia areata, eczema, and very rarely in lichen planus and fungal infections. In alopecia areata the hair is usually severely affected, and in eczema there is usually involvement around the nails accompanied by ridging of the nails. Onycholysis may also occur in fungal infections and eczema. In the absence of skin lesions it is difficult to be certain whether the onycholysis is due to psoriasis or comes into the category of idiopathic. The other common causes of thickening and breaking of the nail plate, from which psoriasis has to be distinguished, are ringworm fungal infections and *Candida albicans* infection. The latter is invariably associated with chronic paronychia of the posterior nail fold and a greenish discolouration of the nail plate.

The arthropathy of psoriasis has to be distinguished from rheumatoid arthritis, gout and other disorders affecting the joints. This can usually be done by the appropriate serological, biochemical and radiological investigations. Rheumatoid arthritis is the commonest disease that has to be distinguished and this can be done by the absence of the rheumatoid factor in psoriatic arthropathy.

Investigations   In the vast majority of patients psoriasis is easily diagnosed by the clinical appearances of the eruption and the sites involved, and no tests are necessary.

Biopsy   This is helpful if the diagnosis is in doubt, psoriasis having a characteristic histological appearance.

Mycology   Examination of specimens of nail and flexural psoriasis may be necessary to distinguish the disorder from fungal infections.

Immunology   If arthropathy is present the presence or absence of the rheumatoid factor should be ascertained.

Radiology   This is necessary if there is joint involvement.

Aetiology   The exact cause of psoriasis is unknown. However, there is good evidence that genetic factors are important in the disease. At least one-third of patients give a history of a first or second degree relative with psoriasis. One school of thought is that psoriasis is inherited as a dominant gene, but that in the majority of persons, the disorder remains latent and there are no clinical manifestations of the disease during the life time of the subject. There are certain known precipitating factors, e.g. psychological stress, streptococcal infections, trauma to the skin, vaccination. However, these factors only apply in those persons genetically determined to be susceptible to psoriasis.

The lesion of psoriasis is characterized by rapid proliferation of epidermal cells and failure of maturation of these cells. Another school of thought has been that psoriasis is a disorder of 'uncontrolled' mitosis of the epidermal cells. However, it is likely that this proliferation is secondary to other changes in the skin, and there is now accumulating evidence that biochemical changes probably mediated by altered immunological responses may be responsible for initiating and maintaining the lesions.

Treatment   Each patient must be assessed individually prior to commencing therapy. It must be stressed that at the present time there is no cure for psoriasis, and the patients should be told this. If the disease is minimal and stable, i.e. no new lesions are developing, then patients may accept their psoriasis and no treatment is necessary. All treatments, topical or systemic, have potential side effects and this must be remembered when treatment is undertaken.

Not all treatments will be effective in psoriasis. This seems to depend on what is termed the 'activity' of the disease. If the disease is very active (as suggested by new lesions appearing, and the fact that the disease is extensive), then treatments may fail and if successful, there is a high relapse rate. If this is the case then some form of maintenance treatment will be required. If no new lesions are appearing, chronic or stable psoriasis, then the treatments are usually more effective.

Topical   The more potent the topical steroid the more effective
corticosteroids   it is in clearing psoriasis. As a general rule, weak topical steroids, i.e. hydrocortisone, are not effective in clearing the lesions. Thus the most potent topical steroid clobetasol propionate, should be used for lesions on the trunk and limbs. Ointments are better than creams and should be used twice daily. If clobetasol propionate is going to be effective it will be so

within two or three weeks. It is inadvisable to continue with strong topical steroids indefinitely because of the hazards of these drugs (see Chapter 9). There is also some evidence that topical steroids become less effective with continual use and thus short, intermittent courses are a better approach. If psoriasis involves the face or intertriginous areas then a moderate strength topical steroid should be used, as the risks of side effects of topical steroids are greater in these areas.

Coal tar and ultraviolet light — The less purified the coal tar the more effective it is in clearing psoriasis. The coal tar may be used in a paste or ointment. It is usual to start with 5% crude coal tar and increase to 10%. The tar preparation should be applied daily and covered with tube gauze. A first degree erythema dose of ultraviolet light is given prior to the application of the tar preparation. It usually takes about four weeks to clear psoriasis with this regime. The treatment is 'messy' and time consuming, and many patients will only tolerate the treatment as an in-patient.

Dithranol — This is usually used in a paste, the best being Lassar's paste. It is necessary to start with a concentration of 0.1% and this may be gradually increased to 2.0% if necessary, providing there is no burning of the surrounding skin. However, 0.5% dithranol is often effective in clearing psoriasis. The paste is applied daily and covered with tube gauze dressings. The treatment usually takes three or four weeks. The disadvantage of dithranol is that it stains the clothes and sheets a permanent purple colour, and the skin surrounding the psoriasis a similar colour, but only temporarily. Dithranol is an irritant to normal skin and will burn the skin if it is too strong. Dithranol is often reserved for in-patient treatment and should only be used on an out-patient basis when supervised by those experienced in its use.

Cytotoxic drugs — These have to be used systemically. Cytotoxic drugs should only be considered when the disease is active, i.e. widespread, and there is a rapid relapse after topical treatment. The cytotoxic drugs which have been used in psoriasis are numerous but the most effective is methotrexate. This should be given weekly as a single dose either orally or intramuscularly. A small test dose of 10 mg should be given in the first instance, and providing this is well tolerated, then the dose should be increased to 25 mg. The usual maintenance dose is 25–40 mg per week, to keep the patient clear of the disease. There are numerous side effects which may occur with methotrexate, some of which are serious and some not. Headaches, nausea and lethargy are common symptoms for 48 hours after the administration of methotrexate. The serious side effects include suppression of the bone marrow, gastrointestinal ulceration and hepatic damage which may lead to cirrhosis. Methotrexate therapy should be supervised by a specialist familiar with its use.

PUVA   This stands for psoralens + UVA. Psoralen is a drug which is extracted from a plant which grows in N. Africa but can also be synthesized. It is a photosensitizing agent. UVA is long wave ultraviolet light. By using lamps which only emit UVA and not middle and short wave ultraviolet light the burning effect of ultraviolet light is omitted. The best results are obtained with psoralens taken orally, and then 2 hours later the patient is irradiated with UVA in specially designed apparatus. The rationale of the treatment is still obscure but the psoralens are activated in the skin by UVA. The treatment is carried out 3–4 times a week until the patient is clear, and then maintenance treatment is usually given weekly if required, to stop recurrence.

PUVA treatment is highly effective and pleasant to the patients and one of the side effects is a deep tan. The disadvantages are the fact that it is time consuming, patients having to travel to hospital, but more serious is the possibility of the treatment being carcinogenic if used long term. Only time will tell if the treatment does in fact produce skin malignancies.

Ultraviolet light   It has been known for many years that ultraviolet light will clear psoriasis. The stronger the light the more effective it is. However, one of the hazards is that patients will burn. The latter effect is due to the short and middle wave ultraviolet light. At the Dead Sea the short and middle wave ultraviolet light is absorbed by the water vapour, as the water evaporates from the sea and patients therefore do not suffer sunburn. Thus a special unit for the treatment of psoriasis has been developed at the Dead Sea. It takes approximately four weeks to clear psoriasis. More recently commercial 'solarium' lamps have been used in the treatment of psoriasis, and these emit UVB (middle wave ultraviolet light) and UVA. If the light is carefully monitored so that the patients do not burn, these lamps alone will clear psoriasis, but this usually takes about six weeks.

Systemic corticosteroids
These drugs are capable of clearing psoriasis, but should only be used in certain circumstances as there is a 'rebound' of the psoriasis when the drug is stopped. Systemic steroids may occasionally be necessary in erythroderma or generalized pustular psoriasis.

Aromatic retinoids
A group of new drugs are being developed from retinoic acid, which is vitamin A acid. These drugs are still at an experimental stage but they have an action on epithelial tissues and some appear capable of affecting the psoriatic process. These drugs are not yet available for routine use.

Scalp
Many of the topical preparations are not suitable for treatment of the scalp, mainly because it is difficult to wash them out of the hair, or because they may burn the surrounding skin as in the case of dithranol. Topical steroid lotions have been developed for use in the scalp but they are not as effective as steroid ointments. It is usual therefore in resistant psoriasis to use special preparations for the scalp, and these are a mixture of coal tar and keratolytics – one commonly used is: liquid coal tar 10%; sulphur 5%; salicylic acid 5%; coconut oil 40%; emulsifying ointment 40%.

Nails
Treatment for psoriasis of the nails is limited. If the fault is in the nail matrix then intralesional steroids administered by a 'Dermo-jet' are sometimes helpful. If the problem is in the nail bed underlying the nail plate, then no treatment is available.

Psoriatic arthropathy
The treatment of psoriatic arthropathy is the same as that of rheumatoid arthritis. In the mild form, salicylates should be given, and other anti-inflammatory drugs such as phenylbutazone are helpful in the more severe stages. Gold and cytotoxic drugs are

reserved for the more severe forms of the disorder. Systemic steroids are best avoided, particularly if skin lesions are present, as there may be a rebound of these when the dose of steroids is reduced.

The localized form of pustular psoriasis on the palms and soles is resistant to topical therapy. A treatment which does clear it, but not cure it, is tri-amcinolone 4 mg b.d.; if the disease is incapacitating it is probably justified. More recently some success has been claimed with PUVA, but more treatments than for other forms of psoriasis are required, and more frequent attendance is necessary to maintain clearance.

Generalized pustular psoriasis is a disease which may prove fatal. Admission to hospital is necessary. The disease may go into remission without any specific treatment, but if this is not so then systemic steroids, methotrexate or PUVA may have to be given. The response to these treatments is variable, and it cannot be claimed at present that one is superior to the others.

Natural history and prognosis

There are very few satisfactory studies on the natural history of psoriasis. The reported spontaneous remissions vary from 20 to 40%, but these tend to be for hospital patients who may be the more severely affected individuals. As a general rule the more extensive the disease the more likely it is to be persistent. Guttate psoriasis particularly following streptococcal infections has a good prognosis, the eruption tending to clear after 3 months. Generalized pustular psoriasis is one of the forms of psoriasis which may prove fatal. This occurs in the acute stages. However, if it clears the patients usually revert to the original plaque type variety of psoriasis, but relapse into the pustular form of the disease is common. Erythrodermic psoriasis has a poor prognosis and tends to be persistent.

Psoriasis of the nails and scalp is like psoriasis elsewhere except it is less amenable to treatment. The involvement of these sites may undergo spontaneous remission in the same incidence as psoriasis elsewhere.

Whether psoriasis clears or persists appears to depend on what is termed the activity of the disease. If active then the prognosis is poor and the disease persists. Undoubtedly however, the disease may change from active to inactive states and vice versa. Rapid recurrence after clearance with treatment implies active disease and a poor prognosis.

Psoriatic arthropathy, like rheumatoid arthritis, may be mild and self-limiting, or it may be severe and lead to permanent deformity before burning itself out.

The localized form of pustular psoriasis tends to be persistent, and hence has been termed the recalcitrant eruption of the palms and soles.

38 PURPURA

Purpura is a distinctive clinical sign which has many causes (see Table 38.1). It is caused by extravasation of red blood cells into the dermis.

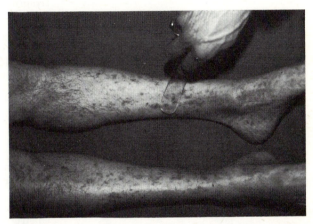

Figure 38.1 **Purpura on the legs; the lesions do not blanch on pressure**

Presentation Purpura occurs at any stage of life, from birth to old age. Each cause has its own peak incidence and sex distribution.

The legs are affected more commonly than any other area of the body because of stasis in the blood vessels there. Purpura can occur anywhere on the skin and mucous membranes.

The lesions are well circumscribed, initially purple but later become reddish-brown (Figure 38.1). They do not blanch on pressure, e.g. with a glass slide. They vary in size from a few mm, petechiae (Figure 38.1), to lesions several centimetres in diameter, ecchymoses (bruises) (Figure 38.2). They may

Table 38.1   The causes of purpura

Thrombocytopenia	Drugs
	Hypersplenism
	Idiopathic thrombocytopenic purpura
	Infections
	Leukaemias and lymphomas
	Marrow aplasia
	Marrow infiltration
	Systemic lupus erythematosus
	Uraemia
Abnormal blood constituents	Cryoglobulinaemia
	Disseminated intravascular coagulation
	Drugs
	Dysproteinaemias
	Infections
Abnormal blood vessels	*Old age
	*Scurvy
	**Steroids (endogenous and exogenous)
Inflammation of blood vessels	**Vasculitis − cutaneous
	− cutaneous − systemic
	− Henoch−Schönlein purpura
Altered local environment	**Eczema
	**Stasis − venous insufficiency
	− postural
	Oedema
	Obstruction
Capillaritis **	
Deficiency diseases	

* Described in detail
** Described elsewhere

be flat, but if due to an inflammatory cause, e.g. vasculitis, they may be papular, and in severe forms bullous (Figure 38.3) or ulcerated.

Purpura may be part of a systemic disease and signs of that disease will be present.

Differential diagnosis   Erythema may be distinguished by blanching on pressure.

Diagnosis and investigations   Purpura has many aetiologies and these must be sought.

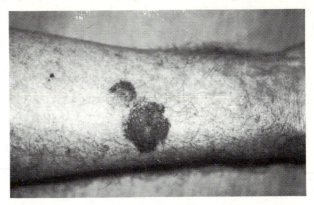

Figure 38.2   Ecchymosis of senile purpura

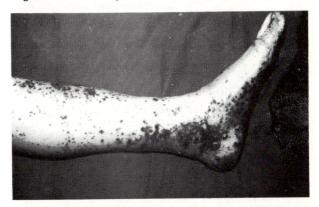

Figure 38.3   Vasculitic purpura; the purpura has become bullous, crusted and ulcerated

The following tests are essential to distinguish the cause; platelet count, full blood count and differential, clotting studies, plasma protein electrophoresis, cryoglobulins, RA latex, ANF and DNA bindings.

Aetiology   Purpura may result from deficiency of platelets, or abnormal function of them, abnormal constituents of blood, or lack of normal constituents, defects of blood vessel walls, altered local environment causing increased permeability, and inflammation of blood vessel walls as in vasculitis and capillaritis.

The main causes of purpura are shown in Table 38.1. Many cases are idiopathic.

Treatment   The treatment of purpura is that of the underlying disease.

Natural history and prognosis	The outcome of purpura varies from spontaneous remission to death; this is determined by the cause.

SENILE PURPURA

This common condition has no pathological significance. Steroid induced purpura has a similar appearance and aetiology.

Presentation	This occurs in old age. Both sexes can be affected, but more women reach the appropriate age. The arms and legs are affected, particularly the backs of the hands. Large purple bruises result from minor trauma (Figure 38.2). The skin is very thin and lacks supporting tissue.
Differential diagnosis	The other forms of purpura may cause confusion, but the involvement of the arms and backs of hands and presence of aged skin are very suggestive of senile purpura. Scurvy should be considered (see below).
Diagnosis and investigations	A full blood count, platelet count and protein strip should be done.
Aetiology	The lack of collagen within the dermis and degeneration of the walls of small blood vessels makes the blood vessels rupture on minimal trauma with consequent extravasation of blood.
Treatment	There is no specific treatment. The arms and legs should be protected from trauma as much as possible.
Natural history and prognosis	Senile purpura persists until the grave.

VITAMIN C DEFICIENCY

Deficiency of vitamin C (ascorbic acid), usually known as scurvy, is a rare but treatable cause of purpura.

Presentation	Scurvy occurs mainly in the malnourished old, whose diet lacks fresh fruit and vegetables. It can also occur in bottle fed infants.

Scurvy occurs mainly in the malnourished old, whose diet lacks fresh fruit and vegetables. It can also occur in bottle fed infants.

There is no sex difference.

The skin lesions are found anywhere on the body, the gums are also affected. There is purpura, consisting of perifollicular petechiae and also ecchymoses in response to minor trauma. Haemarthroses occur. The gums become swollen and tender, and bleed easily. Wounds heal slowly.

There is also osteoporosis and anaemia.

Differential diagnosis

Senile purpura may be confused with scurvy, but the perifollicular haemorrhages are found only in scurvy.

Diagnosis and investigations

The Hess test is positive.

A full blood count and platelet count should be performed. An ascorbic acid saturation test confirms the diagnosis. Often a therapeutic trial of vitamin C is easier to administer.

Aetiology

The purpura, poor wound healing and gum changes are all due to deficient collagen formation.

Treatment

Ascorbic acid should be administered in a dose of 1 g b.d. The patient must be educated to eat a diet containing adequate amounts of ascorbic acid in fruit and vegetables.

Natural history and prognosis

Complete recovery occurs on administration of ascorbic acid. Untreated scurvy can be fatal.

39 PYODERMA GANGRENOSUM

Presentation This is a rare but distinctive disorder. Males and females are equally affected. The disease mainly occurs in adults of any age and is rare in children. The typical lesion begins as a small, tender, red nodule or pustule which rapidly breaks down to form an ulcer. The ulcer slowly increases in size and may eventually be 15–20 cm in diameter. More often the lesion stops increasing in size after it has reached 4–5 cm. The outline of the ulcer is irregular with an

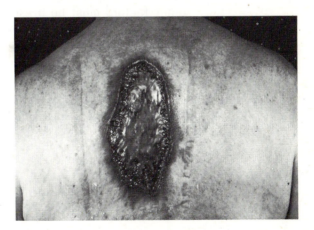

Figure 39.1 Large ulcer with reddish-blue edge in pyoderma gangrenosum

overhanging reddish-blue edge (Figure 39.1). The ulcers may be solitary or multiple although there are very rarely more than ten. The ulcers may heal spontaneously or leave an atrophic scar. The most common sites to be affected are the trunk and buttocks.

Differential diagnosis

Chronic infections may present with persistent ulcers and these have to be distinguished by the appropriate investigations. Very large and solitary basal cell carcinoma on the trunk may present as a large ulcer, but the rolled, pearly edge should give the correct diagnosis.

Investigations

A biopsy should be performed. Full bacteriological and mycological investigations should be carried out including culture of biopsy material if the diagnosis is in doubt. Because of the association with ulcerative colitis, sigmoidoscopy and barium enema should be performed.

Aetiology

Two diseases are associated with pyoderma gangrenosum; these are ulcerative colitis and rheumatoid arthritis. How the skin lesions are produced in these disorders is unknown but it is generally assumed that it has an immunological basis, and the skin lesions may be due to immune complexes. However, pyoderma gangrenosum is rare in both ulcerative colitis and rheumatoid arthritis, and so other factors must be present to produce the skin lesions. Pyoderma gangrenosum may also occur with no underlying disease. Occasionally the lesions are found in debilitated subjects, but no one single deficiency can be shown to be the cause.

Treatment

Cleaning of the ulcers and sterile non-adhesive dressings are used. Systemic steroids are sometimes helpful but not always. Fresh frozen plasma infusions have proved helpful in some patients. Any underlying deficiencies must be corrected. If ulcerative colitis or rheumatoid arthritis is present then treatment of this disease may heal the lesions and stop the development of new ones.

Prognosis and natural history

If the disease is related to ulcerative colitis or rheumatoid arthritis, then the skin lesions often parallel the course of these illnesses. If no underlying disease is found, the course of the skin disorder is variable. It may persist for years with lesions showing spontaneous healing, but new ones developing. Occasionally, however, the disease will burn itself out after one or two years. There are no known complications from the skin lesions.

40 PYOGENIC INFECTIONS

STAPHYLOCOCCAL INFECTIONS

Presentation Cutaneous infection with staphylococcus is very common, either as the primary cause of skin infection or as a secondary invader. *Staphylococcus aureus* is one of the most common causes of cutaneous infections, and it is frequently harboured in healthy individuals in the so-called carrier sites, i.e. nose, axillae, perineum and groins, and this plays a major role in the spreading of the infection. The carrier rate is highest in infancy, even on normal skin, and is low between the ages of 2 and 5. During school age it becomes high, and falls in adolescence. In closed communities, hospitals and institutions, the carrier rate is high.

Skin infection by staphylococcus involves males more than females and the highest incidence is in the first and fourth decades. Recurrent cutaneous infection may occur in diabetes mellitus, nutritional deficiency, alcoholism, systemic corticosteroid therapy, reticulosis and other disorders which affect the body's defence mechanisms.

Folliculitis Folliculitis is an infection in the opening of the hair follicle, although the lesion may extend deeper than the orifice. Clinically the lesions are discrete small pustules which heal without scarring. A similar clinical picture may be produced by chemical or physical damage to the skin but the pus may be sterile. Folliculitis is more common in male adults and the sites of predilection are thighs, buttocks, legs, neck and beard area.

Furunculosis A furuncle is a necrotic infection of a hair follicle caused by *Staphylococcus pyogenes*. Furuncles are most common in young adults; males are affected more than females. Diabetes mellitus, malnutrition, impaired immunity and atopy are predisposing factors. Clinically the lesions are painful, small follicular red papules which enlarge and become pustular and necrotic and discharge pus. The lesion heals with scarring. Lesions may be single or multiple, and most commonly involve the face, neck, buttocks and anogenital area.

Differential diagnosis Acne is the commonest condition in young adults to distinguish from furunculosis. Hidradenitis suppurativa is confined to the axillae and groins. Secondarily infected herpes simplex and zoster can be distinguished by the sites and history.

Carbuncles A carbuncle is infection of a group of adjacent hair follicles with involvement of the surrounding connective tissue, accompanied by an inflammatory reaction. It is most common in the middle aged and elderly male. Diabetes mellitus, malnutrition and impaired immunity are predisposing factors.

Clinically it is a very painful erythematous, deep-seated lesion with multifocal pustules draining pus. The lesions heal with scarring. The commonest sites of involvement are the back, neck, legs, thighs, hips and shoulders.

Differential diagnosis Anthrax has haemorrhagic blisters and satellite vesicles. Syphilitic gumma is painless and there is no constitutional upset. Pyoderma gangrenosum and deep fungal infections must be considered if the lesions fail to respond to antibiotics.

Sycosis Sycosis is a subacute chronic infection by *Staph. pyogenes*. It involves the whole hair follicle with its subsequent destruction.

Clinically sycosis presents as follicular erythematous papules and pustules which may coalesce to produce raised plaques, covered with pus. Sycosis may last for years, without treatment. Healing takes place with scarring. The site of involvement is usually the beard area, but it may occur on the scalp, axillae and genital area.

Differential diagnosis Impetigo produces a more superficial infection. Fungal infections particularly a kerion have a more acute course, but may produce a similar lesion. Lupus vulgaris produces a reddish-brown plaque, but no pustules.

Investigations The lesions produced by staphylococci are diagnosed by the clinical picture, but a *swab* for bacteriology will reveal the organism.

Treatment Folliculitis may require no treatment, but topical antibiotics or antiseptics will clear the infection. In the deeper infections systemic antibiotics should be used. The antibiotic chosen will depend on the sensitivity of the organism. Penicillin and erythromycin are the drugs of choice. In recurrent furunculosis, underlying causes should be excluded. The carrier sites must be treated with topical antiseptics.

STREPTOCOCCAL INFECTIONS: ERYSIPELAS

Presentation Erysipelas is now seen mainly in the newborn, young children and the elderly. The incubation period is 2–5 days. The clinical picture is characterized by sudden onset of pyrexia, malaise, headache, vomiting and discomfort at the site of the lesion.

Within 24 hours the affected areas become a painful, erythematous, indurated, oedematous plaque, with well defined and raised edges (Figure 40.1). Vesicles may be present in the margin of the lesions which spread peripherally. The oedema in facial lesions may be severe and cause closure of the eyelids. There is regional adenitis. The common sites of involvement are the face, ears and lower legs in adults, the abdominal wall in infants, and the face, scalp and limbs in children.

Differential diagnosis Cellulitis is mostly confined to subcutaneous tissue with ill defined borders in contrast to erysipelas which involves the skin.

Herpes zoster infection of the fifth cranial nerve, especially the ophthalmic branch, causes pain a few days prior to the onset of the lesions which are unilateral, grouped blisters.

Contact dermatitis may have a similar appearance, but there is no raised edge to the lesion.

Erysipeloid occurs mostly on the hands as a well defined purplish plaque with central healing. Constitutional upset is mild. Erysipeloid usually occurs in persons handling fish, pigs and poultry.

Angioedema presents as swelling around the eyes but there is no constitutional upset.

Investigations
Bacteriology
Streptococci may be found in the vesicles in the advancing edge of a lesion.

Blood count
A blood count will show a polymorphonuclear leukocytosis.

Serology
There is a rising titre of antistreptolysin O.

Aetiology
Erysipelas is due to Lancefield group A streptococci. Poor general health and damaged skin are predisposing factors.

Treatment
Penicillin is the drug of choice and produces rapid recovery.

Prognosis
Erysipelas is a self-limiting disease and clears without treatment in 1–2 weeks, with desquamation of the skin. There is a tendency for erysipelas to recur in the same area. Recurrent attacks may cause chronic lymphatic obstruction with ensuing lymphoedema. Other rare complications include meningitis, endocarditis and local abscess.

IMPETIGO

Presentation
Impetigo is a superficial infection of the skin caused by streptococci or staphylococci or both. It is common throughout the world, and its incidence is higher in warm climates and during the summer. The infection occurs at any age, but is most common in children.

The clinical manifestations differ, depending on the causative organisms.

Streptococcal impetigo
The cutaneous manifestation consists of an eruption of transitory small vesicles and vesicopustules on an erythematous base. The vesicles rupture and produce superficial erosions with yellowish exudate. The lesions enlarge peripherally.

Staphylococcal **This presents as flaccid bullae on normal skin. The**
impetigo bullae quickly rupture and give rise to yellow
crusted lesions (Figure 40.2). The eruption in impetigo
is asymmetrical. In neonates impetigo presents as
large erosions.

The lesions of impetigo may be single or multiple
due to auto-inoculation. In severe cases there may
be regional adenitis and constitutional upset. The
lesions enlarge peripherally and there may be central healing. Lesions heal without scarring. The sites
of predilection are the face and exposed areas.

Differential In herpes simplex there is a history of a preceding
diagnosis burning sensation and the vesicles and pustules do
not rupture so early.

Secondarily infected eczema has a preceding
history of the eczematous eruption.

Pemphigus may also present as erosions with
crusts. Pemphigus occurs mainly in the middle aged
and elderly, and may be associated with oral ulceration.

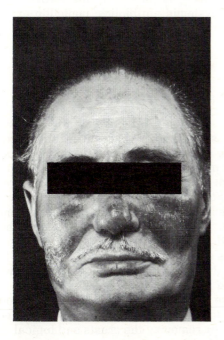
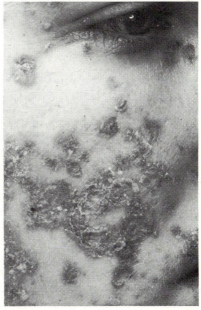

Figure 40.1   Erysipelas   **Figure 40.2   Impetigo**

Investigations The diagnosis can be confirmed by bacteriology.

Histopathology of the lesion shows a blister or erosion beneath the horny layer, and above the granular layer, with a collection of neutrophils in the lesion. The bacteria may be seen in the lesion.

Aetiology Impetigo may be caused by either staphylococci or streptococci or both. Staphylococcal impetigo is caused by *Staph. aureus*. This type of impetigo is seen in temperate climates including the UK.

Non-bullous impetigo is caused by *Strept. pyogenes* or both *Strept. pyogenes* and *Staph. aureus*. The non-bullous type of impetigo is more common in the USA and warm countries. Poor hygiene and malnutrition predispose to the infection.

Prognosis Lesions heal without scarring; without treatment there is eventual clearing of the lesions. Complications are rare, but include cellulitis, nephritis, and septicaemia.

Treatment Topical antibiotics such as fusidic acid and neomycin will clear most lesions. The alternative treatment is with systemic antibiotics; penicillin or erythromycin are the drugs of choice.

ECTHYMA

Ecthyma is a pyogenic infection of the skin with adherent crusts beneath which ulceration occurs. Trauma such as excoriations and insect bites, poor hygiene and malnutrition are predisposing factors. The causative agent is similar to impetigo, i.e. *Strept. pyogenes* or *Staph. aureus* or both. The lesions begin as small vesicles or vesicopustules on an erythematous base, which break down and produce a punched-out ulcer with adherent crust.

The lesions enlarge and may reach a size of a few centimetres. Removing the crust shows an ulcer with a granulating base deep in the dermis.

Lesions are usually multiple and most commonly occur on the lower legs. Ecthyma occurs at all ages. Treatment is by removing the crusts and topical and systemic antibiotics.

41 REITER'S DISEASE

Presentation Reiter's disease is a syndrome of urethritis, conjunctivitis and arthritis, and it may also involve the skin and oral mucosa. Characteristically it is a disorder of males (Figure 41.1). The commonest age group to be affected is 15–25 years and it is very rare in persons under the age of 10, and the elderly (Figure 41.2).

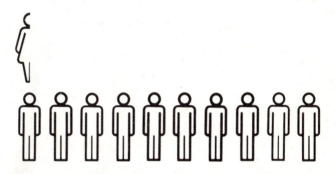

Figure 41.1   Reiter's disease is a disorder predominantly of males

The first sign of the disease is the urethritis followed within two weeks by conjunctivitis and arthritis. The skin lesions may appear at the same time as the conjunctivitis or a few weeks later, and occasionally, months later. The skin is only involved in a small proportion of patients. The initial lesion is a red macule which then changes colour to yellowish-orange and the skin thickens considerably, forming a hyperkeratotic plaque (Figure 41.3). New lesions may develop subsequently and merge together with the older ones. Occasionally the lesions become pustular. On moist areas, i.e. the genitalia, erosions may

351

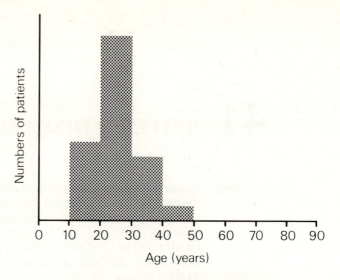

Figure 41.2   Age of onset of Reiter's disease

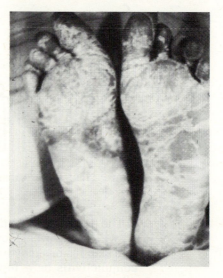

Figure 41.3 Thick hyperkeratotic plaques in Reiter's disease

form and small brown papules appear. If the nails are involved there is gross thickening with subungual hyperkeratosis and the nails may eventually be shed.

The commonest sites to be affected are the palms

and soles. Lesions may appear elsewhere on the body, particularly the legs, umbilicus and scalp. Occasionally the disease becomes widespread with generalized involvement, so-called erythroderma as in psoriasis.

Mucosal lesions occur in approximately a third of patients. Characteristically a circinate balanitis develops. The initial lesion may be a small blister which ruptures to form an erosion. New lesions develop and coalesce so that a circinate lesion forms. The corona of the glans and foreskin are involved. In the circumcised individual a hard crust develops on the glans, and resembles the lesions on the soles.

In the mouth the palate is the commonest site to be affected, but the tongue, buccal mucosa and lips may also be involved. The typical lesion is a red plaque surrounded by a whitish area. Occasionally the lesions present as painless ulcers.

The arthritis is usually asymmetrical and characteristically affects the lower limbs, particularly the knees, ankles, midtarsal and metatarso-phalangeal joints. Involvement of the sacro-iliac joint is also common.

Apart from conjunctivitis, iritis and keratitis may also occur.

Differential diagnosis The skin lesions have to be distinguished from psoriasis on the palms and soles, and if psoriatic arthritis is also present, then it may be difficult to distinguish between the two diseases. The balanitis resembles seborrhoeic eczema with or without secondary monilial infection. If the mouth is involved Behcet's disease has to be considered, but joint involvement is not common in Behcet's disease, and a history of arthritis is lacking in Behcet's disease. Erythema multiforme, the Stevens–Johnson type, may be similar to Reiter's disease in that the genitalia and mouth are involved but if skin lesions are present they are different, and should distinguish between the two disorders.

Investigations
Urethral smears Patients should be seen by a venereologist and their urine and urethral smears examined. Threads will be present in the first specimen of urine passed if micturition has not taken place for at least four

hours. The urethral smear will show pus cells but no organisms. Swabs should be taken to exclude gonorrhoea.

Rheumatoid factor

Blood should be taken to see if the rheumatoid factor is present; it is absent in Reiter's disease.

Mycology

If a balanitis is present, swabs should be taken to exclude monilial balanitis.

Aetiology

Most cases of Reiter's disease follow non-specific urethritis. A small proportion follow dysentery. The infecting organism in non-specific urethritis is a chlamydia, but there is also a proportion of patients who have non-specific urethritis due to non-chlamydial organism, and in these the infecting organisms are not known. It would appear that Reiter's is an immunological reaction, in certain predisposed individuals, to the organisms which cause non-specific urethritis and dysentery. Both non-specific urethritis and dysentery are common diseases and yet Reiter's disease is extremely rare. The underlying factors which predispose to Reiter's disease are not known, but it has been suggested that some patients are potential psoriatics because of the similarity of the skin lesions and the arthritis which occurs in psoriasis.

Treatment

The non-specific urethritis is treated with a two or three week course of tetracycline or erythromycin. The arthritis is managed as in rheumatoid arthritis with salicylates or phenylbutazone in the first instance, and if this is not helpful then gold, systemic corticosteroids, or other immunosuppressive drugs may have to be used. The skin lesions are treated similarly to those of psoriasis with potent topical corticosteroids in the first instance. If these drugs are not successful then other measures as used in psoriasis (Chapter 37) should be considered.

Natural history and prognosis

The disease is usually self limiting and has a good prognosis. The skin lesions last from 2 to 10 months. The arthritis tends to clear after 3 months. The ocular lesions also tend to clear. Occasionally the arthritis and iritis recur, and the former may lead to permanent disability. Very rarely when the skin lesions develop into erythroderma the disease may prove fatal.

Patients with HLA-B27 often progress to ankylosing spondylitis.

42 ROSACEA

Presentation Rosacea is a disease of young adults and middle aged persons. However, it may also present for the first time in elderly persons (Figure 42.1). It is three times as common in females as in males (Figure

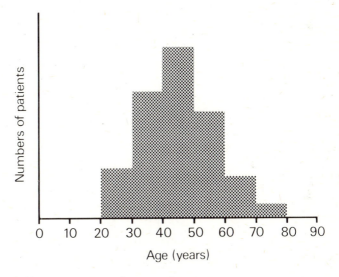

Figure 42.1   Age of onset of rosacea

42.2). Rosacea is a disorder which affects the face (Figure 42.3). It usually begins as flushing attacks and then persistent erythema develops. Subsequently telangiectasia, papules (Figure 42.4) and finally pustules may appear. Rosacea may affect all the face or only parts, e.g. forehead, cheeks or chin. Occasionally papules and pustules may form without background erythema. Rosacea is usually but not always symmetrical.

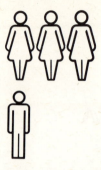

Figure 42.2   Rosacea is more common in females (3 : 1)

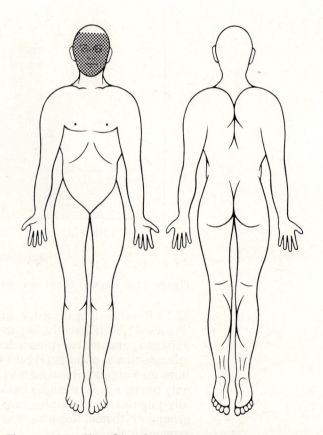

Figure 42.3   Site of involvement in rosacea

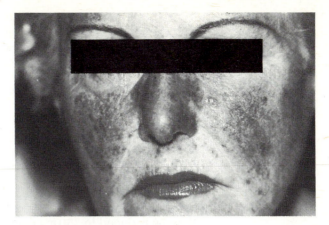

Figure 42.4   Erythema and papules in rosacea

Sometimes considered a variant of rosacea is a condition termed rhinophyma. However, rhinophyma is a disorder of men and is not always associated with changes of rosacea elsewhere on the face. Rhinophyma is enlargement of the nose due to hypertrophy and hyperplasia of the sebaceous glands and connective tissue.

In addition to the skin the eye may be affected in rosacea. There may be blepharitis, conjunctivitis and in some instances, keratitis. The latter is a specific change and associated with corneal vascularization. The eye changes may precede the skin changes, and are present in over half the patients who have rosacea.

Differential diagnosis   The commonest disease to be distinguished from rosacea is acne. The presence of comedones enables the diagnosis of acne to be made, and telangiectasia and general background erythema are not found in acne. Systemic lupus erythematosus which may present as generalized erythema of the face does not have papules or pustules. The carcinoid syndrome may begin as flushing attacks and eventually give rise to persistent erythema.

Perhaps the commonest condition to mimic rosacea is produced by the long term use of potent topical steroids on the face, usually in the treatment of eczema. The face becomes red with telangiectasis and pustules tend to develop when the topical steroid is stopped.

Investigations   There are no investigations that need be carried out in the management of rosacea. The clinical diagnosis is usually obvious, and a skin biopsy need only be performed if there is any doubt about the diagnosis.

Aetiology   The causes of rosacea and rhinophyma are unknown. There is no evidence whatever that dietary factors or an abnormality of the gastrointestinal tract, which have been incriminated in the past, play any part in the aetiology of rosacea.

Treatment   Systemic tetracyclines are the most effective treatment. The dose is 250 mg b.d. until the condition has cleared, usually after 2–3 months. The dose should then be reduced to 250 mg daily for a further period of 6 weeks. If there is no recurrence then the tetracycline may be discontinued. However, in two-thirds of patients the condition will return within 6 months of stopping treatment, and the tetracycline will have to be taken again. These patients will require maintenance therapy of tetracycline 250 mg daily or on alternate days until the disorder goes into spontaneous remission.

Tetracyclines also improve the eye lesions of rosacea but only partially help rhinophyma, which usually has to be dealt with by a plastic surgeon if it is disfiguring.

In the few patients in whom tetracyclines are not helpful, metronidazole 200 mg b.d. may clear the condition. The duration of treatment is the same as for the tetracyclines and maintenance therapy will be necessary.

Prognosis   In the majority of patients rosacea tends to last for a few years, approximately 5–10, after which time the condition clears and no further treatment is required. Occasionally the disease will last longer. Tetracyclines are not a cure and do not seem to shorten the duration of the disease, but they can suppress it adequately. Rhinophyma is persistent once it forms and has to be dealt with surgically.

43 SARCOID

Sarcoid is a disease affecting many organs. There is great variation between patients with regard to which organs are affected and the severity of the disease.

Presentation Sarcoid is rare is childhood. Young adults between the ages of 20 and 40 are usually affected. Women are affected more commonly than men. Although all races are susceptible to sarcoid it is rare in Asians. The incidence is highest in Northern temperate countries. It is common among American negroes but rare in African negroes.

It is a multisystem disorder.

The skin There are several types of cutaneous lesions:

Erythema nodosum This is a common manifestation of sarcoid (see page 507) (Figure 43.1).

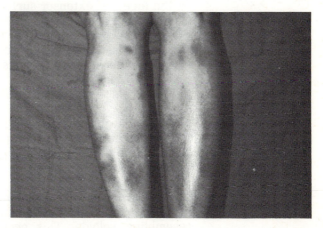

Figure 43.1 Erythema nodosum in acute sarcoid

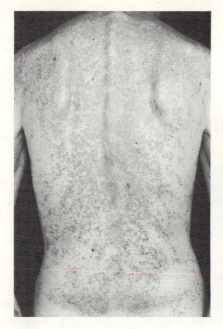

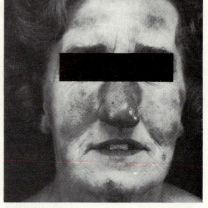

Figure 43.2 Numerous papules in acute sarcoid

Figure 43.3 Lupus pernio: infiltration of nose, ear lobes and plaques on cheeks, chin and forehead

Papular lesions

These present as crops of numerous small papules on the face and extensor surfaces of the limbs, and elsewhere (Figure 43.2). They may become confluent. Deep papules may be palpable in the subcutaneous tissues. The skin is normal in texture, but they are often yellow, or purplish-red in colour. They resolve with scarring.

They are associated with a good prognosis.

Nodular lesions

These are larger than papular lesions. They arise on the face, trunk and proximal portions of the limbs. They can be superficial or deep. They are yellow or purplish in colour.

Scar sarcoid

This arises in old scars, immunization or venepuncture sites. The scars become infiltrated and purple, resembling keloids. This occurs in acute active disease.

Plaques	These occur on shoulders, buttocks, and thighs. Large indurated plaques develop. Their association is with chronic disease and a poor prognosis.
Annular sarcoid	This is confined to the head and neck. The lesions have a peripheral scaly edge and central hypopigmented scarred area. They are associated with chronic disease and a poor prognosis.
Lupus pernio	This affects poorly perfused peripheral areas, i.e. nose, ear lobes and fingers. These areas become swollen and indurated, with a deep purplish-red colour (Figure 43.3). The phalangeal bones may contain bone cysts due to sarcoid granulomas, and the nasal bones may be eroded. Lupus pernio is a sign of a bad prognosis.
The lungs	The intrathoracic lymph nodes are commonly involved, particularly the hilar nodes. This is often asymptomatic. Pulmonary infiltrates are more serious and may progress to pulmonary fibrosis. Bronchial stenosis and obstruction can be troublesome.
The eyes	Anterior and posterior uveitis, conjunctivitis, and dry eyes all occur.
The kidneys	Hypercalciuria and hypercalcaemia can give rise to nephrocalcinosis and renal failure.
Nasal lesions	Erosion of the nasal bones, nasal discharge and obstruction are common, particularly in negroes.
The lymphoreticular system	Lymph nodes are frequently enlarged. Hepatosplenomegaly may occur.
Joints	Arthralgia and acute arthritis can occur.
The bones	Bone lesions occur in nose and fingers in association with lupus pernio.
The nervous system	Cranial nerve palsies are common. Central nervous system involvement is a rare but serious complication.
The heart	Cardiac involvement is unusual but sometimes fatal.
Sjogren's syndrome	This occurs in sacroid.

Constitutional symptoms	Fever, malaise and weight loss occur.

Specific syndromes are seen in sarcoid. These are: (1) Erythema nodosum associated with bilateral hilar lymphadenopathy and arthralgia. This is common in Irish women. This is acute and has an excellent prognosis. (2) Lupus pernio with its combination of skin and bone lesion is a very distinctive and chronic form. (3) Uveoparotid fever (Heerfordt's syndrome) is uveitis with swollen parotids, facial nerve palsies and fever.

There is an increased incidence of lymphomas in patients with sarcoid. |
Differential diagnosis	Cutaneous sarcoid may resemble lupus erythematosus, tuberculosis, leprosy and granuloma annulare. Other signs of systemic disease reveal the diagnosis. Biopsy is essential.
Diagnosis and investigations *Biopsy*	Skin biopsy shows the typical sarcoid granulomas. Other biopsies can be taken from liver, lymph nodes, lungs and conjunctiva.
Cell mediated immunity	As shown by delayed skin tests, cell mediated immunity is depressed.
Mantoux test	This is negative.
Kveim test	This is positive.
Blood tests	There may be a leukopenia or lymphopenia. Hypergammaglobulinaemia is common. Serum calcium and liver function tests should be done.
Urine tests	Urinary calcium must be measured.
Respiratory function tests	These are mandatory.
X-ray	Nose and hand X-rays may be helpful. Chest X-ray is mandatory.
Aetiology	The cause of sarcoid is unknown. There is defective T-cell function but it is not known whether this is involved in the pathogenesis, and if it is primary or secondary.

Treatment Most cases do not require treatment. The cutaneous lesions may respond to intralesional steroids; systemic steroids are not always effective. Systemic steroids are given for severe constitutional symptoms: deteriorating lung function, uveitis, hypercalcaemia, neurological and cardiac disease.

Natural history and prognosis Sarcoid may be an acute or asymptomatic disease resolving in a few months or a chronic and serious disease extending over many years. Some patients recover with serious sequelae, e.g. impaired vision, respiratory or renal function. Many make a full recovery. The mortality is 5%; those dying do so from pulmonary or cardiac disease.

44 SCLERODERMA

Scleroderma is also known as systemic sclerosis because the process involves many different systems.
The disease is very variable both in terms of systems
affected and severity.

Presentation
Scleroderma may commence from childhood onwards, but most commonly between 30 and 60. Men
are affected later than women. Women outnumber
men 4 : 1 (Figure 44.1). All races are affected but it
seems to be most common in negroes.

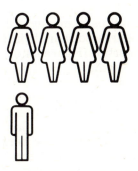

Figure 44.1 Sex ratio in scleroderma

It is a multisystem disease, but in some patients
only a few systems will be involved.

Cutaneous
lesions
The face and hands are most often affected, the neck
and upper chest next most frequently, the entire skin
may be involved. It is sometimes difficult to define
where the skin becomes normal. The sclerodermat-
ous skin is shiny and often hypo- or hyperpigmented;
it feels hard and is taut and tightly bound down to
underlying tissue. The hypopigmentation may be so
extensive that it gives a picture like vitiligo.

The face assumes a mask-like appearance, it becomes immobile, opening of the mouth is restricted, the nose becomes beaklike (Figure 44.2), and the lower eyelid cannot be pulled down. Macular telangiectasia may be numerous (Figure 44.3).

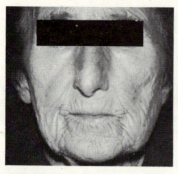 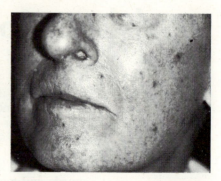

Figure 44.2 Scleroderma showing pinched nose and mouth

Figure 44.3 Macular telangiectasia on the face

The hands are nearly always involved. The usual picture is of sclerodactyly. The fingers are shiny, tapered and permanently flexed. There is pulp atrophy, depressed scars from ischaemia, and often loss of fingertips (Figure 44.4). The nail folds show abnormal capillaries and nail fold infarcts. The nails show the changes of ischaemia, discolouration, brittleness and longitudinal ridging; there may be beaking due to pulp atrophy and pterygium inversus. The nails may be shed. Calcinosis cutis due to deposits of calcium in the dermis may be marked, and is usually located on the fingers (Figure 44.5); they discharge through the skin and can be very uncomfortable.

The fingers are sometimes swollen and shiny, often red, and called 'sausage fingers'.

The whole hands may be involved.

Raynaud's phenomenon This is the most common presentation of scleroderma, but it may be many years before further features develop.

Gastro-intestinal tract The entire gastro-intestinal tract can be involved. The gums become abnormal, and the mouth may be dry because of Sjogren's syndrome. Oesophageal involvement occurs in 75% of patients, there may be

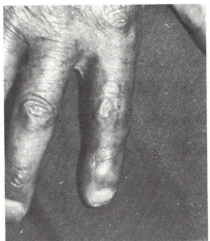

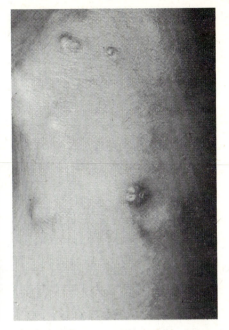

Figure 44.4   Fingers in scleroderma, showing tight shiny skin and loss of fingertip

Figure 44.5   Calcinosis cutis, showing subcutaneous deposits of calcium

reflux, abnormal peristalsis and aspiration. Small intestinal disease causes stagnant loop syndrome and malabsorption. The colon is a frequent site for scleroderma, which causes characteristic diverticulae; perforation of these leads to peritonitis.

The liver   Primary biliary cirrhosis occurs more commonly than usual in patients with scleroderma.

The kidney   Renal involvement manifest by proteinuria and hypertension is a very bad prognostic sign. Most patients with hypertension die within a year.

The heart   Cardiac involvement causes heart failure and dysrhythmias; the latter can cause sudden death.

The lungs   Pulmonary fibrosis occurs, and predisposes to lung cancer. There may also be external restriction of movement and aspiration pneumonia.

The joints   Acute arthritis may occur as part of scleroderma.

Sjogren's syndrome Sjogren's syndrome is found as part of scleroderma. The patient may notice dry eyes and mouth.

CRST syndrome CRST syndrome is a variant of scleroderma. It comprises calcinosis cutis (C), Raynaud's phenomenon (R), sclerodactyly (S) and macular telangiectasia (T); in addition the oesophagus is usually involved. It has a very good prognosis and serious visceral involvement is rare.

Differential diagnosis The clinical appearance of scleroderma is unique. The scleroderma-like changes occasionally seen in mixed connective tissue disease or dermatomyositis occasionally cause diagnostic problems, but the rest of the clinical picture and serology should differentiate it.

Diagnosis and investigations
Skin biopsy Biopsy is rarely necessary but is characteristic. Immunofluorescence is negative.

Blood tests The ESR is raised in the acute phase. Renal function should be assessed and malabsorption looked for. The ANF is often present in very high titres and is usually nucleolar in pattern. RNA antibodies are present.

Chest X-ray Chest X-ray, in combination with respiratory function studies, show the extent of pulmonary involvement.
Barium swallow and barium meal are both diagnostic as the abnormalities of scleroderma are unique.

Aetiology It is speculated that the basic defect is either some auto-immune phenomenon or an abnormality of collagen.

Treatment The huge number of diverse treatments tried emphasizes the failure of any to alter the course of the disease. Steroids may dramatically worsen the hypertension.
The hands should always be kept warm, and smoking discouraged, to preserve the fingers. Attenuated androgens, e.g. stanozolol, may alleviate the Raynaud's.

Natural history and prognosis The prognosis is very variable; life expectancy can be a few months or over 30 years. Fifty per cent are dead within 5 years. They die from renal failure, cardiac dysrhythmias and intestinal perforation. The morbidity from the Raynaud's phenomenon is considerable.

45 SELF-INDUCED DERMATOSES

DERMATITIS ARTEFACTA

Presentation Dermatitis artefacta is self-inflicted skin lesions, and is more common in patients with personality disturbances. Lesions may occur at all ages and in both sexes, but are more common in young and middle aged females (Figures 45.1 and 45.2).

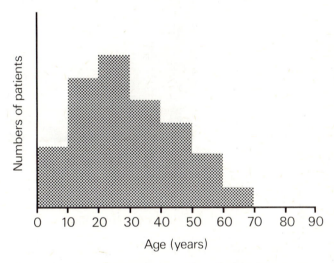

Figure 45.1 Age distribution of dermatitis artefacta

The lesions are characterized by sudden onset and bizarre and irregular configuration. The morphology of the lesions depends on how they are produced, e.g. punctate ulcers (Figure 45.3) by digging the skin with the nails, linear cuts and ulcers (Figure 45.4) from sharp instruments, necrotic ulcers and blisters by caustic chemicals and heat.

371

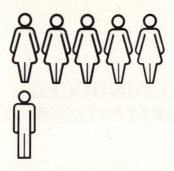

Figure 45.2 Dermatitis artefacta is more common in females (5 : 1)

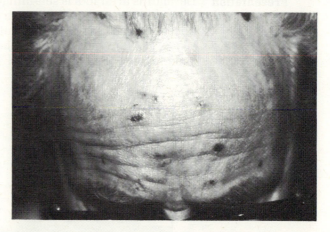

Figure 45.3 Ulcers on the forehead in dermatitis artefacta

The lesions are in a region of easy access, and may be single or numerous.

Differential diagnosis Bacterial infections may produce bizarre lesions, but the diagnosis can be established by bacteriological studies.

Necrotic ulcers occur in vasculitis, which is most commonly seen on the legs. A biopsy may be necessary to establish the diagnosis. Porphyria cutanea tarda may present with erosions in exposed areas which may be confused with dermatitis artefacta.

Investigations Biopsy shows necrosis and inflammation. Swabs are necessary to exclude bacterial infections.

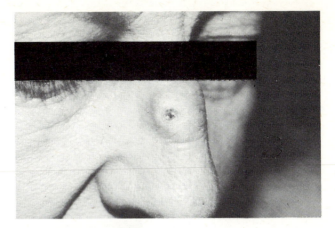

Figure 45.4 Dermatitis artefacta: solitary ulcer with surrounding thickening of the skin

Aetiology   Dermatitis artefacta is most commonly seen in persons with personality disorders. Occasionally it is seen in other psychiatric illnesses. Dermatitis artefacta is also seen in malingerers as a way of avoiding work.

Treatment   The skin lesions should be treated symptomatically. If new lesions appear or the old ones fail to heal, occlusive bandages are useful as they heal the lesions and confirm the diagnosis. Although patients are often in need of psychiatric help this is often refused by the patient.

Prognosis   The prognosis often depends on the underlying psychological state. If the patient refuses help then the dermatitis artefacta may persist indefinitely. Patients frequently discharge themselves from the skin clinic when told that it is suspected that the lesions are self-induced, only to reappear at another skin clinic. Severe scarring may result from some of the lesions if the damage is deep.

NEUROTIC EXCORIATIONS

Presentation   Neurotic excoriations are self-induced lesions due to scratching or picking the skin. The condition is seen

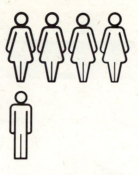

Figure 45.5 Neurotic excoriations are commoner in women (4 : 1)

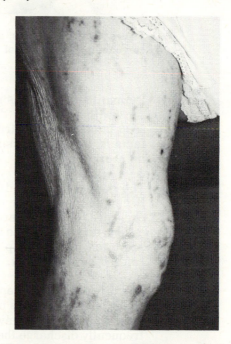

Figure 45.6 Linear lesions in neurotic excoriations

in both sexes, but is more common in young and middle aged women (Figure 45.5).

Clinically the lesions are characterized by linear excoriations (Figure 45.6) or small crusted ulcers. The patient admits to picking or scratching the skin, and complains of irritation. The lesions may leave scarring. The sites of predilection are the upper back, shoulders, face and arms.

Differential diagnosis Pruritus due to internal causes is not associated with a rash, and often the skin is not excoriated in this instance, but if it is, the damage is considerably less than in neurotic excoriations. Pediculosis pubis or corporis may cause irritation of the trunk, and the lice and nits should be looked for. Scabies may cause generalized irritation with a minimal eruption but burrows will usually be found on close inspection. Occasionally dermatitis artefacta may have similar lesions, but the patient will not admit to producing the lesions.

Investigations None are necessary if the diagnosis is made with certainty. If in doubt, causes of pruritus (see chapter 36) should be excluded.

Aetiology Neurotic excoriations are seen in patients with underlying psychiatric illness, which may be minor or part of a more serious illness.

Treatment Symptomatic treatment with bland topical preparations. If the problem persists, psychiatric assessment is indicated.

46 SKIN TUMOURS (BENIGN) AND NAEVI

The distinction between benign tumours and naevi is arbitrary. It can be argued that so-called naevi, which are attributable to developmental abnormalities, are benign tumours. Conversely, lesions which are obviously benign tumours, e.g. granuloma pyogenica, could also be due to a developmental predisposition, although not obvious on histological examination, or by accepted criteria. However there are areas where there is obvious overlap and thus it is convenient to consider naevi and benign tumours together. All the cell types in the skin may present as benign tumours, or naevi, although some are more commonly affected than others.

MELANOCYTIC NAEVI

Presentation
This is the most common type of naevus and is often referred to as a 'mole'. The abnormality affects the melanocytes of the epidermis and also cells derived from Schwann cells. Over 95% of Caucasians have one or more melanocytic naevi. These naevi are not usually present at birth; they begin to appear during childhood and may appear at the time of adolescence, and some in early adult life (Figure 46.1). They may also appear for the first time during pregnancy and when patients take the contraceptive pill. After middle age no new naevi appear, and they disappear in old age. The sexes appear to be equally affected although some studies have reported a higher frequency in females in childhood.

Melanocytic naevi have a wide variety of presentation, and this is probably dependent on what stage in their evolution development stops. The naevus

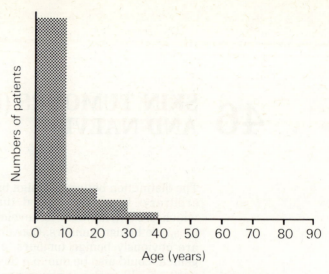

Numbers of patients

Age (years)

Figure 46.1   Age of onset of melanocytic naevi

begins as proliferation of the melanocytes in the epidermis and at this stage the lesions appear as flat pigmented areas, and are sometimes termed the junctional naevus. If no further progression of development takes place the lesion persists as a macular, well circumscribed pigmented area. Pigmentation may be uniform or variable. On the palms, soles and genitalia, the lesion persists as a macular pigmented area and no further change takes place. In the next phase of development the proliferating melanocytes migrate into the dermis and form clumps or columns of cells.

A naevus which has junctional and intradermal components is referred to as a compound naevus. Clinically a compound naevus presents as a small raised pigmented papule, which usually has a smooth surface. Compound naevi often increase in size and in the amount of pigmentation around puberty, and at this stage, coarse hairs may appear growing from the surface of the lesion. If the superficial cells in the dermis proliferate they throw the overlying epidermis into folds, thus giving a surface with numerous clefts.

The final stage in development occurs when the epidermal melanocytes stop proliferating and then the naevus becomes wholly intradermal. In addition, components from Schwann cells in the dermis form parts of the intradermal naevus. When the naevus is wholly intradermal the melanocytes may or may not stop producing melanin. The deeper cells in the naevus usually stop melanin production. An intradermal naevus may therefore present as a pigmented or non-pigmented lesion. It is raised and most frequently dome shaped (Figure 46.2).

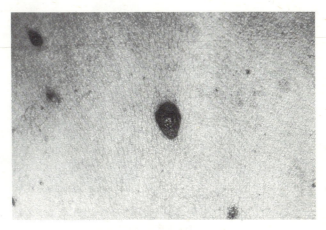

Figure 46.2   Melanocytic naevi

Clinically the size and surface of melanocytic naevi may vary from a few mm to a few cm. The surface may be smooth, but on occasions is clefted. Occasionally naevi may be pedunculated, particularly around the neck, axillae and groins.

There is a very rare type of melanocytic naevus which is present at birth and is termed the *congenital melanocytic naevus*. Compared to other melanocytic naevi which develop after birth, congenital ones are extremely rare. The lesions are raised and have an irregular surface. The size may vary from a few mm to being very extensive involving the whole of an anatomical part such as a limb (Figure 46.3), bathing trunk area, scalp or neck. These lesions are sometimes known as animal skin naevi. These lesions become thicker and hairy in childhood. Occasionally this type of naevus is associated with other severe developmental abnormalities such as spina bifida, when it is over the vertebral column, and hypertrophy or atrophy of the deeper structure when it is on a limb.

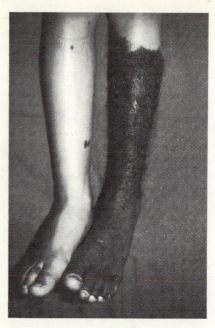

Figure 46.3   Congenital melanocytic naevus involving the lower leg

Differential diagnosis In childhood the melanocytic naevus has to be distinguished from macular or nodular lesions which may occur in urticaria pigmentosa. In the latter the lesions urticate and are usually numerous and occur at an earlier age than naevi. Xanthogranulomas which present in growing children have a more yellowish appearance.

Around puberty the so-called juvenile melanoma may appear. This is usually redder because of an increase in vascularity which does not occur in melanocytic naevi. The lesion grows rapidly for a few months and then remains static in size.

In adults, seborrhoeic warts have to be distinguished from naevi. The former usually appear for the first time much later in life. The surface of seborrhoeic warts is usually rough and clefted. The amount of pigment in a seborrhoeic wart varies from being absent to large quantities giving a black colour. Pigmented basal cell carcinomata usually appear in middle aged or elderly persons and the lesions tend to ulcerate. Occasionally, however, cystic basal cell carcinomata become pigmented, but the pigmentation tends to be irregular, and telangiectasia are usually seen on the non-pigmented areas. Histiocytomata are pigmented dermal lesions and are usually situated deeper in the skin.

The most important distinction has to be made from a malignant melanoma. The latter are extremely rare before puberty. If a pigmented lesion is rapidly growing, changing colour, or showing signs of ulceration, then a malignant process must be considered, although melanocytic naevi can show change in size and pigmentation.

The congenital pigmented naevus has a similar appearance to the pigmented hairy epidermal naevus. The latter however is not present at birth.

Investigations   The only investigation is histological if the lesion is excised.

Aetiology   The cause of the abnormality in the melanocytes and their behaviour is unknown. However, because the lesions are so common, being present in 95% of Caucasians, they should not be considered as an abnormality, but a variation of normal cutaneous reactions. A hereditary factor has been implicated in some instances, particularly when large numbers of naevi occur in successive generations. A hormonal influence has been suggested, because of the naevi which appear around puberty, during pregnancy, or whilst taking the contraceptive pill.

Treatment   The only treatment, if any is required, is surgical excision. If the lesions are extensive, they have to be dealt with by a plastic surgeon. Since nearly all persons have some naevi, they are usually accepted as being normal. However, the commonest reason for removal is cosmetic.

The question is often asked whether melanocytic naevi are more likely to develop into malignant melanomata than normal skin. Although malignant change does occur in pigmented naevi the chance is so small that it can be ignored. There is also no truth in the belief that naevi on the palms, soles and genitalia are more likely to become malignant than lesions elsewhere. The one type of naevus which does have a high risk of malignant change is the congenital pigmented naevus, the risk of malignancy being estimated at nearly 10%.

Prognosis As has already been alluded to, melanocytic naevi may increase in size and vary their pigmentation, particularly at puberty and during pregnancy. Once established in adults they tend not to alter until after middle age when they may begin to involute. The melanocytic naevus is very rare in elderly persons. The risk of malignant change is insignificant (except in the congenital pigmented naevus) and some authorities do not consider it higher than in normal skin. The congenital pigmented naevus does carry a risk of malignant change and should therefore be excised if this is feasible.

JUVENILE MELANOMA

Presentation The lesion usually presents in early childhood, but may appear any time up to middle age. The sexes are equally affected. The lesion is solitary and has a reddish or reddish-brown appearance. The lesion grows rapidly and may reach a diameter of 2 cm, although 1 cm is more common. Initially the surface is smooth, but later becomes rough and scaly. The commonest sites are the face and legs.

Differential diagnosis The lesion has to be distinguished from the ordinary melanocytic naevus. The rapid growth often suggests a malignant melanoma in post-puberty patients. A xanthogranuloma if solitary may have a similar appearance, although it is usually more yellow. In adults, histiocytomata have to be considered, but they are usually smaller and deeper. Dermatofibrosarcomata may have a similar appearance and often the diagnosis can only be made by histological examination.

Investigations Biopsy excision of the lesion for histological examination is indicated if the diagnosis is in doubt. The histology may mimic a malignant melanoma. Therefore an expert opinion is necessary.

Aetiology At present this type of lesion is best considered to be a variant of a melanocytic naevus, although histologically there are different features.

Treatment If the diagnosis is made with certainty and the lesion is relatively small, then no treatment is necessary.

The only way of removing the lesion is by surgical excision.

Natural history and prognosis   Juvenile melanoma is a benign lesion. After an initial growth when it first appears the lesion remains static.

HALO NAEVUS

This is an area of depigmentation around a melanocytic naevus (Figure 46.4). It may form around one or a number of naevi. This phenomenon is seen in childhood or adult life and the naevus gradually disappears after a few months. The area of depigmentation may then repigment. The halo naevus may be

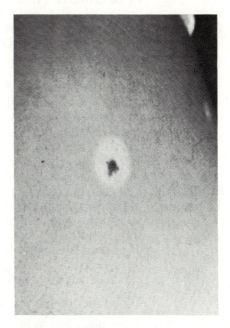

Figure 46.4   Halo naevus: Area of depigmentation around melanocytic naevus

found in association with vitiligo and is thought to be an auto-immune process with antibodies against the melanocytes of the naevus. The lesion is not malignant and no treatment is required.

BLUE NAEVUS

This is so called because it has a bluish appearance. It is however a melanocytic naevus due to adherent melanocytes in the dermis which have failed to arrive at the epidermis. The colour is probably due to the depth of the naevus and subsequent reflection of light.

The lesions are commoner in females. The commonest sites are the backs of the hands, feet and buttocks. The lesion is usually raised and up to 1 cm in diameter. The lesions are benign and treatment is for cosmetic reasons, by surgical excision.

EPIDERMAL NAEVI

These may be present at birth or appear early in infancy or childhood. Occasionally they may appear for the first time in adult life. There is no sex predominance.

The characteristic feature of epidermal naevi is that they have a rough or warty appearance. They may be skin coloured or pigmented. The lesions may be single or multiple, and often have a linear morphology (Figure 46.5). Occasionally they are extensive and affect large areas of the body.

Differential diagnosis   Viral warts exhibiting the Koebner phenomenon may present as a linear warty lesion. The roughened surface of the epidermal naevus usually distinguishes it from other melanocytic naevi. There is a linear form of eczema known as lichen striatus which appears on a limb in a child and lasts for approximately eighteen months before showing spontaneous resolution.

Investigations   If the diagnosis is in doubt a biopsy will be helpful. The predominant change is in the epidermis.

Aetiology   As with other types of naevi, the cause is thought to be a developmental defect. The bizarre linear configuration is difficult to explain.

Treatment   The lesion can only be treated by surgical excision or cryotherapy.

Natural history and prognosis The lesions will persist if untreated. There is a very small risk of neoplastic change. This is suggested by sudden change in a localized part of the lesion.

PIGMENTED HAIRY EPIDERMAL NAEVUS (BECKER'S NAEVUS)

Presentation This is a distinct clinical entity. The lesion is usually first apparent in adolescence. It is predominantly a disorder of males (Figure 46.6). The lesion commences as a localized area of increased pigmentation. After a year or two, coarse dark hairs develop in the area of pigmentation. The affected skin also then becomes thicker and rougher. The most commonly affected area is the shoulder (Figure 46.7).

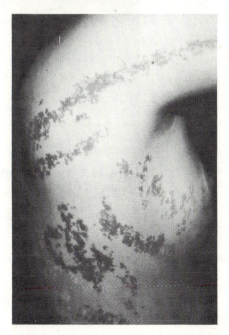

Figure 46.5 Extensive epidermal naevus

Differential diagnosis The condition that may have a similar appearance is the congenital pigmented naevus. The latter how-

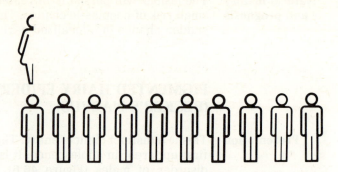

Figure 46.6   Becker's naevus is predominantly found in males

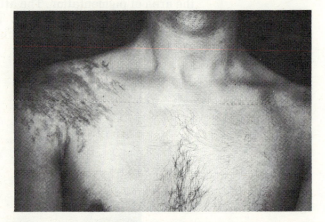

Figure 46.7   Becker's naevus is commonly found on the shoulder

ever usually begins at a much earlier age or is present at birth.

Investigations   If the diagnosis is in doubt a biopsy will confirm it. The principal changes are in the epidermis.

Aetiology   Unknown, but is considered as a development abnormality.

Treatment   As the lesion is usually extensive, treatment is difficult; plastic surgery is the only treatment that may be considered.

Natural history and prognosis   The lesion is persistent.

BENIGN TUMOURS AND NAEVI OF BLOOD VESSELS: MATURE CAPILLARY NAEVUS (PORTWINE STAIN)

Presentation The sexes are equally affected. The lesions are usually present at birth. The naevus may range in colour from pale pink to deep purple (Figure 46.8). The lesion is usually flat but on occasions is slightly raised. The size may vary from a few millimetres to large confluent areas of skin. The commonest sites to be involved are the face and upper trunk (Figure 46.9). This type of naevus is usually on one side of the body and does not cross the midline.

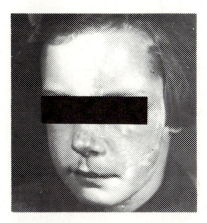

Figure 46.8 Portwine stain (mature capillary naevus)

Differential diagnosis The diagnosis is rarely in doubt. The lesion blanches on pressure as opposed to flat melanocytic naevi whose colour will not change. Occasionally flat capillary haemangiomata are accompanied by vascular abnormalities of the deeper tissues, the most common being the Sturge–Weber syndrome in which there is involvement of the meninges and eye.

Treatment If the lesions are small they may be amenable to plastic surgery. If not the patient should be referred to a person experienced in skin camouflage at the appropriate age.

Natural history These lesions are formed from mature vessels and are persistent throughout life.

IMMATURE HAEMANGIOMAS (STRAWBERRY NAEVUS)

Presentation The lesions are not usually present at birth, but make their appearance at about 4–6 weeks of age. The sexes are equally affected. The lesions commence as small red spots of 1–2 mm and then rapidly enlarge, growing until the child is 6–9 months old. The eventual size may vary from a few mm to several cm, and the lesions are raised (Figure 46.10). Occa-

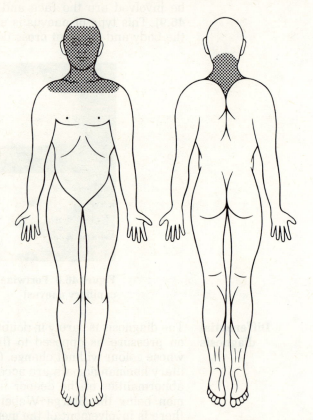

Figure 46.9 Common sites of mature capillary naevi (portwine stains)

sionally there is a deeper subcutaneous component, which is seen as a bluish swelling under the skin surrounding the red, superficial component. These naevi may affect any part of the skin and are frequently multiple.

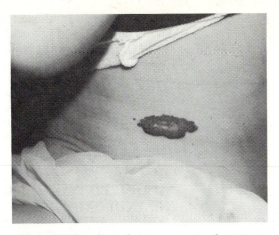

Figure 46.10 Strawberry naevus (immature capillary naevus)

Differential diagnosis

This is not usually a problem, the history being so typical. The mature capillary naevus is flat and present at birth.

Aetiology

The immature haemangioma is derived from angioblastic tissue which fails to establish normal contact with other developing vascular tissue. These islands of vascular tissue then proliferate abnormally and develop into haemangiomas. As with other naevi the cause is unknown.

Treatment

The important point is to stress to the parents that nearly all these lesions undergo spontaneous resolution and are best left alone. If the lesions are still present after the age of 6, then surgery may have to be considered.

Natural history and prognosis

The prognosis of this type of lesion is excellent. After the initial growth period up to the age of 9 months the lesions remain static until the age of 2–3 years. The centre of the lesion then begins to fade and become white and the lesion then slowly regresses in size so that by the age of 5 or 6 it has disappeared, the colour of the skin being normal. If the lesion has been very extensive some puckering of the skin may remain which can be dealt with surgically.

There are a few complications associated with these naevi. If the lesion is on the eyelid it may close the eye and stop the development of binocular vision.

In this instance the lesion should be treated with a small dose of radiotherapy or a short course of systemic steroids. Ulceration of the skin over the tumour may occur because of the abnormal blood supply, but usually heals quickly, as ulceration leads to thrombosis of the vessels and more rapid resolution of the tumour. Occasionally thrombocytopenia occurs. This is due to the tumour trapping platelets. If it is a problem then the naevus is treated with radiotherapy.

ACQUIRED HAEMANGIOMA (PYOGENIC GRANULOMA)

Presentation   This is a distinct entity presenting at any age and the sexes are equally affected. The lesion is a small bright red papule. As the lesion bleeds easily on slight trauma (Figure 46.11) it is often covered by a dark scab. The size varies from 0.5 to 1.0 cm. The initial growth is rapid over a matter of weeks. The lesion then persists without further increase in size. The lesion may occur anywhere.

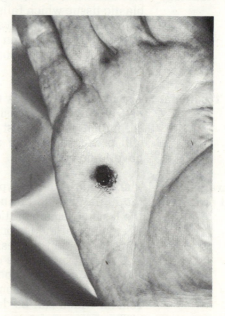

Figure 46.11 Pyogenic granuloma presenting as a haemorrhagic papule on the palm

Differential diagnosis   The lesion may be confused with both benign and malignant neoplasms which bleed. The important lesion that may present diagnostic problems is the malignant melanoma. Viral warts which bleed may also present as papules with a dark scab.

Investigations   The lesion should always be sent for histological examination when removed.

Aetiology   The lesion is a proliferation of capillaries. It used to be thought that it was caused by infective agents – hence the name pyogenic granuloma. However, there is no evidence to support this theory. The exact cause is unknown but it may be an abnormal proliferation of blood vessels in predisposed individuals to trauma.

Treatment   The simplest and most effective treatment is curretage and cautery. This seems to offer a higher cure rate than simple excision and leaves a better cosmetic result.

Natural history and prognosis   The lesions are benign but persist and show no signs of spontaneous remission. They have to be removed for cosmetic reasons and the fact that they bleed easily. There is a recurrence of the lesion in a small percentage of patients, and this is attributed to the fact that the capillaries, which have the ability to proliferate and cause the lesion, are situated deep in the dermis in some lesions and are not destroyed on the initial removal.

GLOMUS TUMOUR

Presentation   The lesions may be present at birth otherwise the lesions present in childhood or adult life. There is no sex predilection. The lesion is a pink or purplish nodule varying from 1 to 20 mm, and is painful, the pain being provoked by pressure or temperature change. The hands and feet are the commonest sites, and they may appear under the nails. The lesions may be solitary or multiple.

Differential diagnosis   Pain is the distinguishing feature, and thus other painful lesions such as leiomyomata and certain sweat gland tumours have to be considered.

Investigations   Histological examination of the excised lesion.

Aetiology   The tumour is composed of angiomatous and neural components, and the latter is the cause of the pain. The lesion is a development defect.

Treatment   Surgical excision.

Course and natural history   The lesion is benign, but excision is necessary because of the pain.

CAMPBELL DE MORGAN SPOTS

Presentation   These lesions are common in middle aged and elderly persons. The sexes are equally affected. The lesions are small bright papules which grow up to 5 cm. They are situated predominantly on the trunk and are usually multiple.

Differential diagnosis   The characteristic appearance and the fact that they are multiple usually make the diagnosis obvious. Multiple pyogenic granuloma may be similar, but these lesions bleed and Campbell de Morgan spots do not.

Aetiology   This is unknown. The lesion is a haemangioma.

Treatment   None is necessary, but if the lesions are a cosmetic embarrassment they can be cauterized.

Course and prognosis   The lesions are benign, but show no signs of spontaneous resolution once they have formed.

SPIDER NAEVUS

Presentation   The lesions are common in children and adults, and are particularly so in pregnant women. The lesion has a small central, raised red papule 1–2 mm in diameter with small telangiectasia radiating from the central papule (Figure 46.12). The telangiectasia may extend up to 1 cm from the central lesion. The commonest site for spider naevi is the face, but they may be found on the upper limbs and upper trunk.

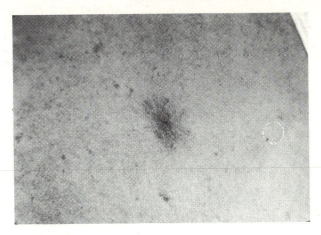

Figure 46.12   Spider naevus

Differential diagnosis
The appearances are so typical that the lesion rarely presents a diagnostic problem. If multiple then hereditary telangiectasia has to be considered, but in this disease there are usually lesions in the mouth. Simple telangiectasia do not have a central papule.

Aetiology
The central part of the lesion is a small arteriole which has enlarged and then gives rise to telangiectasia. Although it has been estimated that this lesion may occur in up to 15% of the population, it is characteristically seen in pregnancy and liver disease. Because of this it has been suggested that oestrogens play some part in the aetiology of the condition.

Treatment
If persistent the lesions can easily be treated by cautery to the central part of the lesion. The best results are obtained by the so-called 'cold point cautery' which has a very fine point and the heat is derived by conduction from surrounding wires, and so it is less hot than an ordinary cautery point.

Natural history and prognosis
The lesions tend to be persistent, except those which occur during pregnancy, in which case many of them will disappear after pregnancy, but may reappear in subsequent pregnancies.

LYMPHANGIOMA

Presentation
There are a number of types of lymphangioma. All are rare and only the commonest type will be discussed.

The lesions may be present at birth otherwise they appear during early childhood. The sexes are equally affected. The lesion consists of a group of small vesicles (Figure 46.13). Frequently there is a haemangiomatous element, so small red spots are seen within the vesicles or there are small red papules between the vesicles. The commonest sites for these lesions to appear are neck, axillary fold, upper trunk and oral cavity.

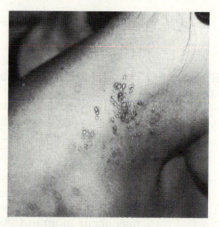

Figure 46.13   Lymphangioma. Small grouped vesicles

Differential diagnosis
If there is a large haemangiomatous element, then a haemangioma may have to be considered. To the uninitiated, molluscum contagiosum may be confused if the lesions are localized, but the lymphangioma is compressible with a glass depressor, while the mollusca are not.

Investigations
None usually, but a biopsy should be carried out if there is any doubt about the nature of the lesion.

Aetiology
The lesion is a developmental abnormality and because of the haemangiomatous element, the lesion is considered to be a hamartoma. There are frequently abnormalities of the deep lymphatics.

Treatment   This is difficult. If the affected area is excised there is frequently a recurrence around the scar. It has been suggested that the deeper abnormality of the vessels must be dealt with by appropriate dissection and destruction of these vessels, but this is not easy and it is too early to assess the long term results. Simple destruction of the vesicles by cautery may improve the result temporarily but if repeated will lead to scarring of the skin. Camouflage procedures may help to improve the appearance but the fact that the lesion is raised makes it difficult to obtain a satisfactory result.

SEBACEOUS NAEVUS

Presentation   This is a relatively uncommon but important condition to recognize. The lesion may be present at birth, otherwise it presents in early childhood. The sexes are equally affected. The lesion has a characteristic yellow colour and is often linear. It is raised and has

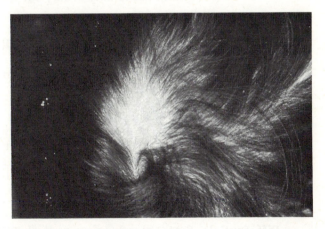

Figure 46.14   Sebaceous naevus. Yellowish plaque with papillomatous surface

an irregular papillomatous surface (Figure 46.14). The lesion may enlarge during puberty. If there is rapid growth of a small area then malignant change should be suspected. The commonest sites to be involved are the neck and scalp. No hair grows in the scalp lesion.

Differential diagnosis   In infancy, ectodermal hypoplasia of the scalp may present as a bald area, but in this instance the skin is white and not raised. On the neck, linear epidermal naevi have to be considered.

Investigations   If the diagnosis is in doubt, a biopsy may be necessary.

Aetiology   Naevus sebaceous is another developmental abnormality. The principal tissues involved are the sebaceous glands, but there is frequently an associated abnormality of other epidermal appendages such as hair follicles and sweat glands.

Treatment   Surgical excision is advisable.

Natural history and prognosis   There is a relatively high risk of malignancy developing in these lesions, usually not until middle age, but occasionally sooner. For this reason the lesions are best excised. The commonest malignancy to develop is the basal cell carcinoma and the incidence is about 20%. Other malignant tumours associated with abnormalities of sweat gland and sebaceous gland tissue may occur, but these are rare.

HAIR FOLLICLE TUMOURS

These are all rare. The one most frequently seen is termed trichoepithelioma.

Presentation   The lesions usually appear at puberty. The typical lesion is a small papule a few millimetres in diameter, which may vary in colour. Some are pink, some skin coloured and others may show brown pigmentation. The lesions are usually multiple and symmetrical. The common sites are the nose, nasolabial folds and cheeks.

Differential diagnosis   Sweat gland tumours are of similar size, but usually predominate around the eyes. The lesions of adenoma sebaceum may have a similar appearance but tend to occur more on the cheeks and begin at an earlier age.

Investigations   A biopsy is necessary to establish the diagnosis.

Aetiology   There is often a family history and thus the abnormality is considered to have an inherited basis.

Treatment If the lesions are few they may be excised. If multiple there is very little treatment that can be offered, although cautery to the lesions does flatten them, and give a more cosmetically acceptable appearance.

Natural history and prognosis The lesions are persistent. There is an increased incidence of malignant change, the neoplasm being a basal cell carcinoma.

SWEAT GLAND TUMOURS: SYRINGOMA

Presentation This lesion is commoner in females than males. They usually appear at adolescence and subsequent lesions appear in later life. The lesions are small papules (2–3 mm), usually skin coloured, but they sometimes have a cystic appearance. The lesions tend to be multiple and symmetrical and the common sites of involvement are the face, around the eyes, the neck and upper chest.

Differential diagnosis The lesions most likely to be similar to syringomata are trichoepitheliomata. The latter usually occur on the nose and sides of the nose.

Investigations A biopsy to establish the diagnosis.

Aetiology Best considered as a predetermined developmental abnormality.

Treatment This is required for cosmetic reasons. If only a few lesions are present surgery may be considered, otherwise cautery to destroy the lesions is the only other treatment.

Natural history and prognosis The lesions persist. There appears to be no increased risk of malignant change.

DERMAL CYLINDROMA

Presentation This is a rare condition but with characteristic features affecting females twice as commonly as males. The lesions first appear in adolescence or early adult life. The lesions are multiple. They begin as firm, small pink papules and gradually increase in size and may reach 5 cm in diameter. The scalp is the commonest site and very rarely they may occur on the face and neck. Occasionally the tumours are pedunculated. They are sometimes known as turban tumours.

Differential diagnosis The tumours are most likely to be confused with neoplasms of the hair follicles.

Investigations Biopsy will establish the diagnosis.

Aetiology The lesions have a hereditary basis, by an autosomal dominant gene. The exact cells in the dermis which give rise to these tumours are unknown.

Treatment Surgery.

Prognosis The lesions are persistent but malignant change is rare.

LEIOMYOMA

These lesions are derived from smooth muscle in the skin.

Presentation The lesions may appear at any age but early adult life is the commonest. The sexes are equally affected. The lesion presents as a reddish-brown firm nodule and may vary in size from 3 to 10 mm. The lesions are usually multiple and grouped. Any part of the skin may be affected but the limbs seem to be more common than elsewhere. One of the distinctive features is that these lesions are painful.

Differential diagnosis Because of the pain the only other lesions that may have to be considered are glomus tumours, but the latter tend to be solitary.

Investigations A biopsy.

Aetiology Unknown.

Treatment Surgical excision on account of the pain.

Natural history and prognosis The lesions are persistent but there is no tendency to malignancy.

SEBORRHOEIC WARTS

These lesions are sometimes referred to as seborrhoeic keratoses or benign basal cell papillomata.

Presentation These lesions are very common. They affect males and females equally and usually first appear in middle age and then increase in number with age (Figure 46.15). The typical lesion is a superficial

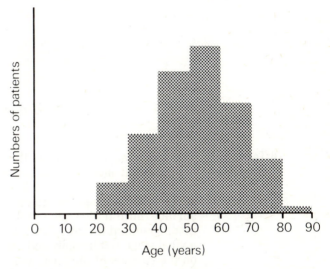

Figure 46.15   Age of onset of seborrhoeic warts

plaque on the skin with a clefted, rough surface with a slightly greasy appearance – hence the name (Figure 46.16). The lesion is usually pigmented, and the amount of pigment may vary from light brown to black. The lesions occasionally are not pigmented. The size of the lesion may vary from a few millimetres to a few centimetres. Rarely the lesion takes a slightly different appearance, presenting as a dome shaped swelling with a smooth surface.

Seborrhoeic warts may affect any part of the skin but they are most common on the face and trunk.

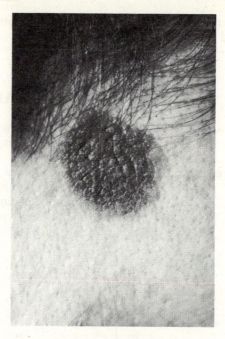

Figure 46.16   Seborrhoeic wart

Differential diagnosis   The lesion most confused with a seborrhoeic wart is a pigmented melanocytic naevus. The seborrhoeic wart usually begins later in life and has the rougher surface. A malignant melanoma usually has a smooth surface, until it ulcerates. If the seborrhoeic wart is non-pigmented it may have the same appearance of a viral wart, but thrombosed capillaries may be seen on the surface of the viral wart as small black dots. A pigmented basal cell carcinoma usually has a smooth surface or a definite ulcer with rolled edges. A crusted pyogenic granuloma may have a similar appearance but there is usually a history of bleeding, which is rare with seborrhoeic warts.

Investigations   Biopsy, or biopsy excision if the diagnosis is in doubt.

Aetiology   Unknown. The lesions are uncommon in Asians and negroes and there is a suggestion that the lesions are sometimes more common in patients who have been exposed to excessive sunlight, but they certainly also occur in non-exposed areas. Despite the name the lesions are not associated with any abnormalities of the sebaceous glands.

Treatment This is only necessary for cosmetic reasons and the lesions are best removed by curettage and minimal cauterization under local anaesthetic. The latter stops the bleeding and there should be no scarring. Cryotherapy may be used but the results are not as good as with curettage.

Natural history and prognosis The lesions show no sign of spontaneous resolution. There is no risk of malignant change.

SKIN TAGS

These are common lesions and are sometimes referred to as fibroepithelial polyps.

Presentation The lesions are more frequent in females (Figure 46.17) 5 : 1. They may appear any time in adult life, but most commonly appear for the first time in middle age. The typical lesion is pedunculated with

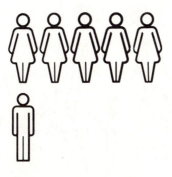

Figure 46.17   Skin tags are more common in females (5 : 1)

a narrow stalk which is attached to the skin at the base of the lesion, and a soft, rounded swelling on top of the stalk (Figure 46.18). The stalk or attachment is 2–3 mm long, and the soft distal swelling or tumour is usually 2–5 mm in diameter. The colour of the tumour may be skin coloured or sometimes pigmented. The lesions are usually mult-

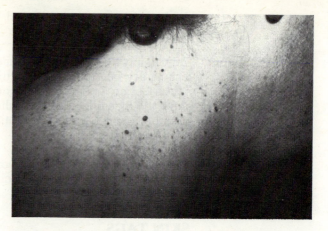

Figure 46.18   Skin tags

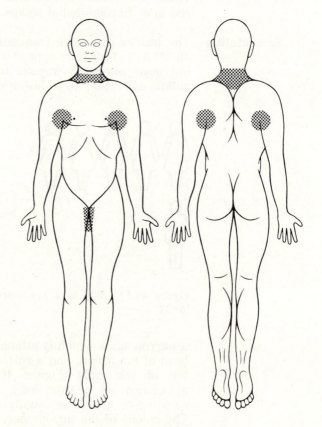

Figure 46.19   Common sites of skin tags

iple and are most commonly found on the neck and axillae (Figure 46.19). They also occur on the upper thighs in obese persons.

Differential diagnosis   Occasionally the lesions may be confused with a melanocytic naevus or the pedunculated lesions in neurofibromatosis.

Aetiology   Unknown.

Treatment   The lesions may be cauterized or snipped with a curved pair of scissors. No local anaesthetic is required for the latter procedure.

Natural history   The lesions are persistent and are not pre-malignant.

MILIA (KERATIN CYSTS)

Presentation   The lesions are common. They may be seen at any age, and are most frequent in females. The typical lesion is a small whitish yellow papule 1–2 mm in diameter. The lesion is superficial and feels firm on palpation. The most common site is the face and around the eyes, although secondary milia may occur at the site of previous damage to the skin, usually following a blister.

Differential diagnosis   Occasionally xantholasma in the early stages may be the same size as milia, but they usually enlarge to form small plaques. Syringomata are usually larger and skin coloured or red.

Aetiology   A milium is a keratin cyst, and they are thought to arise from undeveloped sebaceous glands, or from the proximal part of divided sweat glands. The common variety arise with no preceding skin damage. However, any lesion which produces blisters or superficial damage may give rise to so-called secondary milia.

Treatment   For cosmetic reasons, the lesions may be removed with the point of a scalpel blade. The epidermis is broken and the cyst is then pierced and lifted out on the end of the blade.

Natural history   The lesions persist and show no spontaneous resolution.

KERATOACANTHOMA

Presentation   The lesion is seen principally in middle aged and elderly persons, and the sexes are equally affected. The initial lesion is a small papule with a central keratin or scaly plug. The lesion enlarges rapidly within the space of three months and reaches a diameter of up to 2 cm. At this stage the lesion is a discoid, elevated plaque with a central depression filled with scaly material (Figure 46.20). The colour

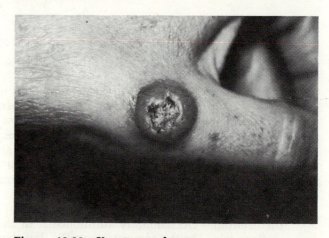

Figure 46.20   Keratoacanthoma

may be slightly red, and the surface is smooth except for the central area. Telangiectasia may be seen on the surface of the rolled edges. The commonest sites to be affected are the exposed areas, namely the face and backs of the hands (Figure 46.21).

Differential diagnosis   The important lesion that has to be distinguished is the squamous cell carcinoma. The rapid growth of the keratoacanthoma may suggest the correct diagnosis. A large and solitary molluscum contagiosum may have a similar appearance in the early stages, but it rarely enlarges to the same size as a keratoacanthoma.

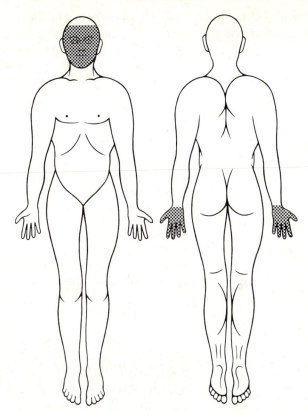

Figure 46.21   Common sites of keratoacanthoma

Investigations   Biopsy is essential in all cases to distinguish the lesion from a squamous cell carcinoma.

Aetiology   As the lesion occurs on the exposed areas, and is rare in dark skinned persons; it is thought ultraviolet light may be the cause of the lesions, although keratoacanthoma is a benign lesion. Other suggestions as to the cause have been contact with other carcinogens such as tar, or a viral aetiology, but there is no proof for the latter.

Treatment   Once the diagnosis has been established by biopsy the best results are obtained by leaving the lesion to undergo spontaneous resolution. Surgery and radiotherapy can both be used but are usually not necessary unless the patient is not prepared to wait for resolution.

Natural history and prognosis This is important. The lesion grows rapidly for 3 months, is then stationary in size for 3 months. It then undergoes spontaneous resolution which takes 3 months. There may be residual scarring. Keratoacanthoma is a benign lesion.

HISTIOCYTOMA

Presentation These are common lesions and are very much more frequent in females (Figure 46.22). They are rare in children but may be seen at any age in adult life. The typical lesion is a small, firm brown nodule which has a smooth surface. The lesion is only just raised above the skin surface. It varies in size from 3 to 10 mm. The lesion may be solitary, but not uncommonly two to three lesions may appear simultaneously. The commonest sites of involvement are the lower legs, but they may occur anywhere, although the face is rarely involved.

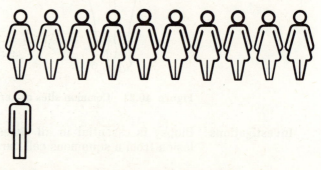

Figure 46.22 Histiocytomata are more common in women (10:1)

Differential diagnosis Because of the brown pigmentation the lesion has to be distinguished from a malignant melanoma. The histiocytoma is usually a 'depressed' nodule rather than an elevated one as in malignant melanoma. Other dermal nodules, such as leiomyoma, neurofibroma, and a simple fibroma have to be considered.

Investigations Histology if the lesion is excised.

Aetiology It is thought that a histiocytoma is an abnormal tissue response to minor trauma such as an insect bite. This is supported by the fact that most lesions are seen in females on the lower legs. There is hyperplasia of histiocytes, vascular and other reticulo-endothelial cells.

Treatment The treatment of choice is surgical excision as this allows histological examination. Other destructive procedures should not be carried out if the diagnosis is in doubt.

Natural history and prognosis The lesions are benign but show no tendency to spontaneous resolution.

KELOIDS

Presentation Keloids may occur at any age, although they are rare in old age. They are commoner in females. They most commonly occur at sites of trauma to the skin, where the dermis has been involved, but spontaneous keloids also occur (Figure 46.23). Keloid forma-

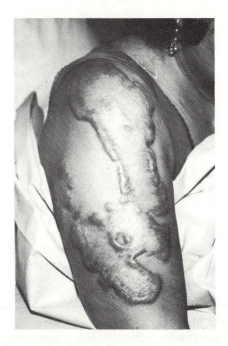

Figure 46.23   Spontaneous keloids

tion becomes evident approximately 3–4 weeks after injury to the skin, and the scar becomes raised and thickened. The growth may continue for many months. After 2–3 months, patients complain of abnormal sensations in the keloid such as pain or irritation. The eventual size, i.e. height and width of the keloid, varies from a few mm to a few cm on occasions. Some parts of the body appear to be more prone to keloid formation, the presternal area, shoulders and neck are the commonest sites both for keloids following trauma and spontaneous lesions. The latter are frequently annular.

Differential diagnosis

If there is a history of recent trauma, then the diagnosis is not usually in doubt. Spontaneous keloids may present problems in diagnosis, and have to be distinguished from granulomatous processes.

Investigations

A biopsy if the diagnosis is in doubt.

Aetiology

Apart from the fact that certain parts of the skin are more prone to keloids, there are other predisposing factors. Genetic factors are important in some individuals, and there is frequently a family history of keloid formation. Keloid formation is very common in negroes; spontaneous keloid formation occurs in people from the Middle East and in negroes, but is rare in white Caucasians.

A keloid is essentially a proliferation of the collagen component of the dermis. The exact cause for this increased formation of collagen is not known.

Treatment

The safest and most effective treatment for keloids is injection into the keloid of corticosteroids. The quicker the treatment is carried out the better the results. The treatment may have to be repeated every 4–6 weeks until satisfactory results are obtained. If the person is known to be predisposed to keloid formation, then infiltration of the wound at the time of operation with corticosteroids should be carried out. Radiotherapy has been used in the past, but because of subsequent risks of malignant change and atrophic scars its use is not recommended.

Natural history and prognosis

Most keloids stop increasing in size after a few months, but a few may continue to enlarge for many years. Spontaneous resolution is rare.

47 SKIN TUMOURS (MALIGNANT) AND PARAPSORIASIS

KERATOSES

It is arguable whether keratoses do in fact progress to true malignant change, and thus in themselves are not really malignant or potentially so.

Presentation The age at which keratoses may first be seen will depend on the colour of the skin, length of exposure, and 'strength' of sunlight to which the subject has been exposed. Keratoses are most commonly seen in middle aged and elderly persons, but are seen in young Caucasian adults who have lived near the equator for any length of time. Keratoses are virtually unknown in negroes and Asians with dark skins. Males and females are equally affected. The typical lesion is a whitish-grey scaly area with a red rim (Figure 47.1). The size may vary from a few millimetres to 2 cm. The majority of lesions are 0.5 cm. If the scale is removed the base is red and shiny and bleeds easily. The commonest sites are the exposed areas, i.e. face and backs of the hands, and the scalp in bald men (Figure 47.2). They are also seen on the legs, arms and trunk if these areas have been exposed to prolonged strong sunlight.

Differential diagnosis If the lesions are large they may be confused with Bowen's disease; the latter is usually less scaly and is seen as a solitary and larger red patch. Large keratoses on the face have to be distinguished from discoid lupus erythematosus. With keratoses there are usually other signs of prolonged exposure to the sun, such as telangiectasia, wrinkles and lentigos. A non-pigmented seborrhoeic wart may have a similar appearance, but there is usually no erythematous skin around the scaling. An early squamous cell car-

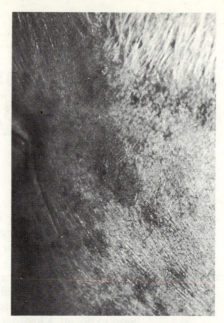

Figure 47.1 Keratosis. Red patch with grey scale

cinoma may have similar appearances to a keratosis, before the stage of ulceration or nodular development.

Investigations If the diagnosis is in doubt a biopsy is necessary.

Aetiology Keratoses are sun-induced. It is a dysplasia of the epidermal cells, and considered by some to be premalignant. The incubation period following prolonged exposure to strong sunlight is about 25 years. Virtually all white persons living for this length of time on or near the equator will have some keratoses.

Treatment If the lesions are numerous or not troublesome to the patient, then they may be left alone as the risk of malignant change is minimal. If treatment is decided upon then the lesions may be treated with topical 5-fluorouracil cream, by cryotherapy or by curettage and cautery. Topical 5-fluorouracil cream is often used when the lesions are multiple and on the face, and an excellent cosmetic result is obtained. It is sometimes not effective on lesions on the backs of the hands.

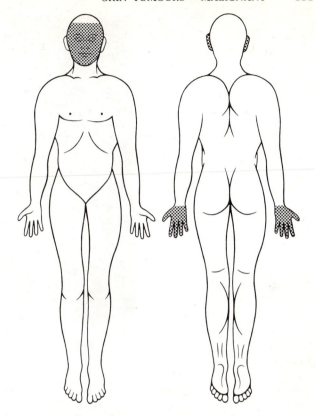

Figure 47.2   Common sites of keratoses

Prognosis   Keratoses will persist if not treated. The most important question is whether they are pre-malignant and will develop into squamous cell carcinomata. Certainly the majority of lesions will not. It has been suggested that squamous cell carcinomata do not arise from previous keratoses and that the lesion is a carcinoma from its inception. At present it cannot be categorically stated that keratoses do or do not develop into squamous cell carcinomata.

BOWEN'S DISEASE (INTRA-EPIDERMAL CARCINOMA)

Presentation   Bowen's disease is usually seen in middle aged or elderly persons. The sexes are equally affected. The initial lesion is a red, scaly patch (Figure 47.3). The

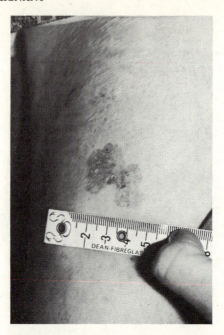

Figure 47.3   Bowen's disease

scale is whitish-yellow. The size of the lesion varies from a few mm to a few cm. The lesion is sharply demarcated from the surrounding skin. On the palm the lesion may show ulceration. The lesions may be found anywhere on the skin.

Differential diagnosis   Bowen's disease may be confused with psoriasis, but in the latter disease the lesions are usually multiple and symmetrical. On the trunk a superficial basal carcinoma may have a similar appearance, apart from the fact that the latter has a pearly edge. If large, a keratosis has a similar appearance.

Investigation   A biopsy should be performed in all instances.

Aetiology   Arsenic can certainly cause the development of Bowen's disease. The commonest source of arsenic was medication thirty and forty years ago, and one is still seeing the results of this therapy in skin clinics. As the use of arsenic has died out, so the incidence of Bowen's disease should fall. Arsenic or arsenicals used in industry are another possible source. Sunlight is also an aetiological factor in some patients. The incubation period after arsenic or sunlight is several years.

Treatment Once a biopsy has been performed the lesion may be treated with topical 5-fluorouracil cream, curettage and cautery, cryotherapy or surgery. Surgical excision gives the best results, as it is thought the process may extend into the skin appendages and be missed by the other methods.

Natural history and prognosis If left untreated the lesion will persist. Bowen's disease may progress to a squamous cell carcinoma but this may not occur for many years. The lesion does not usually progress laterally once it has formed, and may stay the same size for many years.

PAGET'S DISEASE

Presentation There are two types of Paget's disease, one which occurs on the breast, and another in the axillae or anogenital region. The breast disease occurs mainly in women (Figure 47.4) 10 : 1 and is commonest in the fifth and sixth decades. The extramammary disease is also more common in women and affects a similar age group. The lesion is a gradually spreading red, scaly and crusted area. On the breast it starts on the

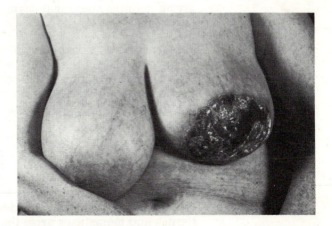

Figure 47.4   Paget's disease

nipple and may be associated with a slight discharge. It then extends to the areola and then skin. Occasionally there may be ulceration of the skin. The lesion is usually sharply demarcated. The lesions in extramammary Paget's disease are similar. The commonest area to be affected is the vulva.

Differential diagnosis   Eczema of the breasts has a similar appearance, and if unilateral it may be impossible to distinguish between the two diseases on clinical grounds. A superficial basal cell carcinoma or Bowen's disease may also give a similar clinical picture. Psoriasis is usually bilateral and symmetrical and this does not present problems, but if solitary it may. Intertriginous eczema and psoriasis are usually bilateral.

Investigation   A biopsy should be performed.

Aetiology   Paget's disease of the breast is due to an intraductal carcinoma of breast tissue. The carcinoma cells migrate into the epidermis, so that an intraepidermal carcinoma is produced. At this stage the carcinoma can be considered to be in situ but at a later stage becomes invasive and behaves like any other carcinoma of the breast. In extramammary Paget's disease it is thought that the carcinoma arises in a duct of an adnexal gland in the skin or mucous membrane, and then extends into skin, giving an intra-epidermal carcinoma.

Treatment   Mammary Paget's disease should be treated like any other carcinoma of the breast, which is by local mastectomy and radiotherapy if necessary. Extramammary Paget's disease is treated by local excision of the affected skin and surrounding mucous membrane if involved.

Prognosis   Paget's disease is a very slow growing tumour and whilst the carcinoma cells remain intraductal or intra-epidermal the prognosis is good once surgery has been performed. Once the lesion invades deeper tissues and metastases arise the prognosis is naturally poor.

ERYTHROPLASIA OF QUEYRAT

Presentation The lesion is an intra-epidermal carcinoma of the penis. It is a disease of adults. The lesion presents as a well circumscribed, raised red patch with a surface which has been described as 'velvety' (Figure 47.5). The initial lesion commences on the glans, and may enlarge slowly to involve the foreskin and surrounding skin. The lesion may ulcerate at a later stage.

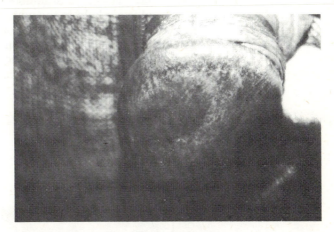

Figure 47.5   Erythroplasia of Queyrat

Differential diagnosis Seborrhoeic eczema of the glans penis may present as a red patch but it usually affects other areas quickly and responds rapidly to treatment. Plasma cell balanitis of Zoon is seen in a similar age group and also presents as a persistent patch on the glans penis. The surface is shiny and moist rather than 'velvety', but the diagnosis can be difficult on clinical grounds alone.

Investigation A biopsy is necessary.

Aetiology The disease does not occur in males circumcised in childhood, so smegma may play some part in the cause of the condition.

Treatment This is with topical 5-fluorouracil cream.

Natural history and prognosis The disease is potentially malignant and may after many years progress to a squamous cell carcinoma.

Fortunately effective topical cytotoxic agents means the disease can be effectively treated without recourse to surgery or radiotherapy.

BASAL CELL CARCINOMA

Presentation This is the commonest form of skin cancer and the lesion may present in a number of ways. The lesion is related to sunlight in the majority of instances and the length of exposure and strength of sunlight will determine at what age the lesion forms. In white persons living near the equator, the lesions will present in the third decade. The lesions most commonly appear in the elderly (Figure 47.6). The sexes are

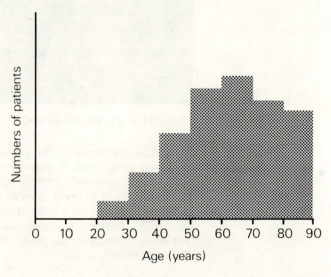

Figure 47.6   Age of presentation of basal cell carcinomata

equally affected. The commonest site is the face (Figure 47.7). Although the lesions are related to sunlight they do not occur on the backs of the hands. They are extremely rare on the limbs even in those persons exposed to long periods of strong sun. They do however occur on the trunk following long exposure to the sun.

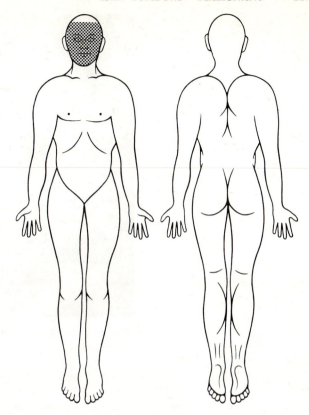

Figure 47.7   Common sites of basal call carcinomata

Ulcerated type   This is the commonest presentation. The lesion has a raised, pearly edge and a central ulcer (Figure 47.8), which is often scabbed. Telangiectasia may be seen in the pearly edge of the lesion. The lesion does not usually ulcerate until it has reached a diameter of 5 mm. The lesion may invade inwards forming a deeper ulcer, with destruction of the underlying tissues, and laterally over the surface of the skin, forming a large ulcer.

Cystic type   The lesion commences as a small cystic papule and gradually enlarges forming a lobulated cystic swelling. The lesion does not ulcerate and may progress to a relatively large size, e.g. 2 cm unless treatment stops its progress. Telangiectasia are classically seen coursing over the surface of the lesion (Figure 47.9).

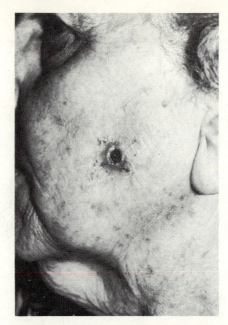

Figure 47.8 Basal cell carcinoma: ulcerated type

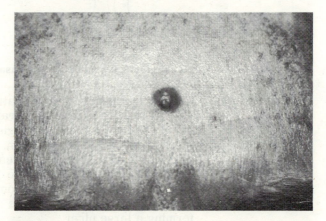

Figure 47.9   Basal cell carcinoma: cystic type with telangiectasia

Morphoeic type   This is so called because the lesions present as a firm red plaque (Figure 47.10). The morphology is due to fibrosis which occurs in response to the basal cell carcinoma, and is an attempt by the body at healing or containing the lesion. The lesion will

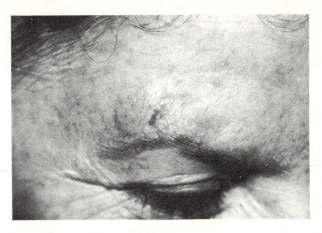

Figure 47.10   Basal cell carcinoma: morphoeic type

slowly increase and its size depends on the stage at which the patient seeks help. The usual size is 1–2 cm on the first consultation.

Superficial type   This type of basal cell carcinoma is most commonly found on the trunk. The lesion presents as a red, scaly patch with a slightly raised pearly edge (Figure 47.11). The edge is usually very narrow 1–2 mm. The superficial basal cell lesion, as its

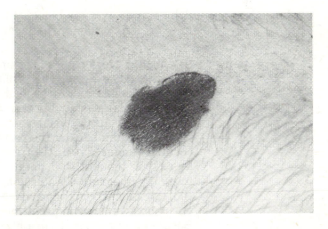

Figure 47.11   Basal cell carcinoma: superficial type

name implies, spreads laterally and not inwardly. It will vary in size depending on how long it has been there when the patient seeks advice. It is usually 2–3 cm long when the patient is first seen. .

Pigmented type — The ulcerated, cystic and superficial types may have varying degrees of pigment present. This may make the diagnosis difficult.

Differential diagnosis — The ulcerated type may have to be distinguished from a squamous cell carcinoma or keratoacanthoma. The telangiectasia over the surface of the edge are present both in the keratoacanthoma and basal cell lesion. However, the basal cell lesion is usually asymmetrical and the ulcer is less deep in a keratoacanthoma. On the periphery of the pinna the basal cell lesion has to be distinguished from chondrodermatitis helicis nodularis. The latter is usually painful. The cystic basal cell lesion has a characteristic appearance and very rarely leads to problems in diagnosis. If the lesion is pigmented then the most important differential diagnosis is a malignant melanoma, and this may be impossible without histological examination. The morphoeic lesion has to be distinguished from morphoea and some forms of granulomatous infiltrates. The superficial basal cell carcinoma may be confused with Bowen's disease, or a patch of eczema or psoriasis. Close inspection of the edge usually gives the correct diagnosis.

Investigations — A biopsy, or excision biopsy if feasible, is necessary in all lesions prior to treatment.

Aetiology — Although the lesions are far more common after prolonged exposure to strong sunlight, the situation of the lesions does not correspond to those parts of the face that necessarily receive the most exposure. Thus the tumour is common on the eyelids, but is uncommon on the back of the hand or forearms which receive similar amounts of ultraviolet light to the face. It is thought that possibly the pilosebaceous unit may in some way be related to the aetiology of the carcinoma, and some have suggested that the carcinoma is derived from the pilosebaceous unit. Basal cell carcinomata are also common in certain naevoid conditions, but the exact significance of this is unknown. Arsenic is related to the superficial type of basal cell carcinoma. X-irradiation is also a cause of basal cell carcinoma after an interval of 15–20 years, and for this reason is best avoided in young and middle aged persons.

Treatment This will depend on the size and type of lesion and the age of the patient. The treatments which are available are surgical excision, radiotherapy, curettage and cautery, and topical 5-fluorouracil cream. If the lesion is larger than 1 cm in diameter, and of the ulcerative or cystic type, then radiotherapy or surgery are the treatments of choice, the deciding factor being age. Radiotherapy should not be used as a rule in patients under 60, as an unsightly scar tends to develop after 5 years. It is a white atrophic area with telangiectasia. Morphoeic basal cell carcinomata are best treated by surgery. Superficial basal cell carcinomata should be treated in the first instance with topical 5-fluorouracil cream; if this is not successful other forms of treatment will usually clear the lesion. If the basal cell carcinoma is the ulcerative or cystic type and less than 1 cm in diameter, curettage and cautery is a simple and successful treatment with a good cosmetic result. The treatment should be performed by a person experienced in the technique, otherwise there is a high recurrence rate.

Prognosis As a general rule basal cell carcinoma has a good prognosis if treated correctly. The ulcerative and cystic lesions may invade deep tissues and eventually cause death. This will however take many years after the first appearance of the lesion. The good prognosis probably depends on the fact that the lesions do not metastasize like other forms of cancer. The recurrence rate after treatment is less than 5% and further treatment usually results in a cure.

SQUAMOUS CELL CARCINOMA

Presentation The lesion usually appears after the age of 60 (Figure 47.12) and is twice as common in males (Figure 47.13). It is often stated that this type of carcinoma does not develop in normal skin, but only

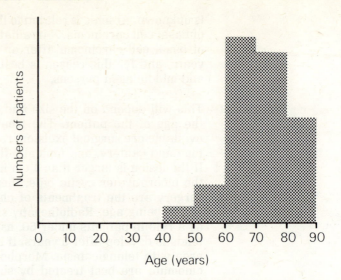

Figure 47.12   Age of onset of squamous cell carcinomata

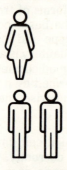

Figure 47.13   Sex distribution of squamous cell carcinoma

in one which has been damaged by a chronic process. The initial lesion may be a small nodule or ulcer with an indurated and thickened edge (Figure 47.14). On the lip the carcinoma may present as a persistent fissure. The lesion gradually enlarges and may continue to be nodular or ulcerative, but the nodular lesions invariably break down in the centre forming an ulcer. The common sites to find squamous cell carcinomata are the exposed areas, the backs of the hands, the face, pinnae and lips (Figure 47.15). In tropical countries the lesions are often found on the lower legs and feet in association with chronic infections.

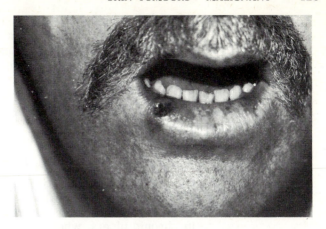

Figure 47.14   Squamous cell carcinoma on the lip

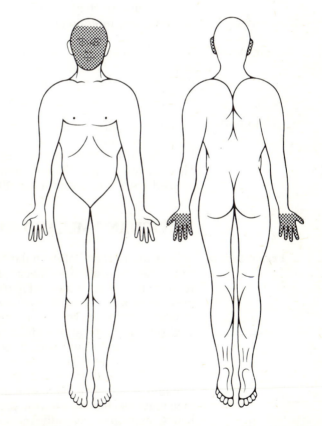

Figure 47.15   Common sites of squamous cell carcinomata

Differential diagnosis   Keratoacanthoma occurs at similar sites and has a similar morphology, but grows more rapidly in the initial stages. Amelanotic melanoma may have the same morphology as a squamous cell lesion. Basal cell carcinoma and chronic granulomata which ulcerate may also give similar clinical appearances.

Investigations   A biopsy is necessary in every case. If the lesion is small an excision biopsy should be performed.

Aetiology   A number of factors would appear capable of inducing this type of lesion. Strong sunlight is certainly the commonest cause. Exposure to industrial carcinogens predisposes to these tumours. They also develop in chronic ulcers, whether they be due to syphilis, tuberculosis, discoid lupus erythematosus, osteomyelitis or old burns. The lesions are very rare in negroes unless they are on the legs and associated with chronic infections.

Treatment   The treatment of choice is surgical excision. Radiotherapy is also effective and can be used in elderly persons in whom an operation may not be advisable.

Natural history and prognosis   Squamous cell carcinomata have the potential to metastasize and thus if not treated, will eventually kill the patient. However, many of the lesions are slow growing and do not metastasize early. The overall cure rate approaches 90% after treatment.

MALIGNANT MELANOMA

Presentation   The lesion is rare before puberty. It may present at any time in adult life (Figure 47.16). It is slightly more common in females (Figure 47.17). The lesion may present as a macular area of pigmentation and extend laterally. The surface may then become slightly irregular and nodular (Figure 47.18). Pigmentation may be uniform throughout the lesion or irregular. At the edge of the lesion the pigment may advance into the surrounding skin in an irregular manner, giving a pigmented halo. Malignant melanoma may also begin as a firm, pigmented nodule. The lesion may grow rapidly in size to several centimetres in a small space of time. Ulceration is not an uncommon feature, and bleeding and scabbing will occur. Very rarely no pigment is present and the lesion then presents as an ulcer or nodule, or plaque in the skin with pinkish-red colour (so-called amelanotic melanoma).

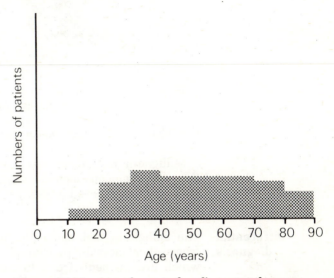

Figure 47.16   Age of onset of malignant melanoma

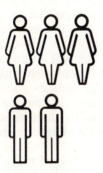

Figure 47.17   Malignant melanoma is slightly more common in females (3 : 2)

Under the nail a malignant melanoma presents as a pigmented area, and the nail may be lifted from the nail bed. If the lesion involves the nail matrix, there may be a linear pigmented streak in the nail.

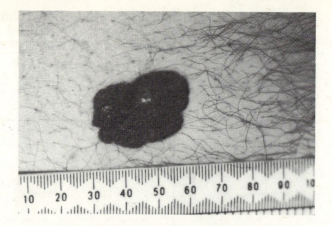

Figure 47.18   Malignant melanoma: irregular surface

Malignant melanoma may appear anywhere on the skin or mucous membranes, but the commonest sites are the exposed areas, particularly the lower leg in females.

Differential diagnosis

The malignant melanoma has to be distinguished from other melanin pigmented lesions, and those which are pigmented due to bleeding. Those with melanin pigment include melanocytic naevi, seborrhoeic warts, and pigmented basal cell carcinomata. The pigmented lesions due to haemorrhage include pyogenic granulomata, basal cell carcinomata, histiocytomata, viral warts and under the nails, subungual haematomata. Not all linear, pigmented lesions in the nail plate imply malignant melanoma. They are seen in benign melanocytic naevi of the nail bed, and are common in negroes. The amelanotic melanoma has to be distinguished from squamous cell carcinomata and granulomatous diseases.

Investigations

There are two schools of thought about a biopsy in malignant melanoma. One feels a biopsy should not be carried out as it disseminates the lesion and adversely affects the prognosis, whilst the other feels the prognosis is not influenced by biopsy. If the diagnosis can be made with moderate certainty and the lesion is relatively small, then an excision biopsy can be performed. If the lesion is large, over 1.5 cm, and the diagnosis is in doubt, then a biopsy is justified rather than performing radical surgery. Frozen sections from a biopsy with a view to going straight on to radical surgery will not distinguish all lesions from a malignant melanoma, i.e. some melanocytic naevi or juvenile melanoma, but frozen sections will distinguish some lesions.

Aetiology

Like most cancers the cause of malignant melanoma is multifactoral. However, one of the factors that has been incriminated in the aetiology is sunlight. The disease is more common in fair skinned people than in the dark skinned, and in negroes the disease is rare on normal pigmented skin, and when it does occur it is on the soles and nail folds. The incidence of malignant melanoma has increased over the last two decades and this has been attributed to increased exposure to sun as a way of life, and possible damage to the ozone layer of the atmosphere by aircraft and the use of aerosols, which allows more damaging rays from the sun to reach the earth's surface.

The question as to whether melanocytic naevi are more likely to develop into malignant melanomata than normal skin has as yet not been answered. There is no doubt that the congenital giant pigmented naevus is more likely to develop into malignant melanomata, but this cannot be said with conviction for other pigmented naevi.

Treatment

Wide excision and a graft is the currently accepted treatment of choice. Excision of the regional lymph nodes is only carried out if there is clinical involvement. Radiotherapy is used in some countries and may be used if the tumour is very large and the patient elderly. Immunotherapy has been used in the treatment of malignant melanoma, both for the primary and secondary lesions, but its exact place and the techniques to be used are still undetermined.

Natural history and prognosis

As a general rule the nodular types of malignant melanoma have a worse prognosis than the flat plaque-like lesions. The clinically nodular lesion often corresponds to the invading tumour histologically. However it is often impossible to predict the course of a malignant melanoma. It has been estimated that 3% of lesions will undergo spontaneous resolution. Others may be excised and secondary deposits occur 20–30 years later. These observations suggest that the host's immunological reactions are important in the prognosis, but as yet these reactions and how to modify them are not known. The overall five year survival rate is now approximately 50%.

LENTIGO MALIGNA (HUTCHINSON'S MELANOTIC FRECKLE)

Presentation

The lesion presents in the middle aged and elderly. The sexes are equally affected. The lesion begins as an irregular flat area of pigmentation and slowly increases in size over the years. The lesion may grow to the size of 5 cm or more. The pigmentation is often irregular. After many years (sometimes even 20) the lesion may become nodular in small areas. Lentigo maligna occurs on the face.

Differential diagnosis

The simple actinic lentigo has a similar appearance in the initial stages, but these are usually smaller and multiple. A flat seborrhoeic wart has to be distinguished, but this usually has a rough surface. A melanocytic naevus begins at a much earlier age. A malignant melanoma is a much more rapidly growing lesion and is nodular from its commencement or at a very early stage compared to a lentigo maligna.

Investigations

The diagnosis is usually obvious on clinical grounds, but if there is any doubt a biopsy should be performed.

Aetiology

Unknown.

Treatment

In the macular stage the treatment of choice is cryotherapy. If a nodular lesion develops this is best excised and the remainder of the lesion treated with cryotherapy.

Natural history and prognosis

The lesion is very slow growing and very rarely do the patients die as a result of it. Even if nodular formation takes place, which is a malignant melanoma histologically, it very rarely metastasizes, and itself is slow growing so the prognosis is different from that of a malignant melanoma. The lesion may persist for 20–30 years without evidence of tumour formation but the lesion has to be considered as pre-malignant although the prognosis is good.

MYCOSIS FUNGOIDES

Presentation The disease usually begins in middle age (Figure 47.19), but may commence in young adults or even the elderly. It is slightly more common in males than

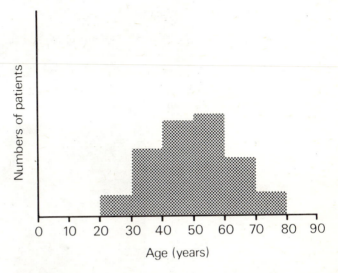

Figure 47.19   Age of onset of mycosis fungoides

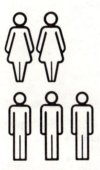

Figure 47.20   Mycosis fungoides more common in males (3 : 2)

females (Figure 47.20). There are a number of different types of lesions. The most common present-ing lesion is a red, scaly patch, and several usually appear in an asymmetrical pattern. The lesion may have a bizarre shape and have a tendency to become darker, developing a reddish-brown colour (Figure

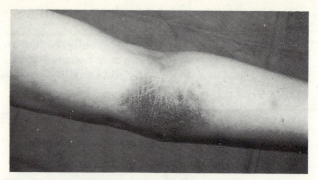

Figure 47.21   Mycosis fungoides: early stage. Reddish-brown scaly patch

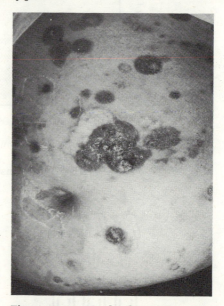

Figure 47.22   Scaly plaques in mycosis fungoides

47.21). The lesions subsequently become thicker or infiltrated plaques (Figure 47.22), maintaining their asymmetrical presentation, but often more numerous as the disease progresses. Finally, frank tumours form which are raised, nodular lesions of varying size. Both the plaques and tumours may break down and ulcerate. Although the scaly patch, infiltrated plaque and nodular lesions are the three types of skin lesion seen, the disease does always begin as scaly patches with progression to plaque and nodules. Mycosis fungoides may begin as plaques or nodular tumours. The lesions may affect any part of the skin, and be solitary or multiple when the disease commences.

Differential diagnosis

The red, scaly patches have to be distinguished from eczema. An endogenous eczema usually is symmetrical, whereas mycosis fungoides is asymmetrical. Both diseases will show clinical improvement with topical steroids, but complete clearing is less likely in mycosis fungoides, and relapse is much higher. Parapsoriasis is a distinct clinical entity, showing oval and longitudinal reddish-brown scaling patches on the trunk; the disorder shows some symmetry. The infiltrated plaques and tumours have to be distinguished from other reticuloses infiltrating the skin, such as sarcomas and Hodgkin's disease, and granulomatous disorders.

Investigations

A biopsy is necessary to establish the diagnosis. A full blood count and chest X-ray should be carried out to see if there is any evidence of spread of the disease, or another type of reticulosis.

Aetiology

Mycosis fungoides is considered to be a reticulosis or lymphoma which starts in the skin.

Treatment

Topical steroids may be helpful in the early, scaly type of lesion; this treatment often clears the inflammatory cells from the skin, improves the clinical appearance, and relieves irritation. However, topical steroids do not clear the abnormal cells from the skin or appear to influence the course of the illness. PUVA (psoralens + long wave ultraviolet) has been shown to be able to clear the early, scaly lesions of mycosis fungoides; it is not effective in the plaques or tumour type of lesion. Whether PUVA alters the natural history of the condition is too early to say. The remissions that have been induced with PUVA may last many months. The tumours and plaques do clear with radiotherapy, but this is usually only given to individual, troublesome lesions. Total body electron beam therapy clears the lesions, but does not cure the disease. Oral cytotoxic drugs have been disappointing in the control of the disease.

Natural history and prognosis

In the majority of patients the disease is slowly progressive over a number of years. More lesions slowly appear and more have a tendency to form plaques and nodular tumours. The duration of the illness is frequently many years, i.e. up to 30, and patients often die from other causes. Eventually the disease may spread to involve the lymph nodes and internal organs and cause death. The most promising treatment is PUVA for the early stages of the disease, and it may be possible to keep the disease under control with this treatment.

PARAPSORIASIS (SUPERFICIAL SCALY DERMATITIS)

This is not a malignant condition and appears to be a distinct entity. It is considered in this section as it is a differential diagnosis of mycosis fungoides and was considered to be pre-malignant in the past.

Presentation   The condition is more common in men; the disease usually begins in middle life but may commence earlier. The typical lesion is reddish-brown and scaly; the shape is finger-like or oval. The lesions tend to be symmetrical and occur on the trunk and limbs.

Differential diagnosis   Eczema, particularly the discoid variety, may have a similar appearance. Eczematous lesions tend to be more exudative and may show blisters. The early stages of mycosis fungoides often have a similar appearance, and this probably accounts for parapsoriasis being previously considered pre-malignant. A biopsy may be necessary to distinguish between the two conditions.

Investigations   A biopsy should be carried out if there is any doubt as to the diagnosis.

Aetiology   The cause is unknown; the condition seems to be more similar to eczema than any other dermatosis.

Treatment   Potent topical steroids often clear the lesions. The lesions tend to clear on exposure to the sun, and PUVA may be a suitable form of treatment if topical steroids are not effective.

Natural history and prognosis The condition is often persistent, but permanent remissions have followed the use of the more potent topical steroids. There is no suggestion that the disease is pre-malignant.

RETICULOSES

Sarcomas may first arise in the skin, or secondary deposits from sarcomas elsewhere, or other reticuloses may appear in the skin.

Presentation The lesions are more common in middle aged and elderly persons, but may occur at any age. The sexes are equally affected. The primary lesions usually begin as deep, red or bluish nodules, and vary in size from a few mm to a few cm. They often occur as groups of lesions confined to one area of the body. The lesions may enlarge and break down and ulcerate (Figure 47.23). They may affect any part of the body. Very rarely a primary reticulosis presents as a generalized red, scaly eruption.

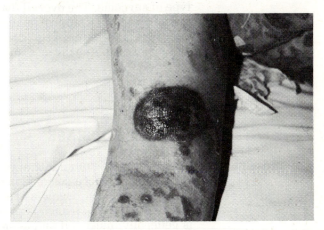

Figure 47.23   Ulcerated plaque in reticulosis

Primary lesions of Hodgkin's disease are extremely rare and present as small nodules in the skin.

Secondary deposits of sarcomas and leukaemias present as firm nodules or plaques in the skin of varying sizes. Infiltration of the nose and ear lobes may occur in chronic lymphatic leukaemia.

Differential diagnosis

The tumour stage of mycosis fungoides may be similar to sarcomas in the skin. Granulomatous disease may also have a similar appearance. The erythrodermic presentation is indistinguishable from that due to eczema or psoriasis. The distinction has to be made by biopsy.

Investigations

Biopsy is essential to establish the diagnosis. Full blood count and chest X-ray will be necessary as screening tests to see if there is any evidence of reticulosis elsewhere in the body.

Aetiology

Unknown.

Treatment

If the lesions are primary then the disease may be treated by radiotherapy and/or cytotoxic drugs. If secondary then the disorder should be treated by a unit specializing in the problem.

Natural history and prognosis

If the lesions are primary, the prognosis is that of a primary reticulosis elsewhere and depends on the type of sarcoma. The overall five year survival at the present time is approximately 50%. Secondary deposits imply widespread disease and will depend on the nature of the disease and what treatment may be available.

SEZARY'S DISEASE

Presentation

This is a disease of middle aged and elderly persons and is slightly more common in males (Figure 47.24). The disease often begins as red, scaly patches, but the classical appearance is erythroderma. The skin is generally thickened and as in the case of erythroderma due to other diseases, there is alopecia and dystrophy of the nails. The lymph nodes are often enlarged. Irritation is a common symptom.

Differential diagnosis

Other causes of erythroderma such as psoriasis, eczema or other reticuloses should be considered. The diagnosis must be made by biopsy.

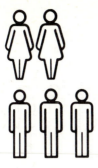

Figure 47.24   Sezary's disease is slightly more common in males

Investigations
Haematology   The diagnosis of Sezary's disease depends on finding Sezary cells in the peripheral blood. The cell is a leukocyte with a large cerebriform nucleus. The Sezary cell is also found in the skin and lymph nodes. There is some debate as to whether this so-called Sezary cell can be found in other skin disorders, or whether it is pathognomonic for Sezary's disease. A full blood count should be carried out.

Biopsy of the skin is obligatory.

Aetiology   Sezary's disease is often considered a variant of mycosis fungoides. The reasons for the variation and the typical Sezary's cells are unknown.

Treatment   Treatment is largely symptomatic. PUVA treatment may be helpful but the experience with this disease is so far limited.

Natural history and prognosis   The disease runs a protracted course over many years. Death usually follows when the disease changes to a leukaemia or a sarcoma.

KAPOSI'S SARCOMA

Presentation   The disease is commoner in men in a ratio of 10 : 1 (Figure 47.25). The disease begins in adult life in Caucasians, but has been described in negro children. The typical lesions are dark blue and initially are macular. They subsequently become papules, nodules or plaques with a scaly thickened surface.

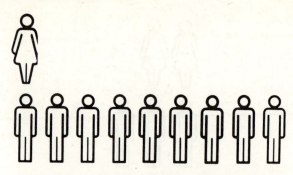

Figure 47.25   Kaposi's sarcoma is more common in males

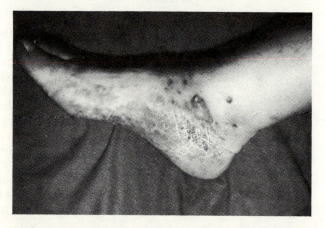

Figure 47.26   Reddish blue papules and scaly plaques in Kaposi's sarcoma

The size varies from 1 to 5 cm. Occasionally the lesions break down and ulcerate. The typical sites for the lesions are on the foot and around the ankle (Figure 47.26). Further lesions may then develop higher on the leg. The foot is invariably swollen. Occasionally the disease may begin on the hands, ears or nose.

Differential diagnosis   In the early stages the individual lesion may have to be distinguished from a pyogenic granuloma, histiocytoma, other types of sarcoma or even malignant melanoma. Once the multifocal nature of the disease is apparent the diagnosis is easily made.

Investigations   A biopsy is necessary to confirm the diagnosis.

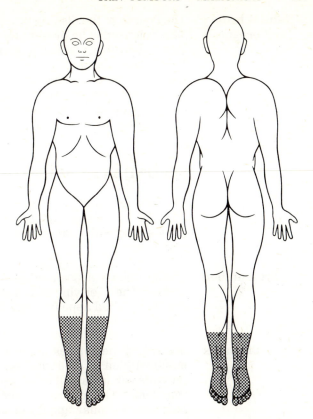

Figure 47.27   Common sites of Kaposi's sarcoma

Aetiology The disease is a proliferation of the vessels and peri-vascular tissue. There is some debate as to whether it is a primary disease of the blood vessels or of the surrounding connective tissue. Current view is that it is primarily a disease of the pericapillary fibro-blasts (and hence it is a reticulosis). The disease is commoner in Southern Mediterranean countries than those in the North. It is common in negroes in central Africa. No specific cause has been estab-lished.

Treatment If the lesions are small and localized, surgery may be considered. If the lesions are large, ulcerating and cause discomfort, radiotherapy will offer symp-tomatic relief. Cytotoxic drugs have been used but the results are not satisfactory for the morbidity of the treatment. The treatments are not curative.

Natural history and prognosis
The course of the disease is very slow in Europeans. The lesions may be present for 10–20 years without internal involvement and patients die of other illness. Visceral involvement when it does occur affects the liver, spleen and other internal organs. Anaemia and lymph node involvement are common in the late stages of the disease. Visceral involvement is more common in negroes.

SECONDARY CARCINOMATOUS LESIONS

The most common primary cancers to metastasize to the skin are breast, kidney and lung. Occasionally intra-abdominal cancers produce deposits in the umbilicus.

Presentation
The secondary deposit in the skin presents as a firm nodule. The overlying skin may be hyperaemic and thus have a red appearance. The lesions are usually 0.5–1.0 cm.

Diagnosis
Secondary metastases to the skin are usually a late manifestation of the disease, but sometimes the patients will not admit to lumps in the breast or other symptoms of the disease. Sarcomas and granulomas may give a similar appearance.

Investigations
If the diagnosis is in doubt a biopsy must be performed.

Treatment
If lesions are solitary and growing in size, and providing the general state of the patient is good, then radiotherapy or surgery may be considered.

Natural history and prognosis
The appearance of secondary deposits in the skin is usually a poor prognostic sign, although hypernephroma may present with a solitary deposit, and treatment of the primary has a reasonably good prognosis.

48 STRIAE

Presentation   Striae are common in adolescence and it has been estimated that they may be present in over a half of all females and a third of males (Figure 48.1) in adol-

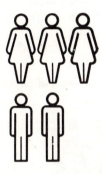

Figure 48.1   Striae are commoner in females (3 : 2)

escence (Figure 48.2). Striae are also seen in obesity, pregnancy, Cushing's disease, and as a side effect of systemic steroids. The initial lesion may be slightly raised and weal-like, and is linear. However, the lesion is not usually straight, but frequently shows curves throughout the length of the lesion. After the initial period of elevation the striae become flat and the surface is slightly wrinkled. On palpation a depression is felt compared to the surrounding skin. Some lesions have a bluish-red colour (Figure 48.3) whilst others are skin coloured. Eventually they become whitish. In the adolescent the common sites in females are the breasts, thighs and buttocks, while in males the lesions are usually found over the lower back and around the shoulders (Figure 48.4). The striae in pregnancy and in Cushing's disease are

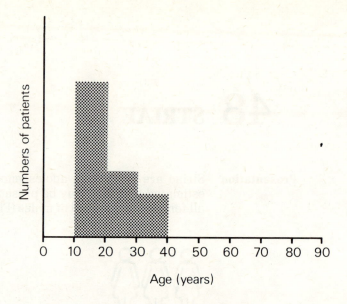

Figure 48.2   Age of onset of physiological striae

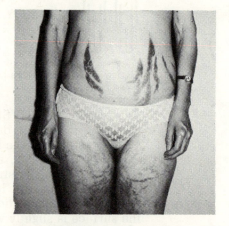

Figure 48.3 Purple striae on the abdomen following prolonged systemic steroid therapy

most frequently found on the abdomen (Figure 48.3). The common sites to see striae after the use of topical steroids are the groins and axillae.

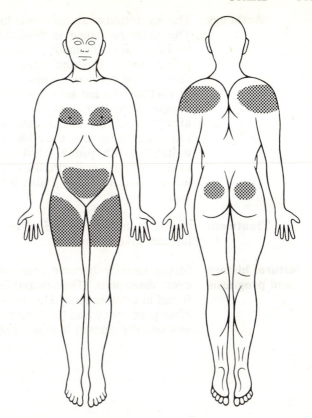

Figure 48.4   Common sites of striae

Differential diagnosis   In the last stages, when there is depression of the skin and wrinkling of the surface there is no difficulty in diagnosing the lesion. However, in the early stages when the lesions may be raised the lesions may be misdiagnosed because this appearance is not usually associated with striae. The fact that the lesions are persistent should distinguish them from urticaria. The Koebner phenomenon in lichen planus may give linear smooth lesions, but they are not usually multiple as in the case with striae.

Investigations   Unless there is other clinical evidence to suggest Cushing's disease no investigations are necessary. If Cushing's disease is suspected then cortisol levels after an oral dose of dexamethasone should be estimated.

Aetiology   The formation of striae is due to damage of collagen. The primary cause is probably hormonal as the lesions are common after puberty, during pregnancy, in Cushing's disease and after systemic and topical corticosteroids. However, raised levels of cortisol are not found in adolescents with striae compared to those who do not have striae. Simple stretching of the skin in itself is not the basic cause, but it may determine the sites of striae in susceptible individuals. In young adult males striae are commoner in those undertaking strenuous manual work as opposed to those following sedentary occupations.

Treatment   There is no known effective treatment once the lesions have formed.

Natural history and prognosis   Striae usually become less conspicuous and may even disappear. This is particularly so in striae found in adolescence. The more severe lesions seen after pregnancy and Cushing's disease may fade but will usually remain to some degree.

49 TOPICAL STEROIDS

Topical steroids have revolutionized the treatment in dermatology over the past three decades. Unfortunately however, these preparations have been used indiscriminately, and have developed a bad name quite unjustly. The reason for this swing against topical steroids results from two factors. Firstly the potencies of the topical steroids that are now available have increased significantly over the last few years, and this has not been realized by many doctors who prescribe these drugs. Secondly, side effects to topical steroids are now becoming apparent. However, these side effects are avoidable if the drugs are used correctly. It is now appropriate to divide topical steroids into weak, moderate, strong and very strong. For the sake of simplicity, the practising doctor should familiarize himself with one topical steroid from each group. An example of a weak topical steroid is hydrocortisone, a moderate strength one clobetasol butyrate, a strong one betamethasone 17-valerate, and a very strong one clobetasol propionate.

The side effects from topical steroids are directly related to the following: (a) duration of use; (b) strength of preparation; and (c) site of application. Site of application is important for two reasons. The thinner the skin, i.e. of the face, the greater the absorption and the greater the risk of side effects. Secondly, in moister areas, i.e. the intertriginous areas, the greater the absorption and therefore the more likely are topical side effects to develop. Systemic side effects from topical steroids are related to the quantity used. Thus, if the disease is widespread, the greater the risk of systemic complications.

Although this section is concerned with the side

effects of topical steroids, this should not minimize their correct use.

Cutaneous side effects   The main side effects are due to the effect of the steroid on the collagen of the dermis. The steroid inhibits formation of new collagen and causes the breakdown of the existing collagen. These actions may present in a number of ways.

Striae   These are most likely to be seen in the intertriginous areas, i.e. axillae and groins (Figure 49.1). They may however occur anywhere.

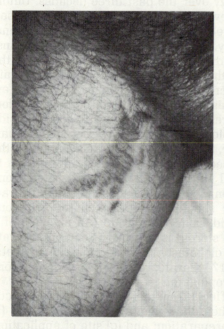 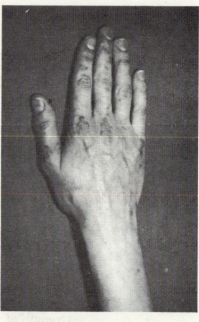

Figure 49.1 Striae in the groin following the use of a potent topical steroid   **Figure 49.2 Thinning of the skin on the back of the hand after long term use of a potent topical steroid**

Atrophy   General thinning of the skin will occur at any site after prolonged use of strong topical steroids. This is usually manifest by the subcutaneous veins being seen underneath the skin which is thin (Figure 49.2).

Telangiectasia   These small vessels are mainly seen on the face, and the face is generally redder (Figure 49.3).

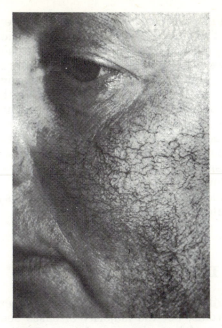

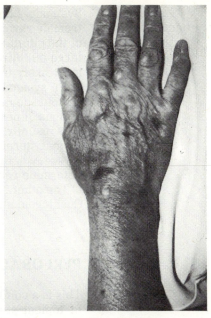

Figure 49.3 Telangiectasia after long use of a potent topical steroid

Figure 49.4 Purpuric lesions due to minor trauma after long term use of potent topical steroids

Spontaneous bruising
Purpuric lesions or ecchymoses arise at sites of minor trauma (Figure 49.4). These are mainly seen as macular purplish patches on the backs of the hands and forearms, but they may appear elsewhere.
These side effects due to atrophy of the collagen are often reversible at least partially, apart from the striae, which will tend to persist although they may become less obvious. Reformation of the new collagen however may take months and even years.

Masking of other dermatoses
If topical steroids are used for fungal or bacterial infections, particularly impetigo, the lesions may lose their characteristic appearance and be difficult to diagnose. If a superficial rash is persisting and spreading despite topical steroids, underlying infection must be considered.

Super-added infection
A hazard of topical steroids is that they suppress the body's defences against infection. Secondary infection, usually with a staphylococcus, may occur with the use of topical steroids.

Systemic side effects of topical steroids

Systemic side effects from topical steroids are extremely rare. The most likely hazard is suppression of the pituitary adrenal axis. Patients who have used large quantities of potent topical steroids are those most likely to be at risk, and appropriate coverage with systemic steroids may be necessary if the patient should be involved in an accident or develop a serious illness. Recovery of the pituitary adrenal axis usually occurs soon after discontinuing the topical steroids. The appropriate tests can be used to see whether suppression has occurred and to determine recovery.

The other side effect which has been reported is a Cushingoid state. This is extremely rare.

PERI-ORAL DERMATITIS

This is a condition which did exist before the advent of topical steroids, but the majority of cases seen today appear to follow the use of potent topical steroids.

Presentation   The disorder occurs in females (Figure 49.5) usually in the third or fourth decades (Figure 49.6). The

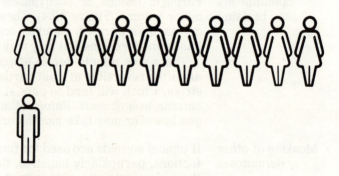

Figure 49.5   Peri-oral dermatitis is predominantly a disorder of females (10 : 1)

topical steroid appears to be used in the first instance for seborrhoeic eczema involving the chin or sides of the nose. Initially the eczema is suppressed, but usually recurs within a few weeks. The next time the topical steroid is used it is found to be less effec-

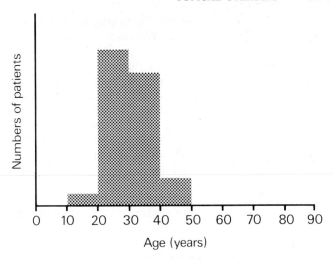

Figure 49.6   Age of onset of peri-oral dermatitis

tive, and the steroid has then to be used continuously to achieve suppression of the rash. When the steroid is stopped the condition quickly flares up and more steroid is required. Eventually small papules and pustules begin to form around the mouth (Figure 49.7) and nose, and these may spread to involve the

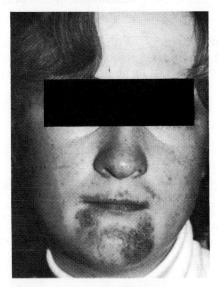

Figure 49.7   Erythema, scaling and papules around the mouth in peri-oral dermatitis

eyelids. Pustulation is often worse when the steroid is discontinued.

Differential diagnosis   Peri-oral dermatitis has to be distinguished from acne and rosacea when the papules and pustules are present. The history of use of a potent topical steroid and localization of the lesions around the mouth suggest the diagnosis. If the disease is very extensive and there is background erythema and telangiectasia it can be difficult to distinguish from rosacea.

Aetiology   The disorder only appears to follow the use of potent topical steroids. Many patients do use potent topical steroids without developing peri-oral dermatitis, and it is therefore considered to be an idiosyncratic response in certain individuals.

Treatment   The topical steroid cannot be stopped suddenly otherwise there is a flare up and worsening of the condition which patients will not tolerate. The strength of steroid should be gradually reduced over a period of 3–4 months. Systemic tetracyclines are helpful in suppressing the papular and pustular component of the eruption. The dose is 250 mg b.d. until the papules and pustules have cleared.

Natural history and prognosis   With appropriate treatment peri-oral dermatitis has a good prognosis. However, only weak topical steroids should be used on the face for any subsequent dermatosis.

50 TOXIC EPIDERMAL NECROLYSIS

Presentation The disease is rare, and is slightly more common in females than males at a ratio of 3 : 2 (Figure 50.1). Toxic epidermal necrolysis may occur at any age but a large proportion of cases are seen in infancy. In infants the condition usually appears after impetigo or a minor infection of the skin. The skin becomes red and tender and these signs usually first appear around the mouth or on the genitalia. The disease then quickly spreads to involve large areas of skin on the trunk and limbs. The erythematous areas then develop an irregular corrugated surface which peels off leaving superficial erosions. The lesions tend to heal spontaneously after one or two weeks. The whole process resembles a burn, and the disease is sometimes referred to as the 'scalded skin syndrome'.

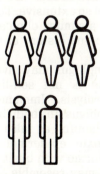

Figure 50.1 Toxic epidermal necrolysis is slightly more common in females (3 : 2)

In adults the inflammation around the mouth and on the genitalia may persist for two weeks before other manifestations appear. The red, tender areas then appear in the groins and axillae and extend

449

over the skin elsewhere. Large flaccid blisters appear (these are not usually seen in the infantile form of the disease), but blisters quickly rupture

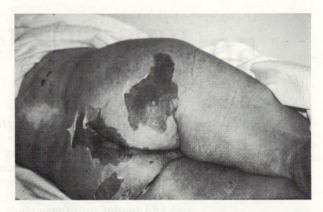

Figure 50.2   Large erosions in toxic epidermal necrolysis

giving rise to extensive erosions (Figure 50.2). As in infants the skin begins to heal within two weeks. The skin lesions are frequently associated with constitutional upset.

Differential diagnosis   In infants widespread impetigo has to be considered. In impetigo 'golden crusts' are usually present and the disease is not so extensive. Thermal and chemical burns may give a similar clinical picture in infants, but there may be no history of this in the 'battered baby syndrome'.

In adults pemphigus may give a similar picture, but the disease is not self-limiting as in toxic epidermal necrolysis. Immunological studies to detect the pemphigus antibody in the skin and blood are not always helpful, as false positives may occur in extensive toxic epidermal necrolysis. Severe erythema multiforme with blisters predominating as the main lesion may resemble toxic epidermal necrolysis. The classical target lesions in erythema multiforme may help to distinguish the two disorders.

Investigations   Swabs should be taken for bacteriological culture and sensitivity, and if a staphylococcus is found, this should be phage typed.

Aetiology   There are two known causes of toxic epidermal necrolysis; one is a staphylococcus, phage Type 71, and
the other is drugs. In infancy and childhood the
cause is usually the staphylococcus. The staphylococcus produces a toxin which causes damage to
epidermal cells with subsequent loss of the upper
region of the epidermis, as occurs in pemphigus. The
drugs which have been reported to cause toxic epidermal necrolysis are barbiturates, sulphonamides
and butazones. Whether other factors can cause
this type of tissue damage is not known, but
occasionally the same syndrome has been reported
with no evidence of a staphylococcal infection or
recent drug intake.

Treatment   If the disease is due to the staphylococcus then the
appropriate antibiotic should be given. While await-
ing the bacteriology results, treatment should be
commenced with systemic erythromycin or flucloxa-
cillin. The antibiotic can be changed if it is subsequently found that the organism is resistant to the
antibiotic given. If it is suspected that the disease is
drug induced, all drugs should be stopped. The treatment otherwise is similar to that for chemical or
thermal burns. Loss of fluid from extensively involved
skin may lead to electrolyte imbalance and dehy-
dration and this must be corrected. Good nursing
and attention to the mouth and eyes are important.
In the drug induced disease, systemic steroids,
starting with prednisone 60 mg daily, appear to dim-
inish the severity of the disorder.

Natural history   Both the staphylococcal and drug induced disease
and prognosis   may prove fatal. There is a higher mortality rate in
the drug induced cases, the mortality rate being
nearly 20%, whilst in the staphylococcal induced
disease the mortality is less than 5%. Death if it
occurs is from fluid loss and secondary infection as
in patients with severe burns.

Both the staphylococcal and drug induced disorders are self limiting, in patients who survive, and
the disease burns itself out within two weeks. There
are usually no residual sequelae such as scarring,
as the disease process is epidermal.

51 TREPONEMAL INFECTIONS

SYPHILIS

Presentation   Usually a sexually transmitted disease, with a very chronic course, which affects all races. There is a higher incidence in males than females (Figure 51.1).

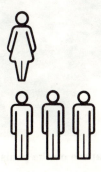

Figure 51.1   Syphilis is commoner in males (3 : 1)

The onset of the disease is highest in the sexually active years, especially between 20 and 24 years. There was a steady decline in the prevalence of the disease after the Second World War, but there has been a slight increase in recent years. Predisposing factors include homosexuality, mobility of population and promiscuity.

The clinical course is divided into three stages. In the primary stage there is localized infection at the site of entry of the treponema and regional adenitis. In the secondary stage there is dissemination of the infection via the blood, and it results in multiple lesions of the skin, mucous membranes and other organs. There is a latent stage between secondary and tertiary stages, when the treponemas are dormant and inactive. There are no clinical symptoms at this stage, but serological tests are positive. This stage may last a few or many years. In the tertiary stage any organ may be involved, and there are specific features.

Primary stage   The incubation period is between 7 and 90 days, but usually 3–4 weeks. The primary lesion or chancre is characteristically a small papule at the site of inoculation which then becomes a painless ulcer (Figure 51.2). The ulcer has an indurated raised

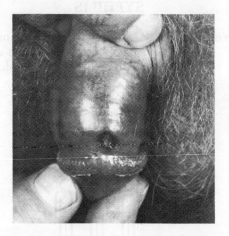

Figure 51.2   Chancre on the penis in syphilis

edge, with a clean and smooth base. The common sites for chancres are on the genital areas, e.g. in males, prepuce, frenum, corona, and occasionally on the shaft or base of the penis; in females, the vulva, cervix, vagina, clitoris and orifice of the urethra. Extragenital chancres may occur anywhere but are most often on the anus, perianal area, fingers, breasts, mouth and tongue. In two thirds of the cases there is unilateral or bilateral, mobile, painless, firm, regional lymphadenopathy. Spontaneous healing takes place in 3–6 weeks with an atrophic scar.

Secondary stage   Lesions in the secondary stage may appear at the same time as the primary lesion, but usually appear between 3 and 12 months later. The secondary stage may be associated with constitutional upset, e.g.

headache, malaise, mild fever, pain in the bones and muscles, generalized lymphadenopathy, hepatitis, arthritis and iridocyclitis. Cutaneous lesions vary greatly and may resemble any type of generalized skin eruption, although they are not itchy and not bullous or vesicular in form. Cutaneous lesions may be monomorphic or polymorphic.

Macular or rosealar syphilide   The lesions are pink, round or oval macules. The eruption is symmetrical on the trunk, limbs, palms and soles. The lesions may be few or numerous, and subsequently may disappear unnoticed or change to the papular syphilide, which mainly affects the face, palms and soles.

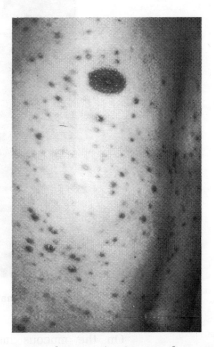

Figure 51.3   Papular eruption in secondary syphilis

Papular syphilide   The lesions are raised, pink or reddish-brown (Figure 51.3) in colour, and may be oval, discoid or annular. The surface of the lesions may be smooth or scaly, and if the latter, is then known as *papulo-squamous syphilide*. The common sites to be involved are the face, head, neck, palms and soles. Other variants of papular syphilide are: *perifollicular* *micropapules; annulopapular lesions* which are papules in annular configuration; and *corymbose syphilide* with a large central papule and satellite lesions around it.

Pustular syphilide   This is an acute form of papular syphilide in which the lesions become pustular and break down and form crusts. Scarring may follow.

Lesions in moist areas   On the genitalia and perianal skin the papules become hypertrophic and are known as condylomata lata (Figure 51.4).

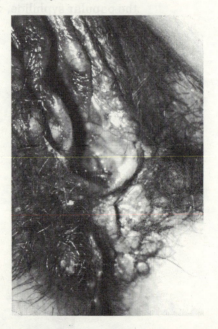

Figure 51.4 Condylomata lata on the perineum and vulva in syphilis

On the mucous membranes, the lesions may appear as white greyish patches or raised, smooth nodules with a tendency to ulcerate.

Patchy hair loss may occur in secondary syphilis. The hair loss is never complete and is often referred to as 'moth-eaten'. The eyebrows and beard may be affected in addition to the scalp.

Latent syphilis   This is the period after the secondary stage lesions have disappeared and patients are asymptomatic.

The serological tests are positive. Once the second-ary eruption has disappeared, patients are no longer contagious.

Tertiary syphilis   Tertiary manifestations may appear any time after two years of contracting the disease. They some-times do not appear for many years, e.g. 30 years. The average time is 6–7 years. The skin lesions are of two types:

Nodular lesions   These start as firm, pink, or red-brownish scaly nodules. They heal centrally and enlarge peripher-ally (Figure 51.5). This enlargement can produce dif-ferent serpiginous configurations. The lesion is superficial and there may be shallow ulceration or pus formation at the periphery. Scars are thin and there is no recurrence of the nodules in the scar tissue. The sites of predilection are the face, scalp, back and arms. The lesions are painless.

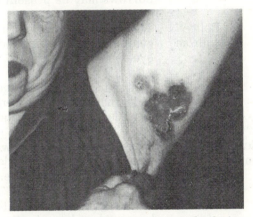

Figure 51.5   Reddish-brown annular lesion in tertiary syphilis

Gummatous lesions   These are deep necrotic punched-out ulcers. They may originate from underlying structures such as bones, or muscles. Spontaneous healing occurs but is only partial. The lesions are painless, single or multiple, and the sites of predilection are the scalp, face, calf and chest.

Mucous membrane lesions   These consist of leukoplakia and gummas which may ulcerate. In addition there may be chronic interstitial glossitis of the tongue.

Differential diagnosis *Primary stage*	The primary stage of syphilis in genital areas must be distinguished from the following diseases.
Lymphogranuloma venereum	This is a small, soft, transient and painless ulcer usually on the genitalia associated with lymphadenopathy in the groin, which progresses to a fluctuant swelling and discharging sinuses. The diagnosis can be confirmed by the Frei Test.
Chancroid	This presents with multiple painful, soft ulcers accompanied by suppurative regional adenitis. Smears from a lesion show *Haemophilus ducreyi*.
Herpes simplex	This presents as a small group of vesicles preceded by a burning sensation.
Scabies	This presents on the genitalia as small papules and there is usually a generalized, irritating rash and burrows may be present on the hands.
Behcet's syndrome	This presents as painful recurrent ulcers on the genitalia. It is associated with oral ulceration and eye problems.
Fixed drug eruption	This may occur on the genitalia and presents as a red area with subsequent blister formation and is often followed by residual pigmentation.
Eczema, lichen planus, psoriasis	These may all present with genital lesions but are usually associated with lesions elsewhere, enabling the diagnosis to be made.
Extragenital chancre	In extragenital chancre the following diseases must be considered: traumatic ulcers; tuberculous ulcers; Herpes simplex; neoplasms; and diphtheritic ulcers.
Secondary stage	In secondary syphilis the following conditions must be considered.
Tinea versicolor	The lesions are reddish-brown, scaly areas predominantly on the chest, back and upper limbs. The palms and soles are spared, and the diagnosis is confirmed by finding the fungus.
Drug eruptions	In the exanthematic form there are bright red papules and macules; the eruption usually affects

the trunk and the lesions may become confluent. A history of drug intake is usually obtained.

Seborrhoeic eczema	The lesions are characteristically reddish-yellow patches in the centre of the chest and back, face and scalp.

Guttate psoriasis	The lesions are small red papules with whitish scales. If the scale is removed, bleeding points are often seen.

Pityriasis rosea	There is frequently a herald patch and the typical lesion is oval with centripetal scaling. The palms and soles are spared.

In addition, granuloma annulare, annular lichen planus, annular sarcoid, fungal infection, and tuberculoid and borderline leprosy may be confused with annular lesions of secondary syphilis. The mucous membrane lesions and condylomata lata must be distinguished from viral warts, haemorrhoids and Herpes simplex infection.

Tertiary syphilis Lupus vulgaris	The lesions of lupus vulgaris are brownish plaques and on diascopy show the apple-jelly nodules. Peripheral enlargement of tuberculosis is slower than that of nodular syphilis. There may be recurrence of the nodules in the central scarred area of lupus vulgaris, but not in syphilis.

Psoriasis	The lesions are pink and scaly and are non-ulcerative.

Bromoderma, iododerma	These are vegetative lesions which may be single or multiple, presenting as dull red, oozing and crusted nodules or plaques, mostly on the face and limbs. They are due to prolonged administration of iodides and bromides.

Leprosy	The tuberculoid and borderline types present as plaques but these exhibit diminished sensation and sweating, with hair loss. Thickening of the nerves is often present.

In addition, varicose or arteritic ulcers may mimic the gummatous lesions. Pyoderma gangrenosum, tuberculous ulcers, deep fungal infections and pyogenic infections may also resemble syphilitic gummata.

Investigations

Due to the many varieties of clinical forms of syphilis especially in the secondary stage, its possibility should be considered as a differential diagnosis in many common dermatoses. The diagnosis should be confirmed by laboratory investigations.

Darkfield microscopy

(a) Examining a smear from the primary chancre or from moist secondary lesions, or abraded dry lesions, by darkfield microscopy may reveal the organisms.

(b) The fluorescent antibody darkfield (FADF) test which will identify the treponema in smears by a fluorescent antibody will demonstrate the treponema.

Standard serological tests (STS)

(a) Complement fixation tests include the Wassermann reaction (WR) and its modifications, e.g. Kolmer test.

(b) Flocculation tests, VDRL, Kahn, PRP.

The STS become positive 7–10 days after the appearance of a primary chancre. The most commonly employed screening test at the present time is the VDRL.

The tests are positive in all patients with secondary syphilis, when the highest titre is present. The titre falls after effective treatment and the test becomes negative in 6–12 months following the primary and secondary stages, but takes longer in the later stage. STS are positive in other treponemal diseases, e.g. yaws and pinta. False positive STS may be present in a very small number of normal individuals. Biological false positive reactions may also occur in a number of febrile illnesses, e.g. malaria, vaccinia, typhus and glandular fever. The titre is usually low and the test becomes negative after three months. Other diseases in which there are false positives are collagen disorders, leprosy and dysgammaglobulinaemia. The tests may be positive for many years. STS may also be positive in pregnancy. When the STS are positive, specific tests must be performed to establish the correct diagnosis.

Specific serological tests for syphilis

These tests are performed with treponema as the antigen.

(a) *Treponema Pallidum* Immobilization (TPI) test with live organisms. An antibody in the patient's serum causes immobilization of more than 50% of *Treponema*. It is specific for treponemal disorders including Bejel, pinta and yaws. After effective treatment in the primary and secondary stages the test becomes negative, but the test may remain positive after treatment of tertiary lesions.

(b) *Treponema Pallidum* Agglutination (TPA) test.

(c) Fluorescent *Treponema* Antibody (FTA) test. This is carried out with the patient's serum and dried *Treponema*. It is a very sensitive test specific for the *Treponema* group, but is not specific for *Treponema pallidum*.

(d) Fluorescent *Treponema* Antibody Absorption (FTA-ABS) test. By absorbing and removing non-specific group antibodies from the patient's serum, and then performing the same FTA test, it is then specific for *Treponema pallidum*. This is the most sensitive and specific test for syphilis. There is rarely a false positive, and it becomes positive earlier than VDRL.

Biopsy   The pathological changes of syphilis are predominantly an endoarteritis and perivascular infiltration with plasma cells and lymphocytes. In primary lesions there is erosion, hypertrophy of the endothelium and *Treponema* are present in the section.

In secondary syphilis, *Treponema* are rarely found except in lesions from moist areas.

In tertiary syphilis there is a granulomatous reaction with epithelioid and giant cells; caseation is marked especially in gummata, and numerous plasma cells are present. Endarteritis and plasma cell infiltration are additional features.

Aetiology   The causative agent is *Treponema pallidum*. Transmission of syphilis is by close contact and is usually sexually transmitted. The organisms can pass through the placenta to the foetus after 4 months of pregnancy. Primary and secondary lesions, especially of the mucous membranes are infectious. In tertiary syphilis the lesions are not infectious.

Treatment   Penicillin is still the drug of choice. Long acting penicillins given by intramuscular injection are used in preference to oral medication. A blood level of penicillin for ten days is considered necessary. Procaine penicillin-G in oil with 2% aluminium monostearate (PAM) 600 000 units every three days for twelve days, or procaine penicillin in watery suspension

600 000 units daily for ten days, are adequate for primary infections.

Treatment for secondary syphilis should be 4.8 megaunits of PAM or 600 000 units of procaine penicillin daily for two weeks. In late syphilis where prolonged treatment is necessary, a minimum of 12 megaunits of procaine penicillin is necessary.

If patients are allergic to penicillin then erythromycin or tetracycline may be given. If erythromycin is used the dose is 20–30 g over a 10–15 day period. With tetracycline 30–40 g over 10–15 days is required. It is advisable for syphilis to be treated in a venereology department so that contacts can be traced, and follow-up of the patient is necessary.

Prognosis In early syphilis, i.e. primary or secondary stage, the cure rate with treatment has been estimated to be 95%. Gummatous and nodular lesions also respond well to penicillin treatment. The progress in cardiovascular and neurological syphilis will depend on the damage to the tissues at the time treatment is given.

YAWS

Presentation Yaws is an infectious, non-venereal disease occurring in hot countries. Poverty and malnutrition are predisposing factors. Yaws affects both sexes but there is a higher incidence in males (Figure 51.6). The onset of the disease is usually in childhood and before the age of 15. The incubation period is usually a month, but may be from two weeks to several

Figure 51.6   Yaws is commoner in males (2 : 1)

months. The disease consists of three clinical stages.

The first stage or primary lesion (mother yaws) starts as a small red papule, which breaks down and becomes ulcerated. The ulcer gradually enlarges and becomes vegetative and papillomatous. In the primary stage the lesions may be solitary, or satellite lesions of a similar appearance may be present. The commonest site of involvement is the legs. There may be regional lymphadenopathy. Mild constitutional upset may be present on onset. The primary lesion heals spontaneously with scarring, after a few months.

The secondary stage may occur a few weeks after the first stage or overlap with it. The lesions are similar to those in the primary stage, but they are smaller in size and are more numerous (daughter yaws) (Figure 51.7). Secondary lesions most com-

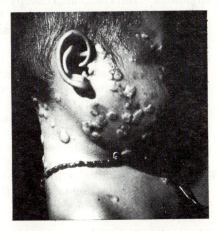

Figure 51.7   Multiple lesions on the face in secondary yaws (Wellcome)

monly occur around the body orifices, the lesions rarely extend to adjacent mucous membranes. There is thickening of the palms and soles. Painful, non-destructive osteitis and periosteitis and generalized lymphadenopathy may be present. Spontaneous healing occurs after several months with little or no scarring.

The late or tertiary stage begins 3–4 years after the onset of the disease. It affects mainly the skin and bones. Gummatous lesions of the skin cause extensive destruction of the skin and underlying tissues, with extensive scarring, pigmentary changes and disfiguration. There is hyperkeratosis of the palms and soles, destructive periosteitis of long bones, synovitis and tendinous synovitis.

Differential diagnosis

Lesions in the primary stage must be differentiated from ecthyma, impetigo, pyoderma gangrenosum, leishmaniasis and syphilis. The secondary lesions may resemble secondary syphilis, pityriasis rosea or psoriasis.

The tertiary lesions must be distinguished from syphilis, leprosy, mucocutaneous leishmaniasis and tuberculosis. Mid-line facial granuloma with lethal necrotizing ulceration and bone destruction of nose and mid-face, must be distinguished from tertiary yaws affecting the face.

Investigations

Darkfield microscopy demonstrates *Treponema pertenue* in the exudate from primary and secondary lesions. Serological tests for syphilis are positive.

Aetiology

The causative agent is *Treponema pertenue*. The disease is transmitted by direct contact with an infected person. The open lesions of primary and secondary stage are filled with *Treponema*. The organisms cannot pass through intact skin, so damage to the skin is necessary before a person can become infected.

Treatment

Penicillin is the drug of choice. 2.4 megaunits of a long acting penicillin (PAM or benzathine penicillin) will produce a cure.

Prognosis

Treated in the primary and secondary stages there should be no sequelae. The tertiary lesions may lead to permanent damage of the bones and unsightly scars.

PINTA

Presentation

A chronic non-venereal disease which is prevalent in tropical areas especially in America. Malnutrition, poverty, lack of hygiene are predisposing factors. It affects all races, male and female equally. The initial onset of the illness is most common in children before puberty.

The incubation period is between 1 and 3 months. The clinical picture consists of an early and late stage, which may overlap.

In the early stage the initial lesion is characterized by a small pinkish lenticular scaly papule, which gradually enlarges and becomes a plaque with raised borders and scales. The lesion becomes hypochromic and there may be satellite lesions which may merge into the primary lesion. Primary lesions may appear anywhere on the skin, but they are more common on the extremities. The secondary lesions appear a few months or a year after the onset of the disease. The lesions seen in the secondary stage are of three varieties; hypochromic, pigmentary, and erythromatosquamous. The lesions are often extensive and may merge, and may lead to atrophy of the skin with a tendency to achromia or hypochromia (Figure 51.8). Hyperkeratosis may occur on the legs, forearms, elbows, knees, ankles, palms and soles. There is no involvement of the internal organs.

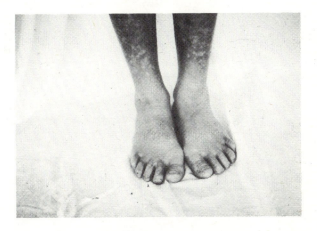

Figure 51.8   Hypochromic lesions in pinta

Differential diagnosis   The initial lesions must be distinguished from psoriasis, eczema and fungal infections. The late lesions will have to be differentiated from disorders with loss of pigmentation, e.g. vitiligo, tuberculoid leprosy and post-inflammatory hypopigmentation following eczema or psoriasis.

Investigations   Dark field examination of the tissue from the early lesions show *Treponema carateum*. Standard serological tests for syphilis, i.e. VDRL and WR, are positive after 2 months. TPI (*Treponema Pallidum Immobilization*) tests are also positive after 2 months.

Aetiology   Pinta is caused by *Treponema carateum*. It is similar to the *Treponema* of syphilis and yaws. Pinta is transmitted non-sexually and the *Treponema* enters the skin at sites of injury.

Treatment   Penicillin is the treatment of choice. Long acting procaine penicillin (PAM) is used and a total of 2.4 megaunits should be given. Tetracycline may be used in patients allergic to penicillin.

Prognosis   The early lesions clear with restoration of pigment. However, the atrophic and achromic lesions of the late lesions persist.

52 TROPICAL INFECTIONS

LEPROSY

Presentation

Leprosy is a chronic infectious disease. It is estimated that 11–15 millions suffer from leprosy, mostly in Asia, Africa and South America. It affects all races; lepromatous leprosy is more common in Caucasians, and tuberculoid leprosy in negroes. Males are affected more than females. Leprosy may present in childhood or adult life. The incubation period is usually between 2 and 5 years. There are different clinical forms of leprosy depending on the state of health, and type of immune response of the host.

Lepromatous leprosy

This is the most malignant form of leprosy and occurs in patients with low immunity to the *Mycobacteria leprae*. It is a generalized infection and progresses gradually if not treated. It may involve the skin, nerves, mucosa of the mouth and upper respiratory tract, reticulo-endothelial system, eyes, bones and testes.

The cutaneous lesions appear first, and they vary from macules and papules to infiltrated plaques and nodules (Figure 52.1). The borders of the lesions are ill defined, asymptomatic with a smooth surface, and with normal sensation and sweating. The sizes of the lesions vary from a few mm to a few cm. They are usually bilateral and symmetrical, and most commonly affect the face and limbs. The lesions may occur anywhere except the scalp, groin, axillae and perineum, and may eventually break down and ulcerate. Other late skin changes include thickening, particularly on the face (leonine facies) and lower legs. The scalp hair remains normal, but hair may be lost at other sites. Ichthyosis may occur in 10% of patients

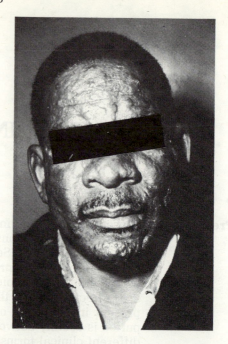

Figure 52.1   Infiltrated nodules and plaques in lepro-matous leprosy

with leprosy and mainly occurs on the legs.

Involvement of the mucous membranes presents as ulceration in the nose accompanied by nasal bleeding and discharge. Lesions of the larynx and pharynx may present as hoarseness or persistent cough.

Peripheral nerve involvement presents as paresis, muscular atrophy, anaesthesia and neurotrophic ulcers. In the late stage the nerves are thickened.

Bone involvement causes destruction of bones, particularly of the nose, leading to saddle nose deformity, the nasal septum, maxillary alveoli (leading to shedding of the teeth), and the phalanges of the hands and feet (leading to the shortening of the fingers and toes).

Eye involvement may cause punctate keratitis, corneal ulceration, plastic iridocyclitis and blindness due to tissue infiltration with *Mycobacteria* and neural damage.

Involvement of the testes leads to impotence, gynaecomastia and eventually sterility.

Tuberculoid leprosy   This is the most benign and localized form of leprosy in patients with high cellular immunity to the *Mycobacteria leprae*. The lesions are limited to nerves and skin. In the purely neural type, there is enlargement of peripheral nerves and there may be pain, paraesthesia, muscular weakness or paralysis.

In the cutaneous form lesions present as sharply defined erythematous or hypopigmented macules with a smooth or scaly surface. There may be papules or nodules present in the periphery of the lesion. An alternative presentation is that of plaques, whose centres become flat and depressed (Figure 52.2). The lesions enlarge peripherally, with

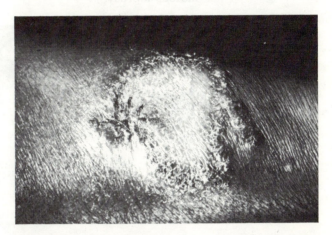

Figure 52.2   Tuberculoid leprosy. Plaque with central flattening

a smooth or rough surface. The plaques are pigmented but the colour may be reddish or violaceous. The cutaneous lesions have impaired sensation (except those on the face) especially to thermal sensation, and the lesions are devoid of hair and do not sweat. There may be multiple lesions which are asymmetrical and their size varies from a few mm to many cm. The lesions may occur anywhere (except the intertriginous areas), but most commonly affect the face, extensor surfaces of the limbs, buttocks and back.

In tuberculoid leprosy there is thickening of the nerves which helps the clinical diagnosis of the cutaneous lesions.

Borderline leprosy
(dimorphous)

Borderline leprosy represents a variety of different types of leprosy. Borderline leprosy occurs when the patient's immune response to the infection is moderate. As in tuberculoid leprosy only the nerves and skin are involved. In the neural form there may be peripheral neuropathy, and the skin lesions are either erythematous or hypopigmented macules or erythematous plaques. The lesions are more numerous than in tuberculoid leprosy. Annular lesions (Figure 52.3) may also occur and these are not found in tuberculoid leprosy. If the patient's immunity is relatively poor, then nodules may occur but these are asymmetrical and less numerous than in lepromatous leprosy.

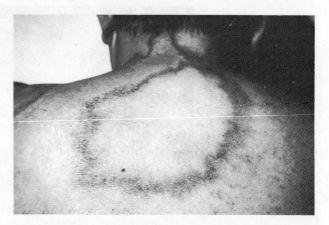

Figure 52.3   Annular lesions in borderline leprosy

Differential diagnosis

There are many different cutaneous lesions which may resemble leprosy due to the different clinical forms of leprosy.

Vitiligo presents with depigmented lesions and there may be some follicular hyperpigmentation; the skin has a normal texture and there is no impairment of sensation.

In pityriasis alba there are hypopigmented discoid scaly lesions, mostly on exposed areas of skin, and it usually occurs in children.

In pityriasis versicolor there are hypo- or hyperpigmented scaly lesions, mostly on the trunk, and mycology tests will show the mycelium and spores.

Post-inflammatory hypopigmentation is especially common in coloured skin, but there is no impairment of sensation in the lesions.

In secondary syphilis when the lesions are macular, they may have a similar appearance to the widespread macules seen in borderline leprosy. In tuberculoid leprosy the plaques have to be distinguished from tertiary syphilitic lesions.

Sarcoidosis may be confused clinically and histologically with the tuberculoid and borderline leprosy. In both these disorders there may be macular, nodular, annular lesions and plaques. peripheral nerves may be affected in sarcoidosis, but the nerves are not thickened.

Cutaneous tuberculosis, especially lupus vulgaris, may resemble tuberculoid leprosy. In lupus vulgaris there are apple-jelly nodules and there is central scarring of the lesion. In addition, the sensation of the lesions is normal and there is no neural involvement.

Leishmaniasis may resemble lepromatous leprosy. Smears from the lesions may show Leishman–Donovan bodies. The late recidivant lesions of leishmaniasis may resemble tuberculoid leprosy.

Yaws and lepromatous leprosy may both cause deformity and destruction of tissues around the nose.

Granuloma annulare has to be distinguished from the annular and nodular lesions of leprosy. Granuloma annulare occurs mainly over bony prominences.

Granuloma multiforme consists of itchy nodules and papules mostly on the upper limbs, and shoulders, and occurs in Nigeria.

Lymphocytic infiltration, mycosis fungoides, alopecia mucinosa, eosinophilic granuloma and other reticuloses of the skin, especially on the face may resemble nodular and plaque lesions of leprosy. A biopsy should distinguish the conditions.

In neurofibromatosis, the multiple neurofibromata may be confused with lepromatous leprosy.

In chronic photosensitivity and atopic eczema with lichenification of the skin, and alopecia of the eyebrows due to scratching, there is pseudo-leonine facies.

Investigations
Sweat test

Intradermal injection of pilocarpine 1 : 100 will fail to produce sweating in tuberculoid lesions due to damage of autonomic nerves.

Histamine test   The normal triple response is abolished due to sympathetic nerve damage. In hypopigmented lesions of tuberculoid and borderline leprosy the delayed reflex erythema is absent.

Skin or nasal smears   Mycobacteria leprae are present in large numbers in active lesions of lepromatous leprosy, but are scanty in borderline and tuberculoid leprosy. Skin smears are made at the edge of active lesions. Ziehl–Nielsen stains will demonstrate the bacilli.

Biopsy   The histology of the lesion depends on the clinical form.

Tuberculoid leprosy   There is a granuloma consisting of epithelioid and giant cells without necrosis. There are no, or very rarely, fragmented mycobacteria to be seen. Involvement of nerves is diagnostic.

Lepromatous leprosy   There is a granuloma in the dermis with large foamy histiocytes (lepra cells) which contain bacilli.

Borderline leprosy   The histology is a mixture of lepromatous and tuberculoid leprosy with granuloma formation. In borderline lepromatous disease a few mycobacteria are present.

The lepromin test   This is not a diagnostic test, but after the diagnosis is established it helps to clarify the clinical type of leprosy, and the state of the patient's immunity. Intradermal injection of standardized lepromin antigen in patients with good immunity produces a cutaneous reaction; it is read either after 48 hours (Fernandez or Dharmenda test) or after 4 weeks (Mitsuda test) depending on the type of antigen used. It is strongly positive in tuberculoid leprosy, and negative in lepromatous leprosy. In borderline leprosy the result depends on the amount of cell mediated immunity in patients to Mycobacteria; a weak positive occurs in borderline lepromatous leprosy, and a moderate reaction in borderline tuberculoid leprosy, but less than tuberculoid leprosy.

The lepra reaction   This occurs when the host–parasite balance is changed. It may be seen with an increase of immunity with high doses of chemotherapy, or due to decrease of immunity, e.g. inter current infections and pregnancy, etc. There are two types of lepra reaction. The first may occur in the three determinate types of leprosy, but the second only occurs in lepromatous leprosy. In the first there is swelling and redness of the skin lesions. The nerves may also be affected with ensuing pain and paresis. In the second type of reaction there are erythematous nodules and plaques, so-called erythema nodosum leprosum, and some of the following may also occur: intermittent fever; the nerves swell and become painful; bone pain; joint swelling; iridocyclitis; acute glottic oedema; orchitis; and lymphadenitis.

Aetiology   The causative agent is *Mycobacteria leprae*. It is an acid-fast and gram-positive organism and difficult to culture. The transmission is by prolonged exposure in susceptible individuals from open cases, and the organisms enter through the skin or nasal mucosa. In patients with lepromatous leprosy the open ulcers and nasal ulcers discharge many bacilli. Other forms only have a few bacilli in the lesions and are probably not infectious. Immunity plays an important part in to whether the disease develops and what type occurs.

Treatment   Treatment depends on the type of leprosy. However, sulphones are still the basis of treatment. In tuberculoid leprosy dapsone is the drug of choice. It is customary to start with a small dose, i.e. 5 mg daily for the first six months to avoid the Type 1 lepra reaction. The dose is gradually increased after six months to 50–100 mg daily. Treatment for tuberculoid leprosy should continue for at least one year after all the lesions have clinically resolved.

Borderline tuberculoid leprosy is also treated with dapsone in a similar manner as that for tuberculoid leprosy. However, it should be continued for life.

In lepromatous leprosy and borderline lepromatous leprosy, rifampicin 450–600 mg is given, with dapsone 100 mg daily, for three weeks. Treatment with dapsone should then be continued for life.

Treatment of the lepra reaction   A number of anti-inflammatory drugs are used to treat the lepra reaction. These include systemic corticosteroids, thalidomide and clofazimine.

CUTANEOUS LEISHMANIASIS (ORIENTAL SORE)

Presentation   Cutaneous leishmaniasis is a localized skin infection prevalent in tropical and subtropical countries. It affects all races and there is no sex predilection. It is most common in children and young adults (Figure 52.4). The incubation period ranges from two weeks to a year. Clinically the lesion appears as a small hard bluish-red papule which slowly enlarges and the ultimate size varies from 0.5 to 5.0 cm. The nodule breaks down and an ulcer forms which is usually covered by a crust (Figure 52.5). The lesion heals spontaneously in 9–12 months, and leaves an atrophic scar.

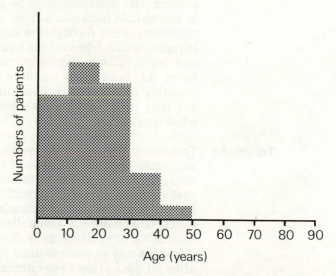

Figure 52.4   Age incidence of cutaneous leishmaniasis

The lesion may be solitary or there may be small satellite lesions which arise from the skin and spread via the lymphatics. Leishmaniasis occurs mainly on exposed areas.

Occasionally small brownish papules and nodules may appear close to or in the scar of an old lesion, once healing has taken place; this is referred to as leishmaniasis recidivans. The small papules eventually coalesce to form a plaque which is chronic and may persist for years.

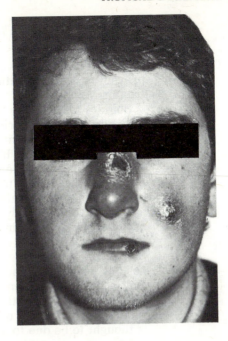

Figure 52.5   Crusted lesions in cutaneous leishmaniasis

Differential diagnosis
In the earlier stages before ulceration, leishmaniasis may be confused with keloids, keratoacanthoma, lepromatous lesions and sarcoidosis. In the later stage when ulceration appears the lesions must be distinguished from malignant neoplasms, tuberculous lesions of the skin, and other infective granulomas. The recidivans lesion may resemble lupus vulgaris, tertiary syphilis and a psoriatic plaque.

Investigations
A smear should be taken from the edge of a lesion for the detection of Leishman–Donovan bodies.

A culture of biopsy specimens on suitable media will grow the organisms.

Biopsy shows a granulomatous reaction with numerous Leishman–Donovan bodies in the macrophages in the early stages.

Intradermal tests with heat killed parasites give a positive skin reaction in 48 hours (tuberculoid type).

Aetiology
Cutaneous leishmaniasis is caused by a protozoon, *Leishmania tropica*. The vectors are sand flies. Leishmaniasis is endemic along the Mediterranean

coast, the Middle East, Central and South America and parts of Central Africa.

Treatment At present this is not very satisfactory and may not prevent scarring. Antimonials form the basis of treatment.

Solitary lesions may be treated with intralesional injections of mepacrine hydrochloride, emetine hydrochloride, trivalent and pentavalent antimonials given for 3–6 weeks. In extensive lesions systemic trivalent and pentavalent antimonial drugs, e.g. Pentostam (sodium stibogluconate) or Glucontine (meglumine antimoniate). The drug may be given either intramuscularly or intravenously. Finally, cryotherapy is sometimes successful in destroying the lesions.

Prognosis Lesions heal spontaneously within a year but scarring occurs. Permanent immunity follows once the lesions have healed, though very rarely there is a recurrence at the site of the original lesion, and this is thought to be due to altered immunity in the host.

53 TUBERCULOSIS OF THE SKIN

Presentation　Tuberculosis of the skin is found throughout the world, although the incidence is gradually falling. It is most commonly seen in communities with malnutrition and poor hygiene.

There are a number of patterns of skin tuberculosis. These depend on the following factors: (a) immunity of the host; (b) whether the infection is primary or secondary; and (c) whether it is primary skin inoculation or haematogenous spread from a distant site.

Primary cutaneous tuberculosis (tuberculous chancre)　This occurs in a patient without previous infection and no immunity. It is most commonly seen in children and infants. Trauma is a predisposing factor. The incubation period is 2–4 weeks. The lesion appears as a small, painless reddish-brown papule which enlarges and then ulcerates. The ulcer is ragged with undermined edges and a ragged haemorrhagic base. In 30% of patients the lesions may appear on mucous membranes. There is regional lymphadenopathy and mild constitutional upset. Spontaneous healing occurs after several months, with scarring. Other forms of tuberculosis, lupus vulgaris or scrofuloderma, may develop as a complication. The commonest sites of involvement are the lower extremities, genitalia and face.

Lupus vulgaris　Lupus vulgaris is a post-primary infection and occurs in patients with good immunity and hypersensitivity to the bacilli. The source of the infection may be from previous skin inoculation at the same site, from direct extension from underlying lymph nodes or joints, or it may be blood borne. The initial lesion is a small brownish papule which gradually enlarges.

477

The well formed lesion is characterized by a reddish-brown nodular plaque, with dermal infiltration (Figure 53.1). The epidermis may be smooth or

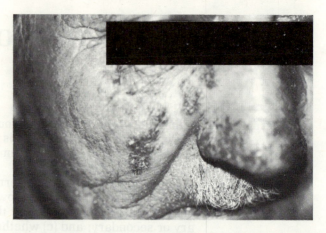

Figure 53.1   Lupus vulgaris. Reddish infiltrated plaque

there may be adherent scales. On diascopy (pressing
a glass slide against the lesion) there is the appearance of so-called apple-jelly nodules; these are small
soft yellow–brown nodules. The lesions heal very
slowly and spontaneously with scarring. There may
be destruction of soft tissue and cartilage leading to
deformity. Scars are thin and atrophic. Recurrence
of lupus vulgaris may occur in the scars and occasionally squamous cell carcinomas develop. The
sites of predilection are the face, nose, cheeks, ear
lobes, neck and adjacent mucous membranes.

Scrofuloderma   This form of cutaneous tuberculosis results from
spread of an infection, e.g. infected lymph nodes,
muscles or bones. The patient's immunity is
variable. Scrofuloderma may occur as solitary or
multiple lesions. The site of predilection is the neck.
The initial presentation is purplish induration
of the skin overlying an infected lymph node. Gradually the induration softens and the area becomes
fluctuant. Subsequently the lesion ruptures to
produce sinuses and ulceration and with undermined edges. There is a purulent discharge (Figure
53.2). Untreated scrofuloderma will last for years
and heals with deformed scars.

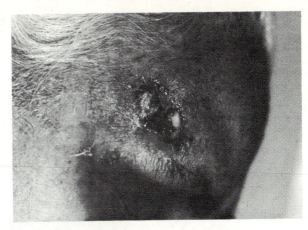

Figure 53.2 Purulent tuberculous ulcer in scrofulo-derma. The skin lesion is secondary to underlying infection of bone

Acute miliary tuberculosis
This occurs in children with active tuberculosis and poor immunity and is due to a haematogenous spread. The condition presents as a generalized symmetrical rash, consisting of dull red, scaling papules or vesicles. There may be a purpuric element or ulceration.

Orificial tuberculosis
This is tuberculosis of the skin adjoining mucosal orifices. It is caused by auto-inoculation of tuber-culosis bacilli. It may be seen in patients with pul-monary, genito-urinary, or intestinal tuberculosis. Patients have poor immunity. The lesions are small nodules which break down to give shallow, small, painful ulcers with undermined edges and a purul-ent discharge. The lesions may be single or multiple. Spontaneous healing is rare. The commonest sites are the mouth, anus and genitalia.

Warty tuberculosis
This occurs in patients with good immunity and is a reinfection. The infection is exogenous, and may be from sputum or as a result of occupational handling of infected material, e.g. in butchers and patholo-gists. It may also arise from auto-inoculation by sputum. The initial lesion is a small reddish-brown papule which enlarges and produces a painless, dull red, firm, warty hyperkeratotic plaque (Figure 53.3), with a serpiginous outline. The lesions persist and

are unchanged for years. Spontaneous healing eventually occurs with scarring. The lesions are usually single. The commonest sites are the hands and buttocks.

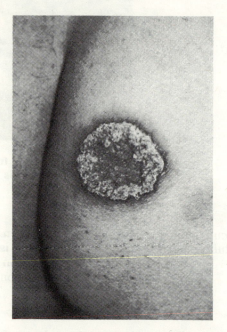

Figure 53.3   Warty tuberculosis on the buttock

Tuberculosis gumma   This occurs in patients with internal tuberculosis who have poor immunity. The lesions arise from haematogenous spread of the bacilli. The initial lesions are subcutaneous nodules which soften and then ulcerate. The latter are bluish ulcers with undermined edges. The lesions are multiple, most commonly occurring on the extremities.

Tuberculides   These are lesions produced by haematogenous spread, but at the time the skin lesions present no clinically active lesion is found. It is postulated that the bacilli may remain in the skin for long periods before certain changes take place allowing the tuberculides to appear in the skin. However, one of the curious facts is that bacilli are not found in the tuberculides, so their nature remains obscure.

Erythema induratum of Bazin This is seen in young and middle aged females. The lesions occur characteristically on the back of the legs. They begin as subcutaneous reddish-blue nodules which may break down and form shallow ulcers with irregular and ragged edges. Spontaneous healing may occur after many years, but scarring is present. Bazin's disease is said to occur in women with fat legs and poor circulation, and lesions usually first appear in winter (see page 505).

Lichen scrofulosorum This occurs in children and young adults. The characteristic site is the trunk. It begins as small yellow–brown, firm follicular papules which develop into rough discoid patches. The eruption becomes extensive for some weeks and then involutes without scarring.

Papulonecrotic tuberculide This occurs in children and young adults. The lesions are symmetrical, multiple painless, reddish-blue papules which enlarge, and then ulcerate to form a necrotic ulcer covered with a crust. Spontaneous healing occurs with scarring. The commonest sites of involvement are the extensor aspect of the extremities, especially knees and elbows, and the buttocks.

Differential diagnosis
Primary tuberculosis Cat scratch fever produces lesions and lymphadenitis similar to primary tuberculosis, but the lesions only last 3–4 weeks.

In sporotrichosis localized lesion may be ulcerative with enlarged lymph nodes. Culture of specimens from a lesion establishes the diagnosis.

The primary lesion of tuberculosis on the genital area may be mistaken for a syphilitic chancre. Warty tuberculosis and scrofuloderma may resemble a primary tuberculous lesion.

Warty tuberculosis Viral warts, solar keratoses and seborrhoeic warts may all resemble warty tuberculosis in certain instances. A biopsy may be necessary to establish the diagnosis. Blastomycosis, sporotrichosis and actinomycosis may all form warty plaques which have to distinguished from tuberculosis. Tertiary syphilis may give rise to scaly plaques with central scarring. Hypertrophic lichen planus on the legs often resembles the appearance of warty tuberculosis. A solitary patch of psoriasis has to be considered when the tuberculous lesion is red.

Lupus vulgaris   The following have to be considered in the differential diagnosis.

Sarcoidosis, especially the plaque form of lesion with superimposed nodules, may resemble lupus vulgaris lesions.

Tertiary syphilis may present with erythematous scaling lesions with nodules and serpiginous edges. There may be central scarring but no recurrence of nodules in the centre.

In tuberculoid leprosy a firm plaque is present which exhibits loss of sensation.

Tropical leishmaniasis presents as a bluish-red plaque which ulcerates, and mostly occurs on exposed areas.

Psoriasis may resemble lupus vulgaris, but it is not infiltrated and the silvery scales and capillary bleeding should distinguish the two conditions.

Bowen's disease, discoid lupus erythematosus and lymphocytoma cutis may also have to be considered in the differential diagnosis.

Scrofuloderma   The following conditions have to be considered: tertiary syphilis, hidradenitis suppurativa, lymphogranuloma venereum, deep fungal infections and malignant skin lesions.

Investigations   The following bacteriological tests may be carried
Bacteriology   out: (a) demonstrations of bacilli in smears or biopsy material; (b) culture; and (c) inoculation of guinea-pigs with material from the lesion. Because of the wide spectrum of disease in tuberculosis of the skin, the tests may give variable results depending on the immunity of the patient and whether the disease is primary or secondary. In primary lesions bacilli are usually found, but in secondary lesions with good immunity the bacilli are not often found.

Tuberculin test   This should be carried out.

Biopsy   The main feature is a granuloma, known as a tuberculoid granuloma with epithelioid and Langhans' giant cells. Caseation may be present.

Aetiology   Skin tuberculosis is due to *Mycobacterium tubercu-* *losis* which reaches the skin by contact with the infected material, haematogenous spread, or extension through the tissues. The type of skin lesion depends on whether the infection is primary or secondary, and the immunity of the patient.

Treatment   The drugs currently used for the treatment of tuberculosis are isoniazid (INH) 5 mg/kg daily, streptomycin 1 g daily, rifampicin 450–600 mg daily, and ethambutol 15 mg/kg daily. The initial treatment is by the combination of INH, rifampicin and ethambutol, or INH, rifampicin and streptomycin. Other regimes may be used if necessary. Initial treatment is for 2–3 months. Treatment is then continued for another 6–18 months and is with two drugs, commonly rifampicin and INH.

Other antituberculous drugs such as viomycin, cyclocerine, PAS (p-aminosalicyclic acid) ethionamide may be used if necessary. Surgical repair of scarred and damaged tissue may be necessary. The skin lesions should show some response to treatment six weeks after starting chemotherapy.

Prognosis   Cutaneous tuberculosis has a good prognosis if treatment is commenced early in the disease. Severe scarring and disfiguration may result if treatment is delayed.

54

URTICARIA, ANGIO-OEDEMA AND DERMOGRAPHISM

Urticaria is a common condition. It is termed nettle rash or hives by the layman.

There are several classifications of urticaria (Table 54.1). Urticaria and angio-oedema differ only in the site of the lesions; those of urticaria are in the superficial dermis, the swellings of angio-oedema are deep in the subcutaneous tissues. Urticaria and angio-oedema may be present together or separately.

Table 54.1 Classifications of urticaria

Duration of *disease*	Acute (minutes – weeks) Chronic (months – years)	
Site	Superficial Deep	Urticaria Angio-oedema
Cause	Allergic Pharmacological Physical Unknown (idiopathic) 80% Pregnancy Contact (very rare)	

Presentation

Urticaria can occur at any age, but mostly commonly presents between the ages of 10 and 40 (Figure 54.1). There is a slight female preponderance. There is an increased incidence of acute allergic urticaria in atopic subjects.

The lesions of urticaria and angio-oedema may occur anywhere on the body. Urticaria particularly affects the limbs and trunk, angio-oedema the periorbital region (Figure 54.2), lips, neck and joints. The mucous membranes may be involved. Involvement of the larynx and lower respiratory tract may be fatal. If the gut is involved, vomiting and abdominal pain may occur.

485

The lesions vary in size from a few millimetres to several centimetres. They are transient and persist for minutes or hours, but resolve within 48 hours. The lesions of urticaria are raised weals: they may be white or red with surrounding erythema (Figure 54.3). When resolving or partly suppressed by treatment there may be erythema only (Figure 54.3). The lesions are intensely itchy. The subcutaneous swellings of angio-oedema are usually skin coloured (Figure 54.2), but may be erythematous. The eyes may close completely (Figure 54.2). The lesions of angio-oedema are rarely itchy.

Several patterns of urticaria can be distinguished by cause, history, and their clinical picture (Table 54.1).

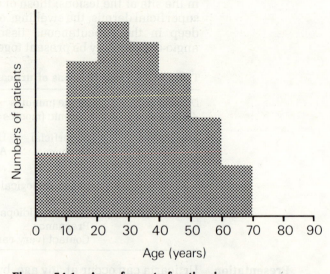

Figure 54.1   Age of onset of urticaria

Acute allergic
urticaria

Acute allergic urticaria is a sudden and dramatic event. It can occur within minutes of administration of the causative agent. It can be very severe and respiratory tract involvement may cause death. It may persist for many weeks or months. The cause is often obvious.

The commonest causes of acute allergic urticaria are shown in Table 54.2. Penicillin and other drugs are important causes. There is a high incidence in atopics who respond in this way to certain foods and drugs, and soon learn to avoid them.

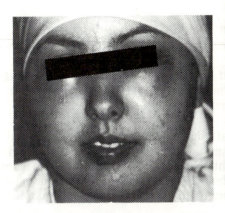

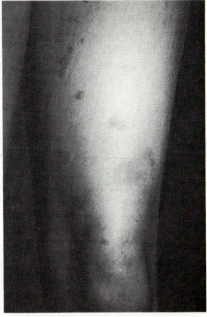

Figure 54.2 Angio-oedema of the face. The whole face is oedematous and swollen

Figure 54.3 Urticaria: the weals are red and raised and there are areas of erythema

Table 54.2 Causes of acute allergic urticaria

Azo dyes	
Drugs	
Foods	– proteins in eggs, fish, fruit
Infections	– bacteria
	parasites
	protozoa
	viruses
	yeasts

Pharmacological urticaria Certain compounds can cause direct release of histamine from mast cells and induce urticaria. This occurs within hours of ingestion. Shellfish, fish and strawberries may cause such reactions, as may salicylates. Penicillin can act by this mechanism. Nettle stings are an example of pharmacological urticaria.

Physical urticaria	There are several types of physical urticaria, which result from changes in the physical environment.
Cholinergic urticaria	This is the most common. It usually occurs in young people in response to sweating induced by exercise or heat. The urticaria occurs on the limbs and trunk and is characterized by small lesions 2–3 mm in diameter.
Cold urticaria	This occurs in response to a fall in temperature. It may be primary or secondary to cryoglobulinaemia.
Solar urticaria	This is evoked by certain wavelengths of light (see Chapter 33, Photosensitivity).
	Heat and pressure may also induce urticaria.
Idiopathic urticaria	This is the most common type of urticaria. It is usually gradual in onset, persists for months or years, and is worse at night. No cause can be found. In some patients psychological factors seem to be important in precipitating urticaria or causing exacerbations of it.
Pregnancy urticaria	Urticaria may develop in the last trimester of pregnancy.
Contact urticaria	This is rare; it occurs at the site of application of certain compounds. The best known example is a nettle sting.
Differential diagnosis	Urticaria may be confused with insect bites, which are distinguished by being grouped and having a central punctum and by their persistence, and with dermographism. The rash of serum sickness is often urticarial, but there are in addition joint pains and haematuria. Drug rashes and vasculitis may have a prominent urticarial component, but this has a long time course. Toxic erythemas are symmetrical and flat or papular.
	Angio-oedema may be indistinguishable from hereditary angio-oedema and sometimes confused with erysipelas.
Diagnosis and investigations	
Skin biopsy	Biopsy shows oedema, but is rarely necessary.

Blood investigations A full blood count should be done, as an eosinophilia suggests a parasitic cause. Cryoglobulins should be sought in patients with cold urticaria. The ANF and DNA binding should be done as SLE may cause urticaria.

Challenge tests It may be useful to confirm that a suspected substance is the cause, and this can be done with a challenge test. The patient is given either placebo or a small dose of the substance under investigation and the response observed. This must *not* be done if there is any history of respiratory involvement or anaphylaxis.

Aetiology The final common path of urticaria is degranulation of mast cells, with release of histamine and other mediators. These cause vasodilation leading to erythema, and increased vascular permeability resulting in oedema and weal formation.

The degranulation may be the result of binding of antigen to cell bound IgE as in acute allergic urticaria, due to direct pharmacological degranulation, or mediated by the axon reflex in cholinergic urticaria. The triggers for degranulation remain obscure in the majority of cases of urticaria.

Treatment
General measures Any identifiable causes should be scrupulously avoided.

Exacerbating agents such as salicylates must be avoided.

When bacterial, parasitic or yeast infections are thought to be the cause they should be treated.

Elimination diets are occasionally of value in chronic urticaria. Diets avoiding azo dyes, tartrazine, certain proteins or fruits have all been of benefit to a few patients.

Drug therapy Antihistamines are successful in suppressing urticaria in many patients. They often need to be given in high doses, and the dose should be increased until symptoms are suppressed, or drowsiness is so great as to interfere with normal life. Long acting antihistamines are particularly useful; sometimes the total dose may be given at night so that the drowsiness is useful. The acute cases usually respond, but unfortunately not all cases of chronic urticaria do so.

The serotonin antagonist, cyproheptidine, is sometimes effective when antihistamines have failed.

Hydroxyzine which combines antihistamine and anxiolytic properties is often very useful. It is the most effective treatment for cholinergic urticaria, but most treatment is ineffective.

Systemic steroids are of value in serum sickness, and are sometimes given in acute severe urticaria. They are not indicated for chronic urticaria.

Adrenalin subcutaneously or intramuscularly may be lifesaving in acute laryngeal oedema due to angio-oedema. Tracheostomy may be required, but will be ineffective if the lower respiratory tract is involved.

Natural history and prognosis   The natural history is very variable. Acute allergic urticaria usually resolves within days or weeks. Very occasionally respiratory tract involvement may be fatal.

Chronic urticaria persists for many years, but its activity often varies, and although it causes discomfort to the patient, it rarely results in severe problems.

The physical urticarias persist for many years, although cholinergic urticaria usually clears after several years.

DERMOGRAPHISM

Dermographism can occur on its own or in association with urticaria, urticaria pigmentosa and vasculitis.

Presentation   It can occur at any age and in both sexes, though it is more common in females.

Any part of the body can be affected. Pressure and trauma result in a weal at the site of the injury (Figure 54.4). The weal takes 5–10 minutes to develop and then slowly fades. There may be slight itching. Pressure from clothing and scratching may produce lesions. It may be associated with chronic urticaria. It occurs in urticaria pigmentosa and may be seen in Henoch–Schönlein purpura.

Differential diagnosis   Dermographism is often confused with urticaria, but is the response to scratching not the cause.

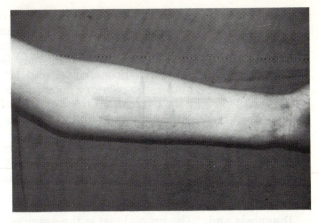

Figure 54.4   Dermographism: weals in response to trauma

Diagnosis and investigations Dermographism is easily demonstrated by firm pressure with a blunt instrument.

Aetiology It is not known why weals are produced in dermographism; histamine is probably the most important mediator.

Treatment Most patients do not require treatment.

Natural history and prognosis Some people have a lifelong tendency to dermographism but the extent of the response is variable. Most troublesome cases become less severe within a few years.

HEREDITARY ANGIO-OEDEMA

This form of angio-oedema, formerly known as angio-neurotic oedema, differs from all other forms of angio-oedema and urticaria in aetiology and prognosis.

Presentation Angio-oedema is usually manifest in late childhood or adolescence but can commence later. Men and women are equally affected. It is familial and the inheritance is autosomal dominant. Sporadic cases occur.

The disease is recurrent, episodes of angio-oedema occurring at intervals of several weeks or months. Any part of the skin or mucous membranes are affected. Subcutaneous or deep swellings arise. These may be initiated by trauma or are spontaneous. They may cause discomfort and pain. The whole respiratory tract may be involved including the small bronchioles, and laryngeal oedema may cause respiratory obstruction and death. The gastro-intestinal tract may also be affected, causing abdominal pain and obstruction.

Differential diagnosis It is distinguished from other forms of angio-oedema with urticaria by the family history, recurrent nature, and respiratory and gastro-intestinal involvement.

Diagnosis and investigation The crucial test is the assay of C_1 esterase inhibitor in the blood. This will be low, or despite normal absolute amounts, lacking in esterolytic activity. The levels of complement components may be low.

Barium studies performed during an attack of abdominal pain show the characteristic appearance of angio-oedema.

Aetiology Initiation of the complement cascade by minor trauma or other stimuli is limited by a feedback system operated via C_1 esterase inhibitor. The absence of this enzyme allows the complement cascade to continue unchecked for long periods, with consequent inflammation and oedema. The mechanism for its cessation in those patients is unclear.

Treatment Acute attacks are terminated by the infusion of fresh frozen plasma to supply C_1 esterase inhibitor. Tracheostomy may be necessary, but if the terminal bronchioles are affected it will be unsuccessful.

Continuous therapy with ε-amino-caproic acid is partially successful in preventing attacks. The use of attenuated androgens has greatly improved the management of the disease. Danazol or stanozolol are continuously administered in the smallest effective dose. Initially the levels of C_1 esterase inhibitor rise, but clinical remission is maintained despite a subsequent fall.

Natural history and prognosis The attacks are recurrent and persist for life. Many patients die from acute respiratory obstruction.

55 URTICARIA PIGMENTOSA

Urticaria pigmentosa is also known as mastocytosis. It is due to abnormal collections of mast cells in skin and other tissues. There are two forms differing in the age group affected, morphology of the lesions and prognosis.

Presentation
Childhood
urticaria
pigmentosa

This may be present at birth or may develop within the first six months of life. New lesions appear throughout the first year. Both sexes are affected.

Any part of the body may be affected. The trunk and limbs are the commonest sites. The lesion may be solitary and is then called a mastocytoma.

The lesions are red brown macules or papules and vary from a few mm to a few cm in diameter (Figure 55.1). Trauma, e.g. rubbing the macules results in urtication and the lesions become erythematous and oedematous (Figure 55.1). In infancy this may progress to bulla formation.

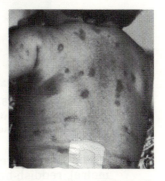

Figure 55.1 Childhood urticaria pigmentosa; large brown macules are present which urticate and blister on rubbing

Dermographism is often present.

Pruritus may be a prominent feature of the lesions.

Other tissues may be involved. The bones, bone marrow, lungs, lymph nodes, liver and spleen and gastro-intestinal tract can all be infiltrated.

Release of hitamine from the mast cells can cause flushing, diarrhoea and tachycardia. Salicylates and other drugs act as histamine liberators, as does trauma to the lesions, e.g. drying the child.

Acquired
urticaria
pigmentosa

This presents at any age, but most commonly between 20 and 40.

The eruption is chiefly on the trunk, upper arms and thighs, but all areas may be involved. The face is spared.

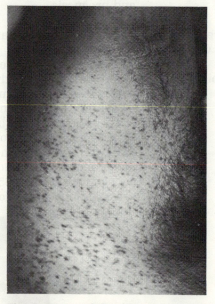

Figure 55.2   Adult urticaria pigmentosa showing widespread small red brown macules and papules

The lesions are small (usually less than a centimetre), reddish-brown macules, papules or nodules (Figure 55.2). Some are telangiectatic. Trauma and rubbing of the lesions causes urtication. Bulla formation does not occur.

Pruritus is a variable symptom; it may be severe or absent.

There is often systemic involvement, with infiltration of bone marrow, bones, lungs, lymphoid tissue, liver and gut. The liver and spleen and lymph nodes may all be palpable.

Histamine release is precipitated by codeine, salicylates, and alcohol as well as by trauma. The flushing, diarrhoea and tachycardias are usually more troublesome to adults than they are to children.

Differential diagnosis	The childhood form may be confused with naevi, the bullous disorders of infancy, and postinflammatory hyperpigmentation.

The adult form may be confused with secondary syphilis (which is transient), freckles and lentigenes.

Diagnosis and investigation	Skin biopsy should be done to confirm the diagnosis. Special stains are required to demonstrate the mast cells. The lesions should not be rubbed prior to biopsy as the mast cells may degranulate and will not take up the stains.

A full blood count and film may show a basophilia.

Bone marrow aspirate and lymph node and liver biopsies may show the presence of mast cells.

Chest X-ray may show infiltration of the lungs. A skeletal survey may show bony lesions. These should not be done routinely in infancy.

Aetiology	It is not known why the mast cells are present in abnormally high numbers. In a very few patients the mast cells proliferate to such an extent that a malignant process supervenes. In most cases they do not behave as malignant cells.

Treatment	The childhood form requires no therapy, other than treatment of secondary infection.

Some adults are troubled by intense pruritus and antihistamines may be of little benefit. PUVA therapy has been helpful to a few patients.

Factors precipitating histamine release should be avoided.

Natural history and prognosis	The childhood form is self limiting. The bullae cease to form after infancy and the lesions gradually involute. Most are completely clear by puberty.

The adult form persists indefinitely, the lesions

becoming more numerous. Infiltration of other organs may be widespread but does not indicate a malignant process. Rarely a mast cell or other leukaemia may arise.

56 VASCULITIS

Vasculitis is inflammation of the blood vessels. The primary event initiating the inflammation may be an abnormality of the blood, the vessel wall, or the tissues adjacent to the vessel. The vessels affected may be arteries, arterioles, capillaries, venules or veins. The small blood vessels with slow rates of flow are usually affected. The stagnant circulation in the capillaries and venules of the legs make these sites of predilection for vasculitis.

The clinical signs depend on the severity of inflammation. The changes range from increased

Table 56.1   Clinical syndromes of vasculitis

Cutaneous
    Chilblains
    Cutaneous vasculitis (leukocytoclastic vasculitis, allergic vasculitis)
    Cutaneous polyarteritis
    Erythema induratum (Bazin's disease)
    Erythema nodosum
    Henoch–Schönlein purpura
    Idiopathic capillaritis
    Livedo reticularis
    Nodular vasculitis
    Panniculitis
    Papulonecrotic tuberculid
    Pityriasis lichenoides
    Waldenström's hypergammaglobulinaemic purpura

Cutaneous–systemic
    Cutaneous–systemic vasculitis (allergic vasculitis)
    Polyarteritis nodosa
    Rheumatoid arthritis
    Systemic lupus erythematosus
    Wegner's granulomatosis

permeability causing oedema, visible as urticaria and blisters, and leakage of red blood cells causing purpura and haemorrhagic blisters, to occlusion of blood vessels with resulting ischaemia and necrosis of the epidermis producing ulceration.

The site of the affected blood vessels, viz. superficial dermis, deep dermis or fat, alters the clinical picture.

There are many characteristic patterns of vasculitis, which have been given names (Table 56.1). These patterns do not represent pathological entities; they are not specific as regards cause. Many agents are postulated to be causes of vasculitis (Table 56.2). Immune complexes are usually invoked as the initiators of the damage. The host response determines the pattern of reaction. The lesions of vasculitis are polymorphic and often vary with time.

Table 56.2   Causes of vasculitis

'Allergic'	Drugs
	Food
	Inhaled allergens, e.g. pollens
Carcinoma	
Connective tissue diseases	Dermatomyositis
	Mixed connective tissue disease
	Polyarteritis nodosa
	Rheumatoid arthritis
	Systemic lupus erythematosus
	Wegner's granulomatosis
Cryoglobulins	
Emboli	SBE
Infections	Bacterial – streptococcal
	– tuberculosis
	Fungal
	Viral
Infestations	
Unknown (the majority)	

Vasculitis can affect all organs. The kidneys, lungs and joints are often affected in addition to skin.

CHILBLAINS

Chilblains, also known as perniosis, are a common reaction to cold. Although troublesome to the sufferer
they are of no serious significance.

They are common in cold countries during winter,
especially in people living in poorly heated homes or
working outdoors.

Presentation All age groups and both men and women are affected.

Chilblains occur on cold, poorly perfused areas,
the fingers and toes, rarely on the ears and nose. In
the obese, areas insulated from the warm core by fat
are involved, e.g. the calves or thighs. Girls who go
riding in winter get deep chilblains of the thighs,
which resemble panniculitis.

Chilblains are evoked by cold. This first sign is
erythema accompanied by itching and burning. They
become purple, papular and may blister and ulcer-

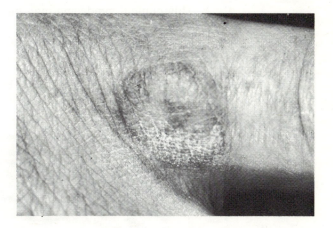

Figure 56.1   Chilblain on the finger

ate (Figure 56.1). Deeper ones form tender subcutaneous lumps, with overlying purple discolouration.
They persist for weeks.

Chilblains may appear throughout the winter.
They cease once spring comes.

Differential Chilblain lupus is distinguished by persistence and
diagnosis the presence of other signs of lupus erythematosus.

Diagnosis and investigations   Skin biopsy shows a vasculitis. It should not be necessary to carry out a biopsy.

Aetiology   Cold induced vasoconstriction causes stagnation of blood in small vessels, with damage to vessel walls.

Treatment   There is no specific treatment. Prevention is by warmth. The whole body as well as the peripheries should be kept warm. Smoking should be avoided as this induces vasoconstriction.

Natural history and prognosis   The severity of chilblains reflects the severity of the winter. Adequate heating and clothing can prevent most occurrences.

CUTANEOUS VASCULITIS AND CUTANEOUS–SYSTEMIC VASCULITIS

This clinical syndrome may be confined to the skin or involve many other organs. It is also known as leukocytoclastic vasculitis, allergic vasculitis or necrotizing angiitis.

Presentation   This occurs chiefly in adults. Both men and women are affected.

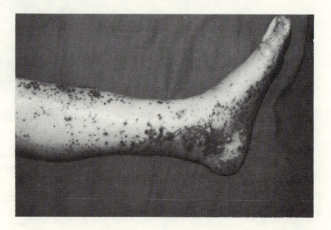

Figure 56.2   Vasculitis: palpable purpura, bullae and crusts on the lower leg

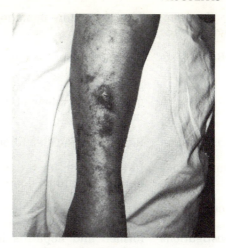

Figure 56.3   Cutaneous vasculitis showing purpura and bullae in the typical site on the lower leg

The chief sites are the lower legs and feet, but the lower trunk, arms and hands are also involved in severe cases. Perforation of the nasal septum may occur, but facial lesions are rare.

The vasculitic lesions commence as palpable purpura, and often progress to haemorrhagic bullae (Figures 56.2 and 56.3), and to necrosis and ulceration. There may be persistent ulcerated nodules. The ulceration is very slow to heal when it is on the lower leg.

Systemic involvement   In this more severe form, in addition to the skin involvement there is involvement of other organs. Arthritis is common. Renal involvement ranges from haematuria to renal failure. Gastro-intestinal involvement causes ulceration, haemorrhage and perforation. The lungs may be affected, with haemoptysis, oedema and infiltration and infarction. Peripheral nerves and the central nervous system are involved in severe cases.

Differential diagnosis   It may be confused with polyarteritis nodosa, rheumatoid arthritis with vasculitis, and systemic lupus erythematosus.

Diagnosis and investigation
Skin biopsy   This shows a leukocytoclastic vasculitis, i.e. many polymorphs undergoing destruction around small vessels.

Immuno-fluorescence	This may show immunoglobulins or C_3 in the blood vessel walls.
Blood tests	The blood count is usually normal, unless there has been great blood loss. The ESR is raised in the systemic form. Serum protein electrophoresis, estimation of immunoglobulins and cryoglobulins should be done.
Renal function	Renal function should be assessed.
Immunology	In the search for a cause, RA latex, ANF and DNA binding should be done.
Bacterial and viral investigations	Streptococcal infection should be sought by throat swab, and ASOT titres. Viral titres should be performed and hepatitis infection sought. Fever and malaise is an indication for blood cultures.
Chest X-ray	A chest X-ray demonstrates pulmonary pathology.

Aetiology

It is presumed that deposition of immune complexes in small blood vessels is the mechanism in many cases. Some drugs perhaps have a direct toxic effect.

Drugs, particularly phenothiazines, barbiturates, and sulphonamides have been implicated. Inhaled or ingested allergens or toxins, or infections may all be causes. Salicylates and anti-inflammatory drugs, e.g. phenylbutazone, can exacerbate vasculitis.

In many cases the cause is not discovered.

Treatment

Treatment of the systemic form must be more aggressive than of the purely cutaneous form, as the prognosis of the former is much worse.

General

Bed rest with elevation of the legs is helpful in the acute stage.

A search should be made for infectious causes.

Specific suppressive therapy

Systemic steroids in high doses usually suppress the vasculitis.

Dapsone has been successful in a few cases.

Fibrinolytic therapy with phenformin 50 μg b.d. and oestrogen (ethinyl oestradiol 50 μg daily) or stanozolol 5 μg b.d. has been successful in some cutaneous cases.

The fulminating systemic form may require cytotoxics, azathioprine, cyclophosphamide or chlorambucil in addition to systemic steroids.

Natural history and prognosis   The cutaneous form may be an episode of a few weeks, but in some cases it is very persistent.

The systemic form can have a similar time course, but may be fatal in the acute stage.

CUTANEOUS POLYARTERITIS NODOSA

This is a variant of polyarteritis nodosa. It is confined to the skin and subcutaneous tissues and has a benign prognosis. There is clinical overlap with nodular vasculitis. A further variant, livedo vasculitis, is described separately (see below).

Presentation   Adults are chiefly affected (see Figure 56.4). It is more common in men.

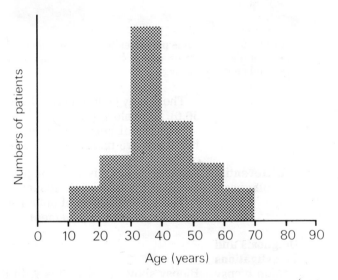

Figure 56.4   Age of onset of cutaneous polyarteritis nodosa

The lesions are often confined to the lower leg and foot, but may occur elsewhere including the arms and breast.

The lesions are painful red nodules which may ulcerate (Figure 56.5). Deeper nodules also occur in the subcutaneous tissue. They persist for many weeks and the ulcers are very slow to heal.

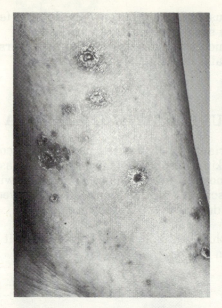 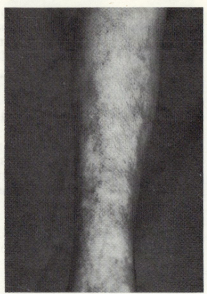

Figure 56.5   Cutaneous polyarteritis: small nodules, many of which have ulcerated on the lower leg

Figure 56.6   The reticulate pattern of livedo reticularis

There may be associated livedo reticularis (Figure 56.6). See below, p. 514.

Superficial nerves and muscles may be involved, but there are no systemic signs.

Differential diagnosis Nodular vasculitis is distinguished by its histology. Panniculitis has much deeper nodules.

The systemic form of polyarteritis is distinguished by the systemic involvement.

Diagnosis and investigations

Skin biopsy Biopsy shows a vasculitis with fibrinoid necrosis of small vessels.

Blood tests These are usually normal.

Aetiology The cause is unknown.

Treatment Treatment seems to have little effect. High dose steroids may cause some improvement.

Natural history and prognosis It is a persistent and troublesome condition often becoming less severe with time. It poses no threat to life.

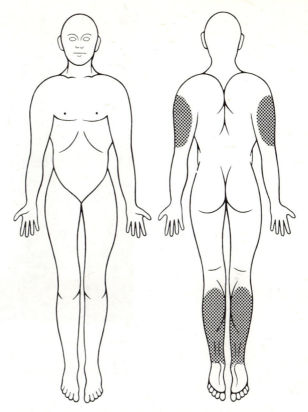

Figure 56.7   Distribution of erythema induratum

ERYTHEMA INDURATUM

Erythema induratum is also known as Bazin's disease.

Presentation It is a disease of young and middle aged adults, though it can occur in children and old age.

Women are most commonly affected.

The sites of predilection are the backs of the calves, but the arms are occasionally affected (Figure 56.7). These are sites overlying fat where the skin is cool.

The lesions are symmetrical and recurrent. They are painful. They commence as soft purplish nodules, which may coalesce or become ulcerated. They heal with scarring (Figure 56.8). They are indolent and persist for three to four months.

There may be signs of tuberculosis.

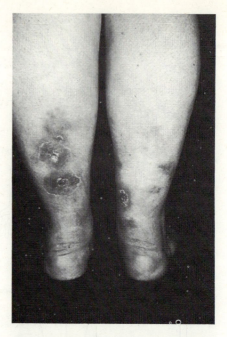

Figure 56.8 Erythema induratum: indolent purple lesions with ulceration on cold fat legs

Differential diagnosis

Erythema nodosum is acute and located on the front of the legs. Nodular vasculitis is more widespread and acute.

Diagnosis and investigations

A full blood count and ESR should be done.
  Mantoux testing, chest X-ray and search for tuberculosis are mandatory.

Aetiology

It was long presumed to be a hypersensitivity to tuberculosis, possibly immune complexes depositing in stagnant blood vessels. In many cases it is impossible to prove that tuberculosis infection is present.

Treatment

Some cases respond to antituberculous therapy. There is usually a good response to systemic steroids.

Natural history and prognosis

Some cases resolve spontaneously after many months. Others persist for years. There are no systemic complications.

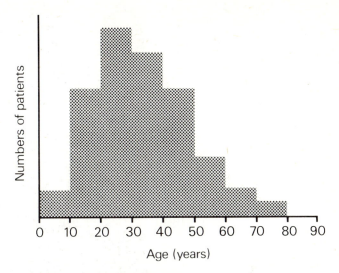

Figure 56.9   Age distribution of erythema nodosum

ERYTHEMA NODOSUM

Erythema nodosum is a distinct clinical entity that occurs in response to many different stimuli. In many cases the cause is unknown.

Presentation   Erythema nodosum occurs chiefly in the young and middle aged (Figure 56.9). Young women are mostly affected.

The lower legs are the chief site; the front of the legs are affected (Figures 56.10 and 56.11). Occasionally the lesions extend to the thighs or upper arms.

The lesions are acute and painful. They occur in crops. They are shiny red nodules (Figure 56.11). These resolve over a few days or a week.

There may be arthritis of the ankles. Symptoms and signs of the causative disease may also be present.

Differential diagnosis   Nodular vasculitis may give a similar picture, but the distribution is less restricted and the lesions less acute.

Diagnosis and investigations
Skin biopsy   Biopsy is rarely necessary.

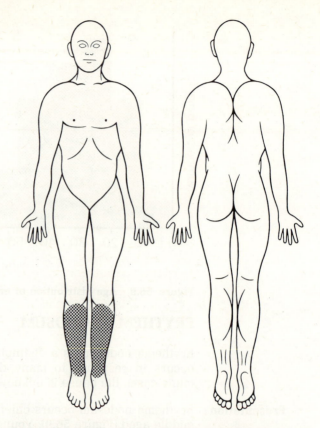

Figure 56.10   Distribution of erythema nodosum

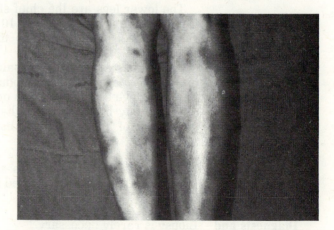

Figure 56.11   Erythema nodosum: acute red nodules on the fronts of the shins

Blood tests   A full blood count should be done, as there may be abnormalities due to the underlying disease. The ESR will be raised if the cause is a bacterial infection, particularly streptococcal infection or tuberculosis, or a sarcoid. The ASOT may be raised.

Bacteriology   A throat swab should be cultured, as should any sputum.

Chest X-ray   This is the most important investigation.

Skin tests   Mantoux testing, and if sarcoid is suspected a Kveim test should be done.

Aetiology   Erythema nodosum occurs in response to many different stimuli.

Infections, particularly streptococcal infections, tuberculosis and more rarely fungal and viral infections, or drugs, particularly sulphonamides, may cause erythema nodosum.

Sarcoid is one of the commonest causes in the United Kingdom. Crohn's disease and ulcerative colitis may cause it.

In some cases no cause is found. It can be regarded as an acute localized vasculitis.

Treatment   In the acute stage, bedrest and analgesics are all that is required as a resolution is usually rapid. Systemic steroids speed resolution of severe cases.

Natural history and prognosis   An attack usually lasts a few weeks. Recurrent attacks may occur. The prognosis is good unless there is some serious underlying disease.

HENOCH–SCHÖNLEIN PURPURA

This was one of the first distinct clinical syndromes of vasculitis to be described.

Presentation   Henoch–Schönlein purpura is incorrectly considered by many clinicians to be a disease of children. Many cases do occur in adults (Figure 56.12). Both sexes are affected, boys more commonly than girls; the sex ratio is equal in adults.

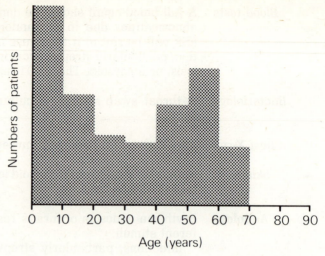

Figure 56.12   Age of onset of Henoch–Schönlein purpura

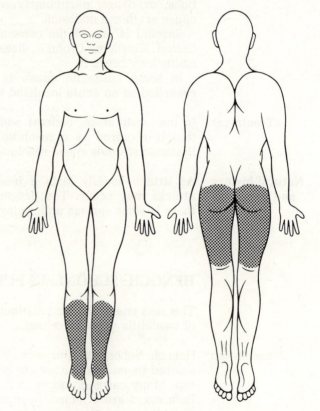

Figure 56.13   Distribution of Henoch–Schönlein purpura

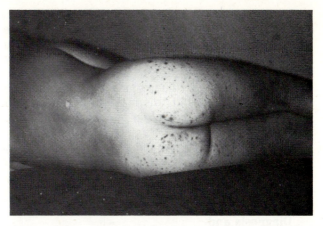

Figure 56.14 Henoch–Schönlein purpura on the buttocks, a classical site

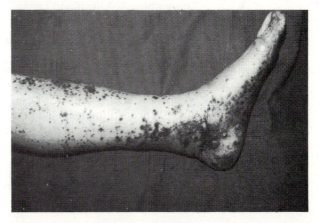

Figure 56.15 Henoch–Schönlein purpura: palpable purpura, bullae and crusted lesions on the lower legs, a typical site

Cutaneous lesions   The lower legs, backs of the thighs and buttocks are the classical sites for Henoch–Schönlein purpura; the elbows and scalp may be involved (Figures 56.13 and 56.14). Any area, but particularly face and joints, may be affected by oedema.

The skin lesions comprise purpura, which may be papular and proceed to bullae (Figure 56.15) and necrosis. Purpura is the hallmark of the disease (Figure 56.15). Urticaria also occurs, as does dermographism. Subcutaneous swellings give rise to local areas of oedema.

Systemic manifestations Arthritis is common. Abdominal pain and melaena often occur during the acute attack. Glomerulonephritis manifests as haematuria, or even renal failure occurs later, sometimes weeks after the acute attack.

There may be signs of a streptococcal infection but this may resolve before the attack of Henoch–Schönlein purpura commences.

Differential diagnosis The haematological causes of purpura do not cause palpable purpura. Other forms of cutaneous systemic vasculitis may give a very similar clinical picture.

Diagnosis and investigations

Skin biopsy Skin biopsy shows a vasculitis. Immunofluorescence may show IgA in blood vessels in the skin.

Renal biopsy IgA deposits may be present in the kidney.

Blood tests A full blood count including platelets must be done. The blood loss may be sufficient to cause anaemia. The ESR will be raised. Urea and electrolytes, and serum creatinine tests, should be done. A raised ASO titre provides evidence of a precipitating streptococcal infection.

Other tests A throat swab should be taken for evidence of streptococcal infection. The urine must be examined for red blood cells.

Aetiology This is a hypersensitivity vasculitis. The identifiable causes are streptococcal infection and antibiotics or other drugs. In many cases the cause is unknown.

Treatment Bedrest is helpful in the acute phase. Moderate dose systemic steroids may shorten the duration of the acute attack. Dapsone is occasionally successful in halting an attack.

Penicillin should be given if a streptococcal infection is found.

Natural history and prognosis Most attacks last a short time, often a few weeks. Occasionally renal failure is so severe that death occurs.

Some patients have recurrent attacks.

IDIOPATHIC CAPILLARITIS

This curious condition is also known as Schamberg's disease or pigmented purpuric eruption.

Presentation This is a condition chiefly of young men.

The lower legs are affected and much more rarely thighs, arms or trunk.

The lesions are discrete discs several centimetres across; rarely they are confluent. They are usually few in number. They consist of small petechiae, which rapidly become reddish-brown giving an appearance of 'cayenne pepper' scattered on the skin (Figure 56.16). The background is often hyper-pigmented and scaly. The lesions are asymptomatic.

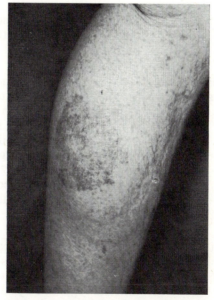

Figure 56.16 Idiopathic capillaritis: localized area of capillaritis with typical 'cayenne pepper' appearance

Differential diagnosis The other forms of purpura are not so localized.

Diagnosis and investigations None are indicated.

Aetiology   The cause and mechanism are unknown. The capillaries are the site of pathology.

Carbromal may produce a similar eruption.

Treatment   There is no treatment.

Natural history and prognosis   The lesions remain unchanged for many years. There may be resolution, or the appearance of new lesions.

The condition is benign and has no systemic complications.

LIVEDO RETICULARIS AND LIVEDO VASCULITIS

Livedo reticularis describes a pattern of dilated blood vessels. This pattern may be physiological or pathological.

Presentation
Physiological   Livedo reticularis is a normal physiological response to cold, and occurs in both children and adults. Women are more often affected than men, because of their distribution of fat.

Cold induces a reticulate pattern of purple dilated blood vessels overlying the fat regions of the legs and arms (Figure 56.17). The fat insulates the skin, and peripheral vasoconstriction causes stagnant blood in dilated capillaries, giving rise to livedo reticularis.

Pathological   There are several localized pathological forms of livedo reticularis. These are called *livedo vasculitis* and *livedo reticularis with summer ulceration*. The latter is regarded by some as a variant of cutaneous polyarteritis nodosa. Women predominate.

There is livedo reticularis of the lower leg and dorsum of the foot. Small painful ulcers arise on the feet and ankles. In some patients the ulceration occurs only in the summer.

There is poor perfusion of the skin and this results in *atrophie blanche*, ivory white patches of atrophied skin with telangiectasia and surrounding hyperpigmentation. Venous stasis can also give rise to this appearance.

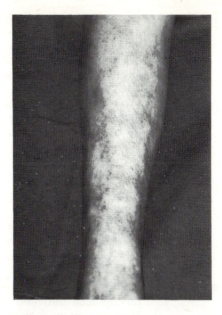

Figure 56.17   Livedo reticularis

Symptomatic	Livedo reticularis is a manifestation of polyarteritis nodosa, rheumatoid arthritis and systemic lupus erythematosus.
Differential diagnosis	Venous stasis and ulceration may cause confusion with livedo vasculitis and atrophie blanche.

Diagnosis and investigations

Skin biopsy	Biopsy is rarely necessary.
Blood tests	All blood tests are normal in livedo vasculitis except that fibrinolysis may be defective. ANF, rheumatoid factor and DNA antibodies should be sought to exclude systemic disease.
Aetiology	Slow flow through small dilated blood vessels as a result of cold or vasculitis gives rise to the pattern of livedo reticularis. Complete sudden cessation of blood flow results in ischaemia and ulceration; gradual cessation causes sclerosis and atrophie blanche.

Treatment   Physiological livedo reticularis requires no treatment.

Livedo vasculitis is resistant to therapy. Fibrinolytics, e.g. phenformin and ethinyl oestradiol and stanozolol, benefit some patients.

Natural history and prognosis   Livedo vasculitis persists for decades. The prognosis of secondary symptomatic livedo reticularis is that of the underlying disease. In systemic lupus erythematosus it may be transient but recurrent.

NODULAR VASCULITIS

Nodular vasculitis is a well recognized clinical entity. There is, however, considerable overlap with other entities and it may not be a homogenous group.

Presentation   Nodular vasculitis is a disease of adults. It usually commences between the ages of 30 and 60 years. Women are more commonly affected than men.

The lesions are located on the lower legs, particularly the calves and sides of the legs. The thighs and the arms may be affected.

The lesions are painful, tender nodules, which may be superficial or deep in the subcutaneous tissue. There is overlying erythema and later hyperpigmentation (Figure 56.18). Ulceration is rare. The nodules resolve slowly over many months.

There are no systemic signs or symptoms.

Differential diagnosis   There is clinical overlap with many other entities. Chilblains are distinguished by their seasonal incidence. Erythema nodosum is much more acute. Erythema induratum is more indolent and overlies fat cold areas. Thrombophlebitis and cutaneous polyarteritis may be difficult to distinguish without histological examination.

Diagnosis and investigations   Skin biopsy shows a vasculitis. Immunofluorescence may show immunoglobulin deposits in the walls of small blood vessels.

Tuberculosis and streptococcal infection should be sought as these can be a source of antigen.

Aetiology   The vasculitis is presumed to be due to deposition of immune complexes. The antigen is rarely identified,

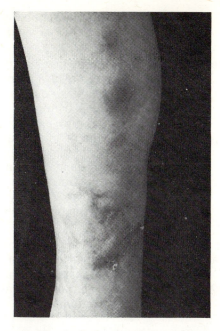

Figure 56.18 The lesions of nodular vasculitis on the lower leg

although in some cases tuberculosis, streptococcal infection or drugs have been implicated.

Treatment Treatment is symptomatic with analgesics and support to the leg. Bedrest is helpful in some cases.

Short courses of systemic steroids in moderate disease (prednisone 20–30 mg daily) may reduce the severity of the acute attacks.

Dapsone or fibrinolytic therapy with phenformin and oestrogen or attenuated androgens has suppressed nodular vasculitis in a few patients.

Natural history and prognosis Nodular vasculitis is a chronic condition lasting for many years. There may be recurrent acute attacks. There are no systemic complications.

PANNICULITIS

Panniculitis is localized inflammation of the fat. It is thought that most cases are primarily a vasculitis of the arteries supplying the fat. There are several different clinical syndromes of panniculitis.

Presentation   Most forms involve young and middle aged women. The areas where there is most fat are involved. The limbs, thighs, calves and upper arms and more rarely the trunk and face are affected. It is often localized and asymmetrical.

Tender nodules appear in the subcutaneous fat. There may be overlying erythema. They resolve slowly over many months. Sometimes there is much overlying fibrosis and an almost scleroderma-like appearance. Atrophy of the fat may cause large depressions of the epidermis.

Weber Christian panniculitis   This affects women between 30 and 60. There are recurrent episodes of fever, anorexia, joint pains, and widespread panniculitis. There may be involvement of visceral fat, i.e. pancreas, intestines and omentum.

Lupus panniculitis   Discoid and systemic lupus erythematosus may cause panniculitis with severe scarring.

Cold panniculitis   This is deep chilblains (see above, p. 499) of the calves, thighs or upper arms induced by cold.

Rothmann–Makai   Children may develop widespread tender panniculitis of the trunk and limbs. This resolves within a year.

Post-steroid panniculitis   This occurs after cessation of high dose steroid therapy.

Panniculitis associated with pancreatic disease   Release of pancreatic lipases in association with acute pancreatitis or carcinoma of the pancreas cause local lipolysis and panniculitis.

Differential diagnosis   Biopsy is necessary to confirm the diagnosis and shows a deep vasculitis and destruction of fat.

Blood tests show that Weber–Christian panniculitis is often accompanied by leukopenia.

The ANF and DNA binding are helpful in distinguishing systemic lupus erythematosus.

Aetiology The aetiology is unknown. The histology often shows vasculitis and this may be the primary pathological event.

A preceding infection or drug is implicated in some cases and this may cause a hypersensitivity reaction.

Treatment No treatment is required for any of the types of panniculitis other than lupus panniculitis (see page 228), and Weber–Christian panniculitis. The latter is best treated by short courses of high dose steroids during the acute attack. Steroids should be withdrawn between attacks.

Natural history and prognosis There may be a single attack or recurrent attacks. Weber–Christian panniculitis may persist for several years. Rarely death may occur from visceral involvement.

PITYRIASIS LICHENOIDES

Pityriasis lichenoides exists in acute and chronic forms, with occasional transition from the acute to chronic form. They are also called pityriasis lichenoides and varicelliformis acuta and pityriasis lichenoides chronica.

Presentation Although it can occur at any age, adolescents and young adults are most frequently affected (Figure 56.19). The male to female ratio is 2 : 1 (Figure 56.20).

The trunk, and flexor aspects of the upper arms and thighs are chiefly affected, but it may be more widespread involving face, hands and feet.

Mucous membranes may be involved in the acute form.

The rash is symmetrical.

Acute form There may be fever and constitutional upset. The initial lesion is a small, red papule, and this becomes vesicular and haemorrhagic (Figure 56.21). Some lesions undergo necrosis and ulcerate. These heal with formation of pitted scars. All stages of the lesions are present.

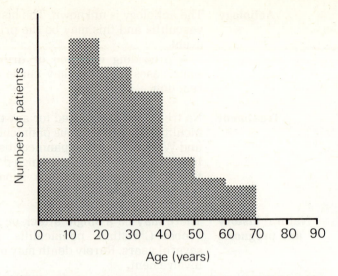

Figure 56.19   Age of presentation of pityriasis lichenoides

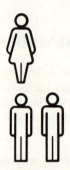

Figure 56.20   Sex ratio of pityriasis lichenoides

Chronic form   There is no constitutional upset. Small red papules are the first sign, these may be purpuric. Later they become scaly. The characteristic lesion is the mica scale; this is a shiny scale attached centrally to a papule, it can be scraped off to leave a slightly brown surface (Figure 56.22). All types of lesion are present together.

The papules slowly resolve and leave hyperpigmentation, or occasionally in dark skinned persons hypopigmentation, which may be the presenting sign.

Differential   The acute form may be confused with acute viral illdiagnosis   nesses, e.g. chicken pox or a vasculitis.

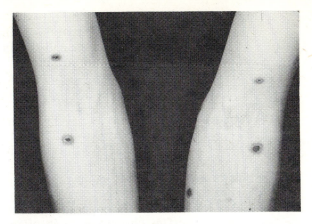

Figure 56.21 Pityriasis lichenoides acuta: the acute necrotic lesions

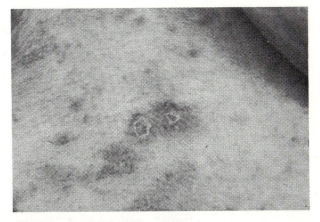

Figure 56.22 Pityriasis lichenoides chronic: the typical small papules with a mica scale

The chronic form may resemble a vasculitis, insect bites, secondary syphilis or if very scaly guttate psoriasis.

Diagnosis and investigations
Skin biopsy

Histology should be done to confirm the diagnosis. Direct immunofluorescence of any early lesion may show IgM or C_3 at the dermo-epidermal junction or in blood vessels.

Blood tests

Immune complexes can often be demonstrated in the blood.

Aetiology   It is considered that pityriasis lichenoides is a vasculitis. The demonstration of immunoglobulin and C_3 in the blood vessels and skin in conjunction with circulating immune complexes, suggest that immune complexes formed in response to some unknown antigen damage small blood vessels.

Treatment   A short course of systemic steroids may curtail the acute attack. Ultraviolet light or PUVA therapy are sometimes successful in healing the chronic forms.

Natural history and prognosis   The acute form may present as a single attack lasting a few weeks, or there may be recurrent attacks. A few cases undergo transition to the chronic form.

The chronic form is often persistent for many years.

There is no effect on the general health.

POLYARTERITIS NODOSA

The systemic disease polyarteritis nodosa is much more severe than the purely cutaneous forms and may be fatal.

Presentation   It is a disease of adults, particularly of the middle aged. Men are affected more frequently than women.

Cutaneous lesions   These are present in 25% of patients. The cutaneous lesions tend to affect the legs. They include livedo reticularis (Figure 56.6), purpura (Figure 56.2) and tender, red nodules (Figure 56.5) and ulcerated nodules.

Systemic manifestations   Malaise and fever are common.

Asthma may be an early symptom. Arthritis occurs. Hypertension, glomerulonephritis and renal failure are common. Abdominal symptoms of pain and malaena arise from liver and gut involvement. Cardiac problems and peripheral neuropathy are frequent.

Differential diagnosis   Cutaneous systemic vasculitis may give a very similar picture. Systemic lupus erythematosus is much commoner in women. Rheumatoid arthritis with vasculitis can also mimic polyarteritis nodosa.

Diagnosis and investigations
Biopsy

Biopsy of skin nodules or kidney will show inflammation, aneurysms and fibrinoid necrosis of small and medium sized arteries.

Radiology

Coeliac axis angiography shows aneurysms and is the *best* diagnostic test.

Blood tests

There may be eosinophilia, leukocytosis and raised ESR. The ANF may be positive.
The Australia antigen is present in 25–40%.

Aetiology

The high proportion of patients with Australia antigen suggests that hepatitis B may be involved in the production of the disease. Immune complexes have been suggested as the mediators of the damage.

Treatment

Steroids in high doses suppress the disease. In severe cases immunosuppressive drugs or plasma exchange may also be necessary.

Natural history and prognosis

Thirty to fifty per cent die within the first year, but if the acute stage is passed the prognosis is good.

WALDENSTROM'S HYPERGAMMAGLOB-ULINAEMIC PURPURA

Presentation

Middle aged women are affected.
The lower legs are the main site; the areas covered by shoes are usually spared. Showers of petechiae appear on the legs. The showers are precipitated by increased venous pressure, e.g. prolonged standing, tight garters etc.
Sjogren's syndrome (dry eyes and mouth) may be present.

Differential diagnosis

Purpura and idiopathic capillaritis may resemble this disease, but the distribution and natural history distinguish it.

Diagnosis and investigations

Skin biopsy shows a vasculitis. Blood tests show the platelet count to be normal. There is a diffuse increase in all gammaglobulins – the hypergammaglobulinaemia of the name. The rheumatoid factor is often positive. Immune complexes may be detected.
Sjogren's syndrome should be sought.

Aetiology This is an immune complex vasculitis. The aetiology is unknown, as is the reason for its relationship to Sjogren's syndrome.

Treatment There is no treatment.

Natural history and prognosis The condition is persistent with recurrent showers of petechiae. There are no serious sequelae.

57 VENOUS STASIS AND ULCERATION

Venous stasis of the legs, whether due to varicose veins, the postphlebitic syndrome, or venous obstruction, causes many skin changes. These are sometimes termed lipodermatosclerosis.

Presentation Middle aged and elderly people, usually women, are affected.

The lower leg is involved, particularly the area on the inner aspect of the ankle.

The changes are purpura and atrophy, sclerosis and hyperpigmentation (Figure 57.1) which may

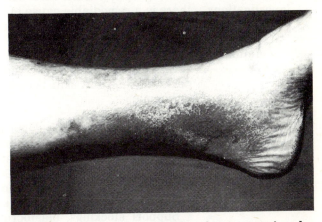

Figure 57.1 **The chronic changes of venous stasis; sclerosis, hyperpigmentation and eczema**

progress to give the appearance of *atrophie blanche* (see page 514). Eczema commonly occurs (see Chapter 11, Varicose Eczema). Oedema is common.

Ulceration may occur (Figure 57.2) initiated by minimal trauma. This is slow to heal and often becomes infected.

525

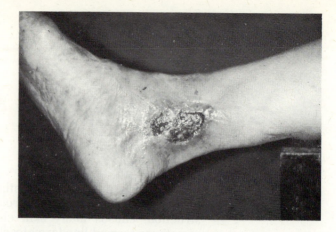

Figure 57.2   Venous stasis has resulted in ulceration at the typical site above the medial malleolus

Differential diagnosis

Vasculitis also causes atrophie blanche and ulceration of the lower leg.

Diagnosis and investigations

Phlebography should be considered to ascertain if there is a remediable cause of venous insufficiency. Ulcers should be swabbed and cultured.

Aetiology

High venous pressure leads to high capillary pressure. The small blood vessels of the skin are poorly perfused, and the skin becomes hypoxic and even ischaemic.

Treatment

Venous pressure and oedema must be reduced by elevation of the leg. This may be done by raising the foot of the bed, sitting with feet up (higher than the bottom) and elevating the legs 90° for one hour each day. Walking with compression to the legs is good. Standing and sitting with the legs down is bad.

Support stockings, elastocrepe or rubber bandages should always be worn when the patient is up.

If possible the cause of the venous insufficiency should be dealt with.

Ulceration requires all the above measures, and careful daily cleansing with, for example, eusol and paraffin. Antiseptic paints such as gentian violet, are helpful to prevent secondary infection. Systemic antibiotics are necessary if there is cellulitis.

Local anaesthetics or antihistamines or topical

antibiotics must not be used as the risk of sensitization is high (see Chapter 11).

Natural history The outlook is poor unless the cause of the venous
and prognosis insufficiency can be removed.

58 VIRAL INFECTIONS

WARTS

Presentation A wart is an epithelial tumour caused by a virus. It is a very common infection throughout the world. The age and sex incidence vary in different clinical forms, but the disorder is rare in infancy, and very common during the school years (Figure 58.1). The highest incidence is between 9 and 16. Genital warts occur usually between the ages of 20 and 50 in the sexually active years. Sexes are equally affected. Plantar warts are slightly more common in females. The commonest sites are the soles, hands, especially the back of hands, around the nail folds in nail biters, and knees (Figure 58.2). Plane warts appear on the face and back of hands. Plantar warts occur

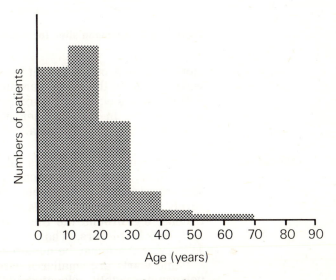

Figure 58.1   Age incidence of warts

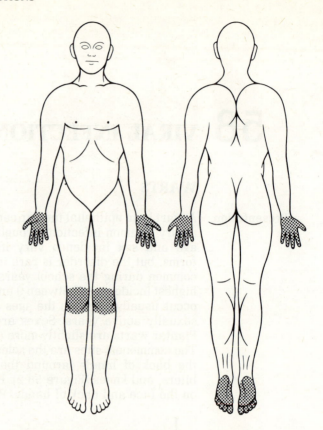

Figure 58.2   Common sites for warts

more commonly on the weight bearing areas. Genital warts occur on the vulva, peri-anal area and penis. Filiform warts occur in the axillary folds, neck, lips and nostrils. In the Koebner phenomenon, warts develop at the site of trauma.

Clinical forms   The common wart (or verruca vulgaris) appears as a small, firm, rounded, elevated tumour with a horny surface, 1–5 mm in diameter (Figure 58.3) and rarely may be larger. Warts may be linear due to trauma, e.g. around the finger nails in nail biters and cuticle pickers. The common wart may be solitary or there may be numerous lesions.

Plane warts are smaller in size, 1–3 mm, with a polygonal, slightly elevated flat top and flesh coloured. They may be numerous and occasionally

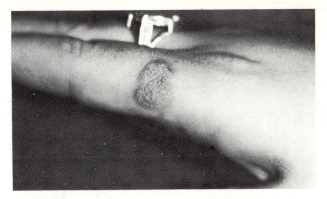

Figure 58.3   A viral wart: raised scaly papule with a defined surface. The black dots are thrombosed capillaries

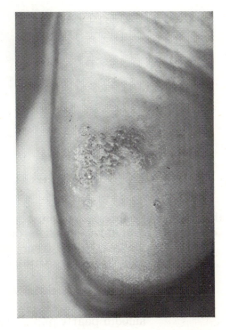

Figure 58.4   Mosaic wart on the sole of the foot

coalesce to cover an area or be linear due to scratching.

Plantar warts are small, deep seated, flat, firm hyperkeratotic lesions. They can be single or multiple and coalesce to form the mosaic wart (Figure 58.4). They occur on the plantar aspects of the feet and may be painful, if situated on a pressure bearing area and may cause difficulty in walking. They are well defined from the normal surrounding skin.

Condylomata acuminata are genital warts, which grow in the mucocutaneous genital areas, especially during the sexually active years. Moisture and trauma are important in inoculation and rapid growth. The lesions are flesh coloured, pedunculated (Figure 58.5) or filiform, or may coalesce to cover the area. They often cause discomfort and irritation.

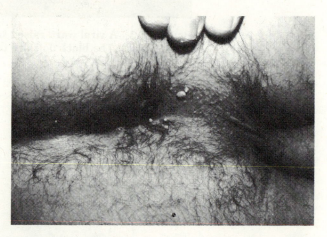

Figure 58.5   Warts on the perineum and perianal skin

Differential diagnosis   Common warts must be distinguished from granuloma annulare, which is dermal, with a normal smooth surface, and from kerato-acanthoma, which is usually solitary with normal epidermis apart from a central horny plug or a crust. Molluscum contagiosum has also to be considered in the differential diagnosis. However, molluscum contagiosum are smooth pearly papules with central umbilication.

Multiple clustered warts may be confused with tuberculosis verrucosa, in which there is dermal infiltration. This form of granuloma gradually enlarges and tends to be a reddish-brown colour and some parts may become necrotic.

Periungual warts may be confused with the fibromata of epiloia. These lesions, however, are smooth and firm and emerge from the nail folds. Subungual warts may be confused with subungual exostosis; the latter, however, is a subepidermal nodule, mainly on the tip of a digit.

Plantar warts may be confused with callosities and corns which usually develop on pressure points, and on paring do not show capillary bleeding points. Callosities are composed of horny material, which is not well defined and in which there is continuation of the epidermal ridges, unlike plantar warts. A wart is more painful on lateral pressure, and a callosity on direct pressure.

Plantar warts may be confused with punctate keratoderma, which is a genodermatosis distributed on the palms and soles, including the digits. Plane warts have to be distinguished from lichen planus, in which the papules are polygonal and are a violaceous colour. In addition lichen planus usually causes irritation, occurs mainly in adults, and tends to involve other parts of the body. In the differential diagnosis of genital warts, condylomata lata should be considered. The latter have a flat surface in contrast to the verrucose surface of genital warts, and there are usually other manifestations of secondary syphilis. Anogenital naevi, malignant melanoma and other tumours may also have to be considered.

Investigations   Warts are easily diagnosed on clinical grounds. However, if there is any doubt, surface paring of a wart with a blade may show black specks (thrombosed capillaries) or bleeding points. Usually there is no need for further investigations.

Aetiology   Warts are caused by a DNA virus of the papova group. The transmission is by direct or indirect contact and auto-inoculation. Genital warts are sexually transmitted. The antigen producing property of common and genital warts may be different. Cell mediated immunity is probably responsible for the ultimate resolution of warts.

Treatment   The treatment of warts depends on the number of the lesions, discomfort, cosmetic disability, and the site of the lesions. The success of treatment depends on the immunity of the patient against the wart virus, and method of treatment. Multiple warts imply poor immunity. Radical treatments should not be used for extensive and multiple lesions.

Salicylic acid, a keratolytic agent, will remove the excess keratin. It is used in varying concentrations, e.g. 3–4% solution for plane warts, and 10% in collodion for common warts, applied daily for one month, and 40% impregnated plaster for plantar warts for 10–14 days. Salicylic acid has a low cure rate and is often used simply to improve the cosmetic appearance of the wart.

Nitric acid and trichloracetic acid can be carefully applied with an orange stick after paring.

Podophyllin, a cytotoxic agent, is used in a 25% solution in spirit or tinct. benz. co. for anogenital warts. The treatment should be carried out weekly. The surrounding skin is protected by Vaseline and the solution washed off 6–8 hours later. 15% podophyllin ointment under occlusive plaster can be used for periungual warts after paring. This should be applied for 6–8 weeks and the plaster should be changed every 3–4 days. Some patients develop a severe reaction to podophyllin which will necessitate cessation of the treatment. Podophyllin treatment must not be used in pregnancy.

Five per cent formalin soaks 15 minutes daily for at least a month can be used for plantar warts. The skin between and under the toes should be protected with Vaseline. Cryotherapy in the form of liquid nitrogen or carbon dioxide snow is effective with a cure rate approximately 70%. The duration of freezing depends on the site of the lesion and its size. Small lesions on thin skin should be treated for 10–15 seconds. Large warts on thick skin, e.g. palms and soles, should be frozen for 30–60 seconds. Within two days a subepidermal blister may form with the wart in the roof of the blister. The wart should disappear within 2–3 weeks of the treatment, if successful. The treatment can be repeated again, with a longer period of freezing, after an interval of 2–3 weeks, if necessary.

Curettage and cautery is the most effective treatment; however, local or rarely general, anaesthesia is necessary. Common plantar warts and anogenital warts may be treated by this method.

Surgical excision and radiotherapy should not be used. Psychotherapeutic techniques including hypnotherapy have been claimed, by some, to be successful, but these must be considered as a final resort. Immunotherapy employing vaccines would seem to be the best hope for the future.

Natural history and prognosis   Warts have a variable prognosis. Some will resolve spontaneously in a few months, others have a much longer course persisting for years, and spreading from one site to another. The average duration of untreated warts is two years. Genital warts often are resistant to treatment and have a high relapse rate. The malignant transformation of warts is doubtful.

MOLLUSCUM CONTAGIOSUM

Presentation   This is a world wide disease affecting any age group, but more prevalent in childhood. There is a higher incidence in males than females (Figure 58.6).

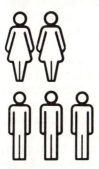

Figure 58.6 Molluscum contagiosum is slightly more common in males (3 : 2)

The lesions may involve any part of the skin, but the more common sites are the trunk and hands and the anogenital area. The genital area is more commonly involved in adults. The mucous membranes may be affected especially the oral cavities. The inoculation period varies from two to several weeks. When the lesions first appear they may be solitary or multiple.

The lesions are dome shaped papules, with a central depression and pore, which causes umbilication and may contain a caseous plug (Figure 58.7). Characteristically the papules are pearl coloured. If left untreated the lesion gradually enlarges to 5–10 mm in diameter. At first the lesions are firm, but soften when mature. New crops of lesions may appear as a

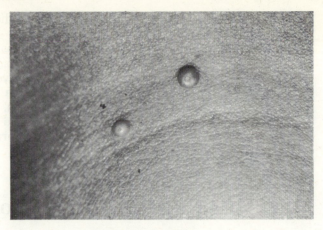

Figure 58.7 Molluscum contagiosum. Pearl coloured papules with a central depression

result of auto-inoculation, and the papules tend to be grouped. Some solitary molluscum may become very large especially after trauma.

Differential diagnosis

A solitary lesion has to be distinguished from the nodulocystic form of basal cell carcinoma. The latter tumour is pearly with telangiectasia on the surface. The surface is uneven as the lesion is often lobulated. There is no central depression.

Pyogenic granuloma is a vascular tumour, which is bright or dark red and partially compressible. It may be eroded and bleeds easily. Kerato-acanthomas may at first simulate a solitary molluscum contagiosum, but the former enlarges to 10–20 mm with a central horny plug.

Multiple lesions may be confused with smallpox or chicken pox, but the latter diseases have a short history and constitutional upset, and the distribution is more widespread and suggestive of the respective disorders.

A lymphangioma may present as a group of vesicles and may resemble molluscum contagiosum. However, in lymphangioma the lesions are compressible and have no central umbilication.

Investigations

The diagnosis can be made on clinical grounds and no investigations are usually necessary.

Aetiology

The lesions are due to a pox virus.

Treatment   The lesions can be removed by curettage and cautery or pierced with a sharpened orange stick dipped in 1% phenol or 1% iodine. They may also be treated with liquid nitrogen or painted with a mixture of 5% podophyllin and 5% salicylic acid in collodion.

Course and prognosis   The disease is self limiting and spontaneous remission usually occurs within a year, but occasionally persists for longer. Transmission is by direct contract.

HERPES SIMPLEX

Presentation   Herpes simplex infection is a common viral disease. The disease is widely distributed throughout the world, but is commonest in communities with low socioeconomic standards of living. Nearly 60% of the population are infected and remain carriers throughout their life. The clinical manifestations of herpes simplex infection can be divided into primary and secondary infections.

The commonest age of onset of the primary infection differs according to the site of the disease. It is rare in the first six months of life due to passive transfer of maternal immunity. From 6 months to 5 years the primary site of infection is most commonly the oral cavity, especially the gums. Between 5 and 14 years the primary infection is usually on the skin around the lips and eyes. Primary genital infection is most likely to present between 14 and 29 years.

The incubation period of the primary infection is usually 4–5 days, but may extend to 20 days. The clinical picture differs depending on the severity of the attack and the location of the infection. In primary infections affecting the gums and mouth, the onset is usually sudden with fever and restlessness. The gums, buccal mucosa and tongue become red and swollen, bleed easily and are painful. One or two days later there is an eruption of small blisters which rupture and produce shallow ulcers. There is regional enlargement of the lymph glands and healing takes place in 2–3 weeks.

The primary cutaneous infection may involve any part of the skin and consists of an area of red and swollen skin with a group of vesicles on the surface.

The vesicles change to pustules which later become crusted. Occasionally the primary infection is on the fingers (herpetic whitlow). There is swelling and redness of the digit and vesicles may be seen. Herpetic whitlow is most commonly seen in doctors and nurses from being in contact with the virus. The primary lesion may involve the eyes and causes keratoconjunctivitis and corneal ulceration. It may also involve the upper respiratory tract and central nervous system and become disseminated and generalized.

Genital herpes simplex is more common in women. The primary infection in the great majority of cases is subclinical and passes unnoticed. However, in some patients the primary infection may cause severe illness. The commonest sites of involvement are the vulva and vagina in females and the penis in males. Other parts of the genital tract and genitalia may be involved. The lesion presents as a group of vesicles which rapidly form pustules and erosions.

In recurrent or secondary herpes simplex infection the initial symptom is a tingling sensation in the affected area. The lesion consists of a group of small uniform vesicles (Figure 58.8) on a red base. The vesicles rapidly change to pustules and then become

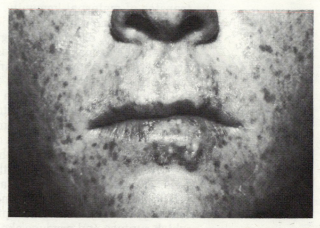

Figure 58.8   Grouped vesicles in the lips in herpes simplex

crusted (Figure 58.9) and normally heal in 7–10 days. In recurrent episodes the lesions usually

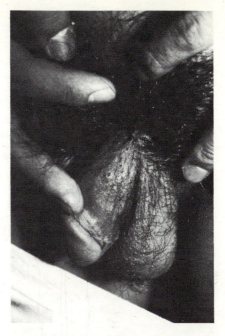

Figure 58.9 Grouped crusted and scabbed lesions in genital herpes simplex

reappear in the same area, and may be accompanied by mild constitutional upset. The commonest sites for recurrent attacks are the mucocutaneous junctions, such as the lips, nose, genitalia (Figure 58.10). Secondary attacks of herpes simplex may be triggered by strong sunlight, winds, high fever, and the viral upper respiratory tract infections.

Eczema herpeticum (see below, Kaposi's varicelliform eruption, p. 547) occurs in individuals with atopic eczema.

Differential diagnosis Impetigo is commonly mistaken for secondarily infected herpes simplex. However, in impetigo there are superficial pustules, erosions and yellow crusts. Contact eczema is usually associated with a history of irritation. In herpes zoster the eruption is usually more extensive occurring in an area of skin innervated by a sensory ganglion. Genital herpes simplex must be distinguished from syphilitic chancre. The

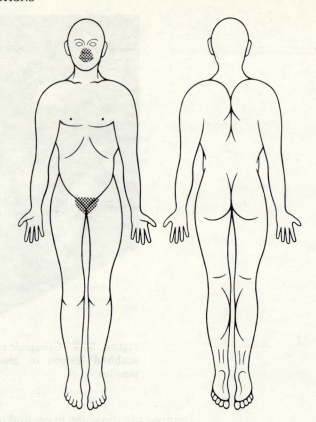

Figure 58.10 The common sites for recurrent herpes simplex infections

herpetic ulcer is superficial and not indurated. Serological tests and dark field examination will differentiate the two diseases. Scabies, *Candida albicans* infection and seborrhoeic eczema are the other diagnoses to be considered. Scabies is characterized by generalized irritation, especially at night, and burrows may be seen on the wrists and hands. A fixed drug eruption will occur at the same site each time the drug is taken and may be mistaken for recurrent herpes simplex. The eruption due to drugs usually has larger blisters than herpes simplex and may show a purplish area before fading completely.

Primary gingivostomatitis should be differentiated from the oral lesions of the Stevens–Johnson syndrome. Isolation of the virus may be necessary to distinguish the diseases. Oral streptococcal infections must also be considered. Moniliasis is very common in infancy, but this is seen as white plaques in the mouth. Mycological tests will establish the correct diagnosis. Aphthous ulcers and Behcet's disease occur in young adults rather than young children.

Investigations None are usually required, but virological studies will establish the diagnosis if necessary.

Tissue culture of fluid from a vesicle will establish the diagnosis within four days.

Serological tests are useful in primary attacks and show a rapid rise in the titre of circulating neutralizing and complement fixation antibodies which start seven days after infection. These reach a peak in 14–21 days and gradually fall to a lower level. There may be slight increase in the antibodies in subsequent attacks. Finally the titre reaches a constant level, except in generalized infection.

Electron microscopy will show the characteristic appearance of the virus, if this facility is available.

Aetiology Herpes simplex in man is caused by the herpes virus hominis. This is a DNA containing virus. There are two types of herpes virus hominis already recognized in man, known as Types 1 and 2. Type 1 causes the facial lesions and Type 2 the genital lesions. Lesions elsewhere in the body may be either Type 1 or 2. Each virus possesses one specific antigen other than the common ones.

After recovery from a primary infection the virus may lie dormant in the cells of the sensory nerves. The virus can be activated by trigger factors, e.g. high fever, exposure to sunlight and wind. These may reactivate the virus and cause recurrent infection.

Transmission of the disease is by direct contact and possibly (although not definitely proven) by droplets. Trauma facilitates inoculation.

Treatment In mild recurrent attacks treatment is not necessary. To speed resolution and prevent secondary infection 10% aluminium acetate solution can be applied. Topical antibiotics are helpful if secondary infection occurs. For troublesome recurrent infections 5–10% idoxuridine in dimethyl sulphoxide limits the duration and severity of the attack. It should be applied with a brush every 2–3 hours in the first 2 days. As yet there is no effective treatment to eradicate the virus completely and prevent recurrent attacks.

In gingivostomatitis 5% idoxuridine in orabase has been claimed to be helpful. In generalized and central nervous system involvement, cytosine arabinoside (Cytarabine) and adenosine arabinoside (Vidarabine) are effective but are relatively toxic. A new antiviral agent, acyclovir, is more effective and has a lower incidence of toxicity. Acyclovir is not available for topical use at present.

Prognosis   In the majority of patients the primary infection is very mild with only slight soreness and the erosions unnoticed. In a small percentage it is more severe with constitutional upset and rarely patients become extremely ill. The primary infection clears in 2–3 weeks. Recurrent attacks are invariably mild and heal within 2 weeks. Herpes simplex heals without scarring providing it does not become severely secondarily infected.

Complications include secondary infection, localized lymphoedema due to recurrent attacks, trigeminal neuralgia and corneal ulcers. The infection may rarely become generalized and involve the central nervous system. Occasionally herpes simplex infections precipitate attacks of erythema multiforme.

The features which precipitate recurrent infections in some individuals are not understood, but certain individuals are susceptible whilst others are not. The frequency of recurrent infections varies from the occasional attack to regular episodes every 6–7 weeks. Recurrent attacks may continue for many years.

HERPES ZOSTER

The eruption is usually characteristically confined to the area of skin innervated by one sensory nerve ganglion, and thus it is unilateral (Figure 58.11). The skin lesions are often preceded by pain in the affected areas. Two to three days later the pain subsides and skin lesions appear and initially are red, oedematous, grouped papules. These change into blisters and in severe cases may become haemorrhagic or necrotic. The lesions usually form scabs after 7–10 days and eventually heal. There may be constitutional upset with the eruption and regional tender lymphadenopathy.

The commonest site of involvement is the chest, followed by the lumbar and cervical dermatomes.

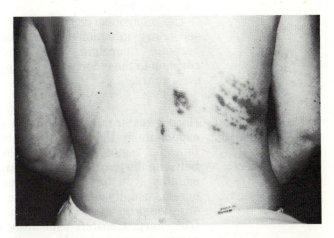

Figure 58.11 Unilateral blisters confined to the area of skin innovated by one sensory nerve ganglion in herpes zoster

In ophthalmic zoster there is involvement of the ophthalmic division of the trigeminal nerve. Lesions appear on the side of the forehead that is affected, there may also be lesions on the side of the nose. The eye complications occur in about 50% of cases and include keratitis, iridocyclitis, and ulcers of the cornea and conjunctiva. Involvement of the ciliary ganglion may give rise to the Argyll Robertson pupil.

Involvement of the maxillary division of the trigeminal nerve, as well as the skin lesions on the cheeks, produces lesions on the uvular and tonsillar areas, and in involvement of the mandibular division there are lesions on the anterior part of the tongue, floor of the mouth and buccal mucosa.

When there is involvement of the geniculate ganglion there is pain in the ear with vesicles on the pinna and in the external auditory canal. Lesions may appear on the anterior two-thirds of the tongue and facial palsy may also occur.

The virus occasionally affects the anterior horn cells of the corresponding sensory ganglion and this results in paresis. Myelitis and encephalitis very rarely occur in herpes zoster infections.

Occasionally the skin lesions become generalized and this is usually due to an underlying disorder associated with abnormal immune responses such as a reticulosis.

The commonest complications of herpes zoster are secondary infection of the skin lesions and post-herpetic neuralgia. The latter is particularly common in the elderly and may persist for months or even years.

Differential diagnosis

Herpes zoster may be confused with herpes simplex especially if the latter is zosteriform and in the thoracic region. Virological tests will distinguish between the two diseases. In contact eczema there is usually a history of the sensitizing agent, and eczema usually causes irritation and there is no constitutional upset. Erysipelas must be differentiated from herpes zoster, especially ophthalmic herpes zoster. In erysipelas the eruption is usually on both sides of the face in contrast to herpes zoster which is confined to one side of the face and does not cross the midline. Vesicles in erysipelas are prominent on the edge of the eruption and there is severe constitutional upset.

Investigations

The most reliable test to establish the diagnosis, if necessary, is to take fluid from an early blister for tissue culture. Blood taken for titration of neutralizing and complement fixation antibodies is not very helpful because of previous chicken pox infection.

Aetiology

Herpes zoster is caused by the herpes virus varicella-zoster (VZ virus). After recovery from chicken pox, the virus remains dormant in the sensory root ganglion. The reasons for activation of the virus in a particular ganglion are unknown. Very occasionally it is due to trauma or disease of the vertebral column in the region of the ganglion. The virus travels down the sensory nerve from the ganglion to the skin. The pain preceding the eruptions is due to involvement of the sensory nerve. Generalized herpes zoster may occur in states of impaired immunity, whether it is due to disease or drugs.

Recurrent attacks of herpes zoster may also occur in patients with impaired immunity. Children and adults exposed to zoster may contract chicken pox if they have not previously had the infection.

Treatment   Only symptomatic treatment is required in most cases. Relief of the pain is with mild analgesics. Topical antiseptics and antibiotics should be used if secondary infection occurs.

Five per cent idoxuridine in dimethyl sulphoxide has been claimed to decrease the severity of the attack. The lotion has to be applied every 4 hours for 2 days as soon as the blisters appear. The treatment is expensive and is not recommended as routine.

Systemic corticosteroids and vitamin B_{12} have been used but there is no satisfactory evidence that either alters the course of the illness or prevents post-herpetic neuralgia.

Eye involvement in ophthalmic zoster should be treated by an ophthalmologist and corticosteroid eye drops are often used.

If systemic involvement or generalized skin involvement occurs, systemic adenosine arabinoside or cytosine arabinoside should be used. However, preliminary studies with a new antiviral agent, a cyclovir, have shown it to be far more effective and less toxic.

Post-herpetic neuralgia is one of the most unrewarding conditions to treat; there are some who believe that none of the present treatments are helpful. It is important to avoid analgesics which are addictive. The treatments which have been used range from ethyl chloride spray to surgical procedures to sever the pain fibres in the spinal cord and destruction of the trigeminal ganglion with alcohol injection.

Prognosis   The skin lesions heal after 2–3 weeks. Occasionally there may be some scarring if the lesions have been severe or if there has been secondary infection. Post-herpetic neuralgia is more common and more persistent in elderly patients, and may last for years.

VACCINIA

Presentation Vaccinia is caused by the virus which is used for the vaccination against smallpox. There may be complications due to an abnormal reaction of the vaccination.

Normal vaccination reaction The normal vaccination reaction begins after three days. On the fourth day there is an irritating papule which within 48 hours becomes vesicular, and by the eighth day is pustular with some local reaction and regional lymph node enlargement. This is accompanied by mild constitutional upset. The pustule develops into a crust and after 3 weeks it sheds and leaves a scar. The rising antibody titre begins from the twelfth day.

Abnormal vaccination reactions Allergic reactions include urticaria, a morbilliform eruption, erythema multiforme, erythema nodosum and purpura.

Eczema vaccinatum or Kaposi's varicelliform eruptions may occur in atopic individuals.

Progressive vaccinia (vaccinia gangrenosum) occurs in patients with impaired immune response, usually due to diseases such as reticulosis. The inoculation lesion does not heal and progresses to a large deep ulcer, and a viraemia causes satellite and metastatic lesions. Without treatment all cases are fatal.

Generalized vaccinia occurs due to delayed response to immunization. There is a widespread eruption 9–15 days after vaccination. The lesions occur in crops and have a centrifugal distribution. They may resolve by the time the primary inoculation lesions heal. It is distinct from Kaposi's varicelliform eruptions.

Congenital vaccinia is generalized vaccinia in the foetus which results from a vaccinial infection in the mother. The infant is stillborn.

Accidental vaccinia results from auto-inoculation or contact with vaccination lesions of other persons. There may be multiple or solitary lesions depending on the immunity of the subject.

Encephalitis occurs in 1 in 10 000 persons vaccinated and occurs two weeks after vaccination.

Differential diagnosis It is very important to distinguish the generalized and progressive forms of vaccinia from modified smallpox, especially in patients who have been vaccinated. The distribution is less centrifugal than in smallpox and patients should be isolated and treated as for smallpox until the virological studies show vaccinia.

Investigations   Virology allows the isolation of the virus by tissue culture. Identification of the virus may be made by electron microscopy. Antibody studies will show rising levels of neutralizing antibodies.

Aetiology   The vaccination response and its complications are due to vaccinia virus. This is distinct from the cowpox and smallpox viruses, and is propagated in eggs or on the skin of animals.

Treatment   In severe cases the patients should be treated with high doses of antivaccinial gammaglobulins and methisazone (Marboran). The initial dose is 200 mg/kg, then 50 mg/kg six-hourly for a further 2 days.

KAPOSI'S VARICELLIFORM ERUPTION

Presentation   Kaposi's varicelliform eruption occurs throughout the world and is due to either the herpes simplex or vaccinia viruses. It occurs in patients who have or have had atopic eczema. It affects both sexes, but possibly more males than females. The commonest age to be affected is in infancy and early childhood, but it may occur at any age. The incubation period is approximately ten days.

The clinical picture is characterized by a sudden onset of an eruption of small vesicles. The disorder usually affects the head and neck (Figure 58.12), but may also involve the skin elsewhere. The vesicles enlarge, become umbilicated (Figure 58.13), and then become pustular. The pustules erode and become crusted and finally heal. There is usually oedema of the skin and subcutaneous tissue, with localized or generalized lymphadenitis. The constitutional upset varies; it may be severe or mild in recurrent episodes due to the herpes simplex virus.

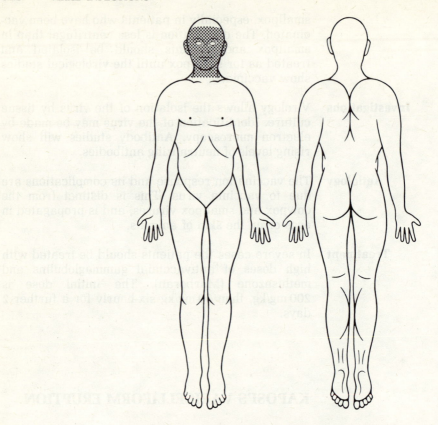

Figure 58.12   The common site for Kaposi's varicelliform eruption

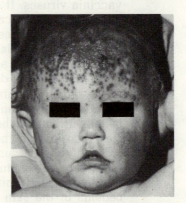

Figure 58.13   Umbilicated vesicles in Karposi's varicelliform eruption

Differential diagnosis The disorder must be distinguished from smallpox which has severe constitutional upset, prodromal signs and centrifugal distribution. Generalized vaccinia has mild or no prodromal signs and there is a previous history of skin disease. In patients with active skin disease the onset of Kaposi's varicelliform eruption may be confused with secondary bacterial infection of the underlying eczema. The constitutional upset and umbilical vesicles may distinguish the disorders, but virological studies should be performed to establish the diagnosis. Occasionally severe chicken pox and erythema multiforme may have similar clinical presentations to Kaposi's varicelliform eruptions.

Investigations Virology studies. Electron microscopy of vesicle fluid and tissue culture are necessary to identify the virus.

Aetiology In certain skin diseases, mainly atopic eczema and rarely pemphigus foliaceus, ichthyosiform erythroderma and Darier's disease, there is a susceptibility to develop a generalized eruption after exposure to the herpes simplex and vaccinia viruses. The skin lesions develop as a result of a generalized viraemia and not from auto-inoculation. The reason for the development of this type of eruption is not known, but it may be due to an altered immune response in susceptible individuals.

Treatment The patient should be isolated from susceptible individuals including nurses. Correction of the fluids and electrolyte abnormality is important. Antibiotics are necessary to control secondary infection. At an early stage it should be determined whether the infection is due to herpes simplex or vaccinia as there are specific anti-viral drugs. Methisazone (Marboran) and hyperimmune antivaccinia gammaglobulin should be given in infections due to vaccinia and acyclovir should be given systemically in infections due to herpes simplex.

With the eradication of smallpox, vaccination is carried out less often and should eventually cease. Until that time atopic subjects should not be vaccinated and they should avoid contact with subjects who have just been vaccinated.

Prognosis   This is an acute self limiting disease and usually clears in 3–4 weeks, in the majority of patients. However, the mortality rate is still nearly 10%. The disease may be complicated by encephalitis.

ORF

Presentation   Orf occurs worldwide especially in sheep, lambs and goats. It is transferred to humans by contact with infected animals or contaminated objects, and is therefore more likely to occur in veterinary surgeons, butchers, and farmers. It is more commonly seen in male adults (Figure 58.14). Incubation period is 5–6 days. The sites of involvement are the hands, forearms, and face (Figure 58.15). The lesion is usually solitary, but occasionally multiple lesions occur.

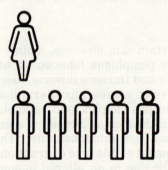

Figure 58.14   Orf is more commonly seen in males (5 : 1)

The initial lesion is 2–3 cm in diameter, red, and haemorrhagic in the centre, surrounded by a greyish-white ring with a surrounding halo of erythema (Figure 58.16). Mild constitutional upset lymphangitis and enlargement of regional lymph nodes may be present. The acute stage lasts 2–3 weeks. The inflammation gradually subsides and spontaneous healing occurs after 6–8 weeks.

Differential diagnosis   Milker's nodules may be similar to orf. However, milker's nodules are usually multiple, but sometimes the two diseases can only be distinguished by laboratory tests. Pyogenic granuloma is sometimes similar to orf in its initial stages. Pyogenic granuloma, however,

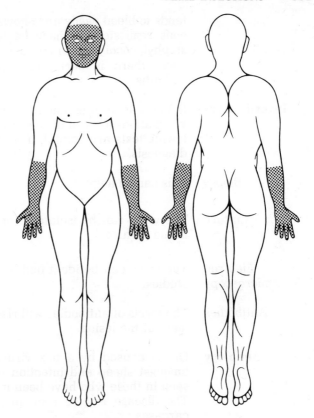

Figure 58.15   Usual sites for Orf

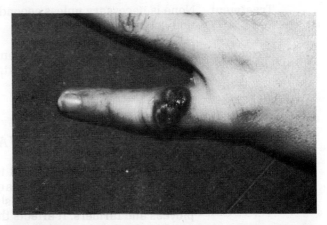

Figure 58.16   Typical lesion of orf. Ulcerated centre surrounded by a greyish-white ring with a surrounding halo of erythema

tends to bleed easily and shows no signs of spontaneous remission. Primary bacterial infections with staphylococci tend to be pustular and with streptococci there is surrounding erythema and even cellulitis.

Investigations   If the diagnosis is made on clinical grounds no investigations are usually necessary. However, the following tests are helpful, if there is doubt about the diagnosis.

Biopsy   This can be helpful.

Culture   The virus can be isolated from vesicular fluids by tissue culture.

Electron microscopy   The virus can be identified by electron microscopy studies.

Antibodies   The levels of antibodies will rise during the development of the lesion.

Aetiology   Orf is caused by a pox virus. Orf is widespread amongst sheep and infection in humans is usually seen in those who have been in contact with sheep. The disease is also seen in persons who handle carcases.

Treatment   None is necessary unless secondary bacterial infection occurs.

Prognosis   Orf is a self limiting disorder and the lesion usually clears within a month. One attack usually confers immunity.

MILKER'S NODE (PARAVACCINIA)

Presentation   The disease occurs throughout the world in agricultural areas. There is an occupational predisposition to the disease in butchers, slaughter house employees and farmers. It affects the sexes equally, the incubation period being 5–7 days.

The sites of predilection are the hands, wrists, arms and face (Figure 58.17). This initial lesions are

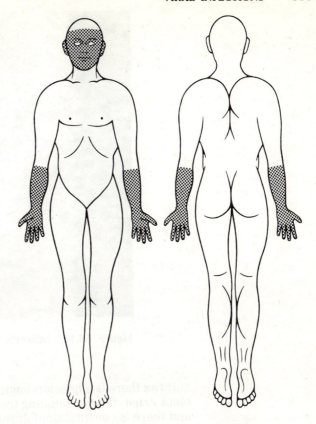

Figure 58.17   Usual sites of milker's nodules

red, itchy papules at the site of inoculation which enlarges to produce reddish–brown, or purplish nodules approximately 1–4 cm (Figure 58.18). There is a red halo and central umbilication. There may be mild pain, constitutional upset, lymphangitis and regional lymph node enlargement. The number of nodules is usually between two and five.

Differential diagnosis Milker's node must be distinguished from orf, which may be difficult on clinical grounds alone, but the latter is contracted from infected sheep or goats. The furuncle is painful and presents as a discharging pustule. Pyogenic granuloma is a vascular tumour and tends to bleed easily. Foreign body granuloma from animal's hair, syphilitic extragenital chancre and anthrax have also to be considered. In

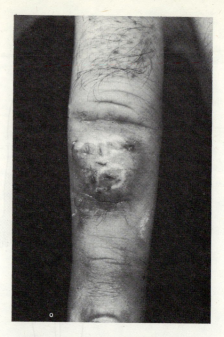

Figure 58.18   Milker's nodule

anthrax there is a haemorrhagic bulla with a central black crust; the surrounding tissues are oedematous and there is constitutional upset, fever and malaise.

Investigations   Diagnosis is made on clinical grounds and previous contact with cows; no investigations are necessary. However, viral culture and haemagglutination tests and electron microscopy of biopsy fragments will confirm the diagnosis.

Aetiology   Milker's node is a viral infection of cows' udders. The virus belongs to the group of pox viruses and the disease is transmitted from cows by direct inoculation.

Treatment   Symptomatic.

Course and prognosis   Milker's node is self limiting and spontaneous remission occurs in 4–6 weeks. There is no scarring. One infection gives life-long immunity to the virus, but there is no cross immunity between milker's node, cowpox and vaccinia.

HAND, FOOT AND MOUTH DISEASE

Presentation   A viral disease with sporadic or epidemic outbreaks throughout the world. Both sexes are equally affected. The disease affects children under the age of ten. The incubation period is about 3–5 days without prodromal symptoms.

The initial clinical manifestations are constitutional upset, mild fever and soreness of the mouth. This is followed by a vesicular eruption but the lesions quickly rupture and cause shallow ulcers on the tongue, gums, and buccal mucosa. The skin lesions which begin at the same time as the oral ones are small vesicles with surrounding erythema on the hands, palms and soles and occasionally the fingers. The lesions resolve in 3–4 days.

Differential diagnosis   Herpangina is also due to a Coxsackie virus but the constitutional upset is more severe. There is usually abdominal pain and vomiting with small painful vesicles at the back of the mouth, tonsils and pharynx. There is no skin involvement.

Primary herpes simplex infections may also present with oral ulceration, but there is usually involvement of the peri-oral skin.

Aphthous ulcers have a yellow base and are not associated with constitutional upset or lesions on the skin.

Investigations   No investigations are usually necessary but the diagnosis can be confirmed by isolating the virus which is Coxsackie A16 or A5 from vesicle fluid, mouth swabs, and faeces. Serological studies show rising titre of neutralizing antibodies. There is also a mild lymphocytosis and monocytosis with atypical cells in the peripheral blood.

Aetiology   Coxsackie viruses A16, A5 and A10 have been shown to cause the disorder.

Treatment   Symptomatic.

Prognosis   A self limiting disease of 4–7 days duration. The lesions heal without scarring. Recurrence is rare. In atopic individuals the eruptions may be more severe and resemble Kaposi's varicelliform eruption.

INDEX